2012
YEAR BOOK OF
MEDICINE®

The 2012 Year Book Series

Year Book of Anesthesiology and Pain Management™: Drs Chestnut, Abram, Black, Gravlee, Lien, Mathru, and Roizen

Year Book of Cardiology®: Drs Gersh, Cheitlin, Elliott, Gold, Graham, and Thourani

Year Book of Critical Care Medicine®: Drs Dries, Zanotti-Cavazzoni, Latenser, Martinez, Rincon, and Zwank

Year Book of Dermatology and Dermatologic Surgery™: Dr Del Rosso

Year Book of Diagnostic Radiology®: Drs Elster, Abbara, Oestreich, Offiah, Rosado de Christenson, Stephens, and Strickland

Year Book of Emergency Medicine®: Drs Hamilton, Bruno, Handly, Minczak, Mullin, Quintana, and Ramoska

Year Book of Endocrinology®: Drs Schott, Apovian, Clarke, Eugster, Meikle, Oetgen, Ovalle, Schteingart, and Toth

Year Book of Hand and Upper Limb Surgery®: Drs Yao, Adams, Isaacs, Lee, and Rizzo

Year Book of Medicine®: Drs Barker, Garrick, Gersh, Khardori, LeRoith, Panush, Talley, and Thigpen

Year Book of Neonatal and Perinatal Medicine®: Drs Fanaroff, Benitz, Donn, Neu, Papile, and Van Marter

Year Book of Neurology and Neurosurgery®: Drs Klimo, Minagar, Gandhi, House, Kevill, Liu, Mazia, Panagariya, Ragel, Riesenburger, Robottom, Schwendimann, Shafazand, Uhm, and Yang

Year Book of Obstetrics, Gynecology, and Women's Health®: Drs Dungan and Shulman

Year Book of Oncology®: Drs Arceci, Bauer, Chiorean, Gordon, Lawton, Murphy, Thigpen, and Tsao

Year Book of Ophthalmology®: Drs Rapuano, Cohen, Flanders, Hammersmith, Milman, Myers, Nagra, Nelson, Penne, Pyfer, Sergott, Shields, Talekar, and Vander

Year Book of Orthopedics®: Drs Morrey, Huddleston, Rose, Swiontkowski, and Trigg

Year Book of Otolaryngology-Head and Neck Surgery®: Drs Sindwani, Balough, Franco, Gapany, and Mitchell

Year Book of Pathology and Laboratory Medicine®: Drs Raab and Bissell

Year Book of Pediatrics®: Dr Stockman

Year Book of Plastic and Aesthetic Surgery™: Drs Miller, Gosman, Gurtner, Gutowski, Ruberg, Salisbury, and Smith

Year Book of Psychiatry and Applied Mental Health®: Drs Talbott, Ballenger, Buckley, Frances, Krupnick, and Mack

Year Book of Pulmonary Disease®: Drs Barker, Jones, Maurer, Spradley, Tanoue, and Willsie

Year Book of Sports Medicine®: Drs Shephard, Cantu, Feldman, Galea, Jankowski, Janssen, Lebrun, and Nieman

Year Book of Surgery®: Drs Copeland, Behrns, Daly, Eberlein, Fahey, Huber, Klodell, Mozingo, and Pruett

Year Book of Urology®: Drs Andriole and Coplen

Year Book of Vascular Surgery®: Drs Moneta, Gillespie, Starnes, and Watkins

2012

The Year Book of MEDICINE®

Editors

James A. Barker
Renee Garrick
Bernard J. Gersh
Nancy M. Khardori
Derek LeRoith
Richard S. Panush
Nicholas J. Talley
James Tate Thigpen

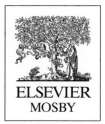

ELSEVIER
MOSBY

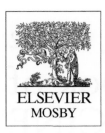

ELSEVIER
MOSBY

Vice President, Continuity: Kimberly Murphy
Developmental Editor: Teia Stone
Production Supervisor, Electronic Year Books: Donna M. Skelton
Electronic Article Manager: Emily Ogle
Illustrations and Permissions Coordinator: Dawn Vohsen

2012 EDITION

Printed and bound by CPI Group (UK) Ltd, Croydon, CR0 4YY

Transferred to digital print 2012

Editorial Office:
Elsevier
Suite 1800
1600 John F. Kennedy Blvd
Philadelphia, PA 19103-2899

International Standard Serial Number: 0084-3873
International Standard Book Number: 978-0-323-08882-4

Editorial Board

Table of Contents

Journals Represented

Journals represented in this YEAR BOOK are listed below.

Alimentary Pharmacology & Therapeutics
American Journal of Cardiology
American Journal of Clinical Nutrition
American Journal of Epidemiology
American Journal of Gastroenterology
American Journal of Kidney Diseases
American Journal of Medicine
American Journal of Respiratory and Critical Care Medicine
American Journal of Surgical Pathology
American Journal of Transplantation
Anaesthesia
Annals of Emergency Medicine
Annals of Internal Medicine
Annals of Surgery
Annals of the Rheumatic Diseases
Annals of Thoracic Surgery
Archives of Dermatology
Archives of Internal Medicine
Archives of Pediatrics & Adolescent Medicine
Arthritis & Rheumatism
Arthritis Care & Research (Hoboken)
Blood
Breast Journal
British Journal of Cancer
British Medical Journal
Cancer
Cancer Epidemiology, Biomarkers & Prevention
Chest
Circulation
Circulation Research
Clinical Gastroenterology and Hepatology
Clinical Infectious Diseases
Clinical Journal of the American Society of Nephrology
Critical Care Medicine
Current Opinion in Pediatrics
Diabetes
Diabetes Care
Digestive Diseases and Sciences
European Heart Journal
European Respiratory Journal
Gastroenterology
Gut
Gynecologic Oncology
Intensive Care Medicine
International Journal of Radiation Oncology *Biology* Physics
Journal of Allergy and Clinical Immunology

Journal of Bone Mineral Research
Journal of Cardiac Failure
Journal of Clinical Endocrinology & Metabolism
Journal of Clinical Microbiology
Journal of Clinical Oncology
Journal of Clinical Rheumatology
Journal of Diabetic Complications
Journal of Emergency Medicine
Journal of Experimental Medicine
Journal of Heart and Lung Transplantation
Journal of Hypertension
Journal of Immunology
Journal of Infectious Diseases
Journal of Neurological Sciences
Journal of Pediatric Gastroenterology and Nutrition
Journal of Rheumatology
Journal of the American College of Cardiology
Journal of the American Medical Association
Journal of the American Society of Nephrology
Journal of Thoracic and Cardiovascular Surgery
Journal of Thoracic Oncology
Journal of Urology
Kidney International
Lancet
Laryngoscope
Metabolism
MMWR Morbidity and Mortality Weekly Report
Nature Medicine
Nephrology Dialysis Transplantation
New England Journal of Medicine
Pediatric Infectious Disease Journal
Pediatrics
Proceedings of the National Academy of Sciences of the United States of America
Rheumatology (Oxford)
Scandinavian Journal of Urology and Nephrology
Science Translational Medicine
Sleep
Spine (Philadelphia, Pa. 1976)
Surgical Oncology
Thorax
Thrombosis Research
Thyroid
Transplantation
United Kingdom National Health Service

STANDARD ABBREVIATIONS

The following terms are abbreviated in this edition: acquired immunodeficiency syndrome (AIDS), cardiopulmonary resuscitation (CPR), central nervous system (CNS), cerebrospinal fluid (CSF), computed tomography (CT), deoxyribonucleic acid (DNA), electrocardiography (ECG), health maintenance organization (HMO), human immunodeficiency virus (HIV), intensive care unit (ICU), intramuscular (IM), intravenous (IV), magnetic resonance (MR) imaging (MRI), ribonucleic acid (RNA), and ultrasound (US).

NOTE

The YEAR BOOK OF MEDICINE is a literature survey service providing abstracts of articles published in the professional literature. Every effort is made to assure the accuracy of the information presented in these pages. Neither the editors nor the publisher of the YEAR BOOK OF MEDICINE can be responsible for errors in the original materials. The editors' comments are their own opinions. Mention of specific products within this publication does not constitute endorsement.

To facilitate the use of the YEAR BOOK OF MEDICINE as a reference tool, all illustrations and tables included in this publication are now identified as they appear in the original article. This change is meant to help the reader recognize that any illustration or table appearing in the YEAR BOOK OF MEDICINE may be only one of many in the original article. For this reason, figure and table numbers will often appear to be out of sequence within the YEAR BOOK OF MEDICINE.

Introduction

This has been an exciting year in Rheumatology. We continue to expand our understanding of the pathogenesis of lupus, rheumatoid arthritis, osteoarthritis, and painful rheumatic disorders. Our broader understanding of these diseases coincides with the development of several new diagnostic/classification criteria. As a specialty, we do better now in our management of vasculitides. We have interventions to offer patients with fibromyalgia, a new therapy for lupus, and the ability to treat rheumatoid arthritis very effectively. Finally, we are intent on identifying early or even preclinical disease to achieve better outcomes. Read on.

R. S. Panush, MD

1 Rheumatoid Arthritis

Risk of atrial fibrillation and stroke in rheumatoid arthritis: Danish nationwide cohort study
Lindhardsen J, Ahlehoff O, Gislason GH, et al (Copenhagen Univ Hosp Gentofte, Denmark)
BMJ 344:e1257, 2012

Objectives.—To determine if patients with rheumatoid arthritis have increased risk of atrial fibrillation and stroke.

Design.—Longitudinal nationwide register based cohort study.

Setting.—Inpatient and outpatient hospital care in Denmark from 1997 to 2009.

Participants.—Entire Danish population aged over 15 years without rheumatoid arthritis, atrial fibrillation, or stroke before 1997. Participants with rheumatoid arthritis were identified by individual level linkage of diagnoses and rheumatoid arthritis treatment.

Main Outcome Measures.—Rates of atrial fibrillation and stroke.

Results.—Of 4,182,335 participants included in the cohort, 18,247 were identified as having rheumatoid arthritis during follow-up, with a mean age at disease onset of 59.2 years and a median follow-up of 4.8 years. A total of 156,484 people, including 774 with rheumatoid arthritis, were diagnosed as having atrial fibrillation (age and sex matched event rates of 8.2 per 1000 person years in rheumatoid arthritis patients and 6.0 per 1000 person years in the general population), with an adjusted incidence rate ratio of 1.41 (95% confidence interval 1.31 to 1.51). In addition, 165,343 people, including 718 with rheumatoid arthritis, had a stroke (7.6 per 1000 person years in rheumatoid arthritis and 5.7 per 1000 person years in the general population), with a resultant rate ratio of 1.32 (1.22 to 1.42). For both atrial fibrillation and stroke, relative risks were increased in all strata based on thirds of sex and age, with higher relative risks in younger patients but higher absolute risk differences in older patients.

Conclusions.—Rheumatoid arthritis was associated with an increased incidence of atrial fibrillation and stroke. The novel finding of increased risk of atrial fibrillation in rheumatoid arthritis suggests that this arrhythmia is relevant in cardiovascular risk assessment of these patients.

▶ I was not aware of this connection. The risk was as much as 40% increased with rheumatoid arthritis (RA). This underscores that RA is a systemic disease with potentially devastating manifestations. It needs to be prevented or identified and treated early and aggressively.

R. S. Panush, MD

Incidence of extraarticular rheumatoid arthritis in Olmsted County, Minnesota, in 1995-2007 versus 1985-1994: a population-based study
Myasoedova E, Crowson CS, Turesson C, et al (Mayo Foundation, Rochester, MN)
J Rheumatol 38:983-989, 2011

Objective.—To assess incidence and mortality effects of extraarticular rheumatoid arthritis (ExRA) in patients with incident RA in 1995-2007 compared to 1985-1994, in Olmsted County, Minnesota, USA.

Methods.—Data on incident ExRA were abstracted from medical records of patients with RA - Olmsted County residents who first met the 1987 American College of Rheumatology criteria for RA between January 1, 1995, and December 31, 2007. Patients were followed until death, migration from Olmsted County, or December 31, 2008. ExRA were classified using the predefined criteria and compared to the corresponding 1985-1994 inception RA cohort (n = 147).

Results.—The 1995-2007 cohort included 463 patients with RA followed for a mean of 6.3 years; mean age was 55.6 years, 69% were women, 67% were positive for rheumatoid factor (RF). The 10-year cumulative incidence of any ExRA (50.1%) and severe ExRA (6.7%) in the 1995-2007 cohort was similar to the 1985-1994 cohort (46.2% and 9.7%, respectively). The 10-year cumulative incidence of vasculitis, but not other features of ExRA, was significantly lower in the 1995-2007 cohort (0.6%) compared to the 1985-1994 cohort (3.6%). RF positivity, erosions/destructive changes, and use of methotrexate, other disease-modifying antirheumatic drugs and systemic corticosteroids were significantly associated with ExRA in the 1995-2007 cohort. ExRA was associated with mortality risk (HR 2.1, 95% CI 1.2, 3.7) in the 1995-2007 cohort. The decrease in mortality following ExRA in the 1995-2007 cohort versus the 1985-1994 cohort did not reach statistical significance (HR 0.6, 95% CI 0.3, 1.2, $p = 0.16$).

Conclusion.—ExRA remains a common complication associated with increased mortality in RA. The occurrence of vasculitis appears to be decreasing in recent years.

▶ Physicians do not see cases of extra-articular disease or vasculitis like we used to. Although this is partly because of recognition and therapy of and for rheumatoid arthritis, others speculated in the 1970s that the nature of rheumatoid arthritis was changing and possibly becoming milder.

R. S. Panush, MD

Observational Studies on the Risk of Cancer Associated With Tumor Necrosis Factor Inhibitors in Rheumatoid Arthritis: A Review of Their Methodologies and Results

Solomon DH, Mercer E, Kavanaugh A (Brigham and Women's Hosp, Boston, MA; Univ of California, San Diego)

Arthritis Rheum 64:21-32, 2012

Background.—Various autoimmune conditions, such as rheumatoid arthritis (RA), have responded to the use of inhibitors of the inflammatory cytokine tumor necrosis factor (TNF). These agents now form the cornerstone of therapy for patients with RA that is severe or refractory to therapy. However, based on their relationship to the immune system, TNF inhibitors may predispose patients to such adverse events as an increased incidence of inflammation and cancer. Mechanistically speaking, TNF inhibition could either enhance or inhibit cancer development. Randomized trials have not provided the evidence needed to clarify this relationship. To collect the needed data, a systematic review of epidemiologic studies of the relationship between TNF inhibitors and cancer was performed, noting both these studies' methodologic attributes and their outcomes.

Method.—PubMed was searched for all English language articles regarding TNF inhibitors and cancer. Eleven articles reported the relative risks (RRs) of cancer associated with TNF inhibitors and 12 included standardized incidence ratios (SIRs), comparing patients with RA against the general population.

Results.—The methodology of the various studies differed widely. Many studies provided only a limited evaluation of important methodologic attributes. Most were of short duration as well. However, the RRs of cancer among patients receiving TNF inhibitors were similar and indicated no increased risk of malignancy associated with TNF inhibitors. Most studies showed a numerically increased but not significant risk for lymphoproliferative cancers and nonmelanoma skin cancers. The increased risk estimates for lymphoma were between 1.1 and 4.9, although most values were nearer the 1.1 level. Considering the studies reporting SIRs, the SIR for all cancers was not increased for patients receiving TNF inhibitors, although the SIRs for lymphoma and hematologic malignancies were increased. The lymphoma SIRs were between 1.8 and 6.0 for those receiving TNF inhibitors and between 1.7 and 5.4 for those in the general RA population. The hematologic malignancy SIRs were between 2.0 and 4.1 for those receiving TNF inhibitors and between 1.7 and 8.8 for those in the general RA population.

Conclusions.—The studies assessed demonstrate little or no cancer risk for persons taking TNF inhibitors for RA. To better characterize the relationship, it is important to standardize the methodology of studies and have long-term follow-up, since many cancers develop very slowly.

▶ No increased risk of cancer could be identified from this meticulous review of the literature. The authors suggest that authors and editors follow standardized methodologic guidelines for new and emerging therapies to make these assessments easier.

R. S. Panush, MD

Antibodies against native collagen and citrullinated proteins precede the development of rheumatoid arthritis with a consecutive pattern
Brink M, Rönnelid J, Hansson M, et al (Umeå Univ, Sweden; Uppsala Univ, Sweden; Karolinska Univ Hosp, Stockholm, Sweden; et al)
Ann Rheum Dis 71:A22, 2012

Background and Objective.—Presence of antibodies against cyclic citrullinated peptides (anti-CCP2) has been demonstrated to precede the development of rheumatoid arthritis (RA) by several years. The RR for developing subsequent RA was increased by the combination of HLA- shared epitopes (SE) and also presence of PTPN22 T variant. The underlying process of why RA-patients develop antibodies against certain citrullinated peptides is largely unknown and here the authors have investigated antibody concentration against thirteen citrullinated proteins, besides anti-CCP2, to elucidate their predictive value in the prepatient phase of RA together with information about HLA-SE, and cigarette smoking.

Material and Methods.—This study comprised 406 individuals, with 717 samples, who were identified before onset of symptoms of RA (median 7.4 years IQR 3.3—12.6 years), as donors to the Medical Biobank of Northern Sweden. 204 of them were also sampled at the time of diagnose, and have been analysed together with 1305 population controls from the Medical Biobank for concentrations of antibodies towards thirteen different citrullinated peptides in plasma; fibrinogen 36—50, fibrinogen 72, fibrinogen 74, fibrinogen α 36—50, fibrinogen α 621—635, fibrinogen β 60—74, fibrinogen 573, fibrinogen 591, α-enolase 1, collagen Type II C1 arginine and citrulline and U1, CCP-1, vimentin 2—17, vimentin 60—75 using the microarray based ImmunoCAP ISAC system (Phadia Diagnostics, Uppsala, Sweden). All samples were also analysed for anti-CCP2 antibodies with ELISA (Euro-Diagnostics). Cutoff levels were set with 98% specificity.

Results.—The three antibodies with highest sensitivity for predicting RA was anti-CCP2 (33.8%), fibrinogen 36—52 (24.3%) and α enolase 1 (24.1%) counting ever being positive in all prepatient samples. On individual and group level, the concentrations of the citrullinated antibodies increased significantly the closer to onset of symptoms the samples were collected. The number of positive samples also increased the closer to disease onset. The predating time for the antibodies to appear (with concentrations above cut-off) varied significantly between them.

Conclusion.—Citrullinated antibodies and antibodies against native collagen appeared many years before onset of symptoms and at different time points. The concentrations increased gradually with few exceptions until onset of symptoms and there was an epitope spreading. Citrullination was an important preceding process for disease development maybe initiated by an earlier non-citrullinated antibody stimulation.

▶ Citrullination and epitope-spreading precedes clinical disease. Available information suggests this is very specific for rheumatoid arthritis and almost always predicts disease.

R. S. Panush, MD

Aggressive therapy in patients with early arthritis results in similar outcome compared with conventional care: the STREAM randomized trial
van Eijk IC, Nielen MM, van der Horst-Bruinsma I, et al (Jan van Breemen Res Inst/Reade, Amsterdam, The Netherlands)
Rheumatology (Oxford) 51:686-694, 2012

Objective.—To compare the effects of aggressive tight control therapy and conventional care on radiographic progression and disease activity in patients with early mild inflammatory arthritis.

Methods.—Patients with two to five swollen joints, Sharp-van der Heijde radiographic score (SHS) < 5 and symptom duration ≤ 2 years were randomized between two strategies. Patients with a definite non-RA diagnosis were excluded. The protocol of the aggressive group aimed for remission (DAS < 1.6), with consecutive treatment steps: MTX, addition of adalimumab and combination therapy. The conventional care group followed a strategy with traditional DMARDs (no prednisone or biologics) without DAS-based guideline. Outcome measures after 2 years were SHS (primary), remission rate and HAQ score (secondary).

Results.—Eighty-two patients participated (60% ACPA positive). In the aggressive group (n = 42), 19 patients were treated with adalimumab. In the conventional care group (n = 40), 24 patients started with hydroxychloroquin (HCQ), 2 with sulfasalazine (SSZ) and 14 with MTX. After 2 years, the median SHS increase was 0 [interquartile range (IQR) 0-1.1] and 0.5 (IQR 0-2.5), remission rates were 66 and 49% and HAQ decreased with a mean of −0.09 (0.50) and −0.25 (0.59) in the aggressive and conventional care group, respectively. All comparisons were non-significant.

Conclusion.—In patients with early arthritis of two to five joints, both aggressive tight-control therapy including adalimumab and conventional therapy resulted in remission rates around 50%, low radiographic damage and excellent functional status after 2 years. However, full disease control including radiographic arrest in all patients remains an elusive target even in moderately active early arthritis. Trial registration. Dutch Trial Register, http://www.trialregister.nl/, NTR 144.

▶ I'm not sure how to interpret this study. There were a lot of variables, and 2 years is not a long time for treatment of rheumatoid arthritis. Maybe aggressive therapy was not as good as touted, but treatments need to be specified not labeled (aggressive means different things to different people). The conventional approach included disease-modifying antirheumatic drugs. Maybe rheumatologists treat patients just as well using clinical judgment (conventional) as with formulaic titration to outcomes/assessments.

R. S. Panush, MD

Assessment by MRI of inflammation and damage in rheumatoid arthritis patients with methotrexate inadequate response receiving golimumab: results of the GO-FORWARD trial
Conaghan PG, Emery P, Østergaard M, et al (Univ of Leeds, UK)
Ann Rheum Dis 70:1968-1974, 2011

Objective.—To evaluate golimumab's effect on MRI-detected inflammation and structural damage in patients with active rheumatoid arthritis (RA) despite methotrexate (MTX).

Methods.—Patients (n = 444) were randomly assigned to placebo plus MTX, golimumab 100 mg plus placebo, golimumab 50 mg plus MTX, or golimumab 100 mg plus MTX (subcutaneous injections every 4 weeks). A subset of 240 patients participated in an MRI substudy. MRIs (1.5T + contrast enhancement) of the dominant wrist and metacarpophalangeal (MCP) joints were obtained at baseline and weeks 12 and 24. Images were scored by two independent, blinded readers for synovitis (0-9 wrist only (n = 240), 0-21 wrist + MCP (n = 223)), bone oedema (osteitis) (0-69) and bone erosions (0-230) using the OMERACT Rheumatoid Arthritis MRI Scoring system.

Results.—Significant improvements in synovitis and bone oedema (osteitis) were observed in the combined golimumab plus MTX groups versus placebo plus MTX at week 12 (-1.77 vs -0.15, $p < 0.001$ wrist + MCP and -2.00 vs 0.19, $p = 0.003$, respectively) and week 24 (-1.91 vs -0.38, $p < 0.001$ wrist + MCP and -1.74 vs 0.71, $p = 0.004$, respectively). Fewer than 10% of patients had a substantial degree of erosive progression (most showed no progression) across all treatment groups (including the control group), precluding adequate evaluation of golimumab's effect on bone erosions.

Conclusion.—Golimumab plus MTX significantly improved MRI-detected synovitis and osteitis (prognosticators of future structural damage) versus placebo plus MTX at weeks 12 and 24. The effect of golimumab on bone erosions could not be determined by semi-quantitative scoring in these RA patients with minimal progression of bone erosions.

▶ In this study, golimumab plus methotrexate proved to be better than placebo plus methotrexate. However, what we'd like to know is how golimumab compares with others in its class (tumor necrosis factor alpha antagonists) or other biologic agents.

R. S. Panush, MD

A plasmablast biomarker for nonresponse to antibody therapy to CD20 in rheumatoid arthritis
Owczarczyk K, Lal P, Abbas AR, et al (Genentech Inc, South San Francisco, CA)
Sci Transl Med 3:101ra92, 2011

An important goal for personalized health care is the identification of biomarkers that predict the likelihood of treatment responses. Here, we tested the hypothesis that quantitative mRNA assays for B lineage cells in blood could serve as baseline predictors of therapeutic response to B cell depletion therapy in subjects with rheumatoid arthritis (RA). In samples from the REFLEX trial of rituximab in inadequate responders to antibodies to tumor necrosis factor-α, a 25% subgroup of treated subjects with elevated baseline mRNA levels of IgJ, a marker for antibody-secreting plasmablasts, showed reduced clinical response rates. There were no significant efficacy differences in the placebo arm subjects stratified by this marker. Prospective testing of the IgJ biomarker in the DANCER and SERENE rituximab clinical trial cohorts and the SCRIPT ocrelizumab cohort confirmed the utility of this marker to predict nonresponse to anti-CD20 therapy. A combination mRNA biomarker, IgJhiFCRL5lo, showed improved test performance over IgJhi alone. This study demonstrates that baseline blood levels of molecular markers for late-stage B lineage plasmablasts identify a ~20% subgroup of active RA subjects who are unlikely to gain substantial clinical benefit from anti-CD20 B cell depletion therapy.

▶ Expect to read a lot more about the importance of biomarkers for disease prognosis and guiding therapy. Here, for example, is identified a marker that predicts nonresponsiveness to therapy intended to deplete CD20-positive cells (rituximab and analogues are used in this fashion for treating rheumatoid arthritis; this may explain why some patients fail to respond as expected).

R. S. Panush, MD

Macrophage positron emission tomography imaging as a biomarker for preclinical rheumatoid arthritis: findings of a prospective pilot study
Gent YY, Voskuyl AE, Kloet RW, et al (VU Univ Med Ctr, Amsterdam, The Netherlands)
Arthritis Rheum 64:62-66, 2012

Objective.—To conduct a prospective pilot study to determine whether macrophage targeting by 11C-(R)-PK11195 positron emission tomography (PET) can visualize subclinical synovitis in arthralgia patients who have anti-citrullinated protein antibodies (ACPAs).
Methods.—Twenty-nine arthralgia patients who were positive for ACPAs but did not have clinical arthritis were studied. High (spatial)-resolution 11C-(R)-PK11195 PET scans of the hands and wrists were performed. For all metacarpophalangeal, proximal interphalangeal, and wrist joints

(i.e., 22 joints per patient), tracer uptake was scored semiquantitatively (0-3 scale) by 2 observers who were blinded with regard to the clinical data. Patients were followed up prospectively for 24 months to investigate the development of clinical arthritis.

Results.—Overall agreement and kappa values for the readings of the 2 observers were, respectively, 97% and 0.91 (95% confidence interval [95% CI] 0.74-1) at the patient level and 99% and 0.81 (95% CI 0.65-0.96) at the joint level. In 4 patients, at least 1 and as many as 5 PET-positive joints (score $\geq$ 1) were found at baseline. Within 2 years of followup, 9 patients had developed clinical arthritis. This included all 4 patients with positive findings on the 11C-(R)-PK11195 scan, who developed clinical arthritis in the hand/wrist region, as identified on PET scans. Of the 5 remaining arthritis patients with negative findings on PET scans, 2 developed arthritis in the hand joints and 3 developed arthritis at locations outside the field of view of the PET scanner.

Conclusion.—Subclinical arthritis in ACPA-positive arthralgia patients could be visualized by 11C-(R)-PK11195 PET scanning and was associated with development of arthritis within 2 years of followup. This indicates that 11C-(R)-PK11195 PET may be useful in determining arthritis activity in the preclinical phase of RA.

▶ Wow. The images from patients with minimal clinically detectable arthritis were impressive. We must not underestimate the burden and extent of disease. These data provide another cogent argument for early recognition and aggressive intervention (for all).

R. S. Panush, MD

Double-blind, randomized, controlled, pilot study comparing classic ayurvedic medicine, methotrexate, and their combination in rheumatoid arthritis
Furst DE, Venkatraman MM, McGann M, et al (Univ of California Los Angeles)
J Clin Rheumatol 17:185-192, 2011

Objective.—To compare classic Ayurveda, methotrexate (MTX), and their combination in a double-blind, randomized, double-dummy, pilot trial in rheumatoid arthritis (RA) for 36 weeks.

Methods.—Forty-three seropositive RA patients by American College of Rheumatology (ACR) criteria with disease duration of less than 7 years were assigned to the following treatment groups: MTX plus Ayurvedic placebo (n = 14), Ayurveda plus MTX placebo (n = 12), or Ayurveda plus MTX (n = 17). Outcomes included the Disease Activity Score (DAS28-CRP), ACR20/50/70, and Health Assessment Questionnaire–Disability Index. All measures were obtained every 12 weeks for 36 weeks. Analyses included descriptive statistics, analysis of variance, χ^2, or Student t test. The unique features of this study included the development of placebos for each Ayurvedic pharmacological dosage form and individualization of Ayurvedic therapy.

Results.—All groups were comparable at baseline in demographics and disease characteristics. There were no statistically significant differences among the 3 groups on the efficacy measures. ACR20 results were MTX 86%, Ayurveda 100%, and combination 82%, and DAS28-CRP response were MTX -2.4, Ayurveda -1.7, and combination -2.4. Differences in adverse events among groups were also not statistically significant, although the MTX groups experienced more adverse event (MTX 174, Ayurveda 112, combination 176). No deaths occurred.

Conclusions.—In this first-ever, double-blind, randomized, placebo-controlled pilot study comparing Ayurveda, MTX, and their combination, all 3 treatments were approximately equivalent in efficacy, within the limits of a pilot study. Adverse events were numerically fewer in the Ayurveda-only group. This study demonstrates that double-blind, placebo-controlled, randomized studies are possible when testing individualized classic Ayurvedic versus allopathic treatment in ways acceptable to western standards and to Ayurvedic physicians. It also justifies the need for larger studies.

▶ Kudos to Dan Furst (and colleagues) for looking at this in a scientific fashion, which is how all these notions must be approached. Many potent agents derive from plants, so the idea that we may yet identify something new and useful is not unreasonable.

R. S. Panush, MD

Deletion of Syk in neutrophils prevents immune complex arthritis
Elliott ER, Van Ziffle JA, Scapini P, et al (Univ of California, San Francisco)
J Immunol 187:4319-4330, 2011

The K/BxN serum transfer model of arthritis is critically dependent on FcγR signaling events mediated by spleen tyrosine kinase (Syk). However, the specific cell types in which this signaling is required are not known. We report that deletion of Syk in neutrophils, achieved using syk(f/f) MRP8-cre(+) mice, blocks disease development in serum transfer arthritis. The syk(f/f) MRP8-cre(+) mice display absent joint disease and reduced deposition of pathogenic anti-glucose-6-phosphate isomerase Abs in the joint (with a reciprocal accumulation of these Abs in the peripheral circulation). Additionally, syk(f/f) MRP8-cre(+) mice manifest poor edema formation within 3 h after formation of cutaneous immune complexes (Arthus reaction). Together, this suggests that neutrophil-dependent recognition of immune complexes contributes significantly to changes in vascular permeability during the early phases of immune complex disease. Using mixed chimeric mice, containing both wild-type and syk(f/f) MRP8-cre(+) neutrophils, we find no impairment in recruitment of Syk-deficient neutrophils to the inflamed joint, but they fail to become primed, demonstrating lower cytokine production after removal from the joint. They also display an increased apoptotic rate compared with wild-type cells in the same joint. Mast cell-deficient c-kit(sh/sh) mice developed robust arthritis after serum transfer whereas c-kit(W/Wv) mice did not, suggesting that previous conclusions concerning the central role of mast cells in this model may need to be revised. Basophil-deficient mice also responded normally to K/BxN serum transfer. These results demonstrate that Syk-dependent signaling in neutrophils alone is critically required for arthritis development in the serum transfer model.

▶ Spleen tyrosine kinase transmits signals intracellularly from B- and T-cell receptors. It is an important therapeutic target in many autoimmune diseases, including rheumatoid arthritis. These experimental studies support its important role in the development and expression of arthritis.

R. S. Panush, MD

What Do MicroRNAs Mean for Rheumatoid Arthritis?

Duroux-Richard I, Jorgensen C, Apparailly F (INSERM U844 and Université Montpellier 1, France; Université Montpellier 1, France)
Arthritis Rheum 64:11-20, 2012

Background.—MicroRNAs (miRNAs) are small noncoding RNA molecules that influence the expression of many protein-encoding genes at a post-transcription level. It is likely that they participate in nearly all the developmental and physiologic processes of the body. However, the function of most miRNAs in mammals is unknown, although an aberrant expression of these molecules can contribute to the pathogenesis of several conditions, such as immune-mediated inflammatory problems. Patients with rheumatoid arthritis (RA) have shown dysregulated expression of a dozen miRNAs in the circulation and inflamed synovium. The current knowledge about miRNA biogenesis and activities shown to be dysregulated in RA was shared, noting potential benefits of the knowledge to patients and clinicians.

miRNA Biogenesis.—Human miRNA genes are found nonrandomly throughout all chromosomes except the Y chromosome, are predominantly seen in introns, and are often noted in cancer-associated genomic regions or fragile sites. Half of the known human miRNAs are in clusters that may be related to their targeting of the same gene or genes involved in the same pathway. miRNA genes are transcribed by RNA polymerase II as monocistronic or polycistronic long primary transcripts called primary miRNA (pri-miRNA). These are processed, then transported to the cytoplasm, where they are cleaved to produce a miRNA/miRNA* duplex, which is unwound into its component strands. The miRNA guide strand is chosen through an unknown mechanism to be incorporated into the multiproteic RNA-inducing silencing complex (RISC) and functions as a "mature miRNA." The passenger strand (miRNA*) is released and degraded. miRNA strands may also regulate gene expression. Efforts have mainly focused on the regulatory functions of miRNA, with less emphasis on regulating miRNA gene expression. In addition, many exceptions to the rules that have been identified are likely.

miRNAs and RA.—Studies have shown upregulation of specific miRNAs in the circulation or in the inflamed joints of patients with RA. These patients have already shown abnormal expression of a dozen miRNAs, most of which are upregulated. The implications of the altered expression of these miRNAs for RA are various. They could serve as a novel class of biomarkers for early disease diagnosis and to predict therapeutic outcomes. They may also help researchers better understand the pathophysiology of RA. In addition, they may suggest or present the opportunities for new therapeutic strategies.

Conclusions.—Although the identification, characterization, and modulation of miRNA expression in patients with RA are of great interest, currently there is little evidence to support miRNAs as candidates for developing immunomodulatory drugs. However, the potential of miRNAs is promising with respect to therapeutic strategies for RA patients. Further study, especially focusing on specificity and safety issues, is needed.

▶ These are small noncoding RNAs that moderate the expression of protein-encoding genes. Many of them are dysregulated in rheumatoid arthritis. We will see whether they prove to be useful biomarkers and elucidate pathophysiology; it did not seem likely that they would be therapeutic targets.

R. S. Panush, MD

Autotaxin expression from synovial fibroblasts is essential for the pathogenesis of modeled arthritis

Nikitopoulou I, Oikonomou N, Karouzakis E, et al (Alexander Fleming Biomedical Sciences Res Ctr, Athens, Greece)
J Exp Med 209:925-933, 2012

Rheumatoid arthritis is a destructive arthropathy characterized by chronic synovial inflammation that imposes a substantial socioeconomic burden. Under the influence of the proinflammatory milieu, synovial fibroblasts (SFs), the main effector cells in disease pathogenesis, become activated and hyperplastic, releasing proinflammatory factors and tissue-remodeling enzymes. This study shows that activated arthritic SFs from human patients and animal models express significant quantities of autotaxin (ATX; ENPP2), a lysophospholipase D that catalyzes the conversion of lysophosphatidylcholine to lysophosphatidic acid (LPA). ATX expression from SFs was induced by TNF, and LPA induced SF activation and effector functions in synergy with TNF. Conditional genetic ablation of ATX in mesenchymal cells, including SFs, resulted in disease attenuation in animal models of arthritis, establishing the ATX/LPA axis as a novel player in chronic inflammation and the pathogenesis of arthritis and a promising therapeutic target.

▶ Autotaxin (a lysophospholipase) catalyzes conversion of lysophosphatidylcholine to lysophosphatidic acid, which results in growthlike responses in almost all cell types. In this study, autotaxin expression was essential for experimental arthritis, suggesting its importance in pathogenesis and potential as yet another therapeutic target.

R. S. Panush, MD

A novel pathogenic role of the ER chaperone GRP78/BiP in rheumatoid arthritis
Yoo SA, You S, Yoon HJ, et al (Catholic Univ of Korea, Seoul, South Korea)
J Exp Med 209:871-886, 2012

An accumulation of misfolded proteins can trigger a cellular survival response in the endoplasmic reticulum (ER). In this study, we found that ER stress-associated gene signatures were highly expressed in rheumatoid arthritis (RA) synoviums and synovial cells. Proinflammatory cytokines, such as TNF and IL-1β, increased the expression of GRP78/BiP, a representative ER chaperone, in RA synoviocytes. RA synoviocytes expressed higher levels of GRP78 than osteoarthritis (OA) synoviocytes when stimulated by thapsigargin or proinflammatory cytokines. Down-regulation of Grp78 transcripts increased the apoptosis of RA synoviocytes while abolishing TNF- or TGF-β-induced synoviocyte proliferation and cyclin D1 up-regulation. Conversely, overexpression of the Grp78 gene prevented synoviocyte apoptosis. Moreover, Grp78 small interfering RNA inhibited VEGF(165)-induced angiogenesis in vitro and also significantly impeded synoviocyte proliferation and angiogenesis in Matrigel implants engrafted into immunodeficient mice. Additionally, repeated intraarticular injections of BiP inducible factor X, a selective GRP78 inducer, increased synoviocyte proliferation and angiogenesis in the joints of mice with experimental OA. In contrast, mice with Grp78 haploinsufficiency exhibited the suppression of experimentally induced arthritis and developed a limited degree of synovial proliferation and angiogenesis. In summary, this study shows that the ER chaperone GRP78 is crucial for synoviocyte proliferation and angiogenesis, the pathological hallmark of RA.

▶ Chaperone proteins assist in the folding, unfolding, or assembly of other macromolecules. This one was shown experimentally to be necessary for synovial proliferation and angiogenesis, and possibly therefore important in pathogenesis of rheumatoid arthritis and perhaps its therapy.

R. S. Panush, MD

2 Systemic Lupus Erythematosus

A phase III, randomized, placebo-controlled study of belimumab, a monoclonal antibody that inhibits B lymphocyte stimulator, in patients with systemic lupus erythematosus
Furie R, BLISS-76 Study Group (North Shore-Long Island Jewish Health System, Lake Success, NY)
Arthritis Rheum 63:3918-3930, 2011

Objective.—To assess the efficacy/safety of the B lymphocyte stimulator inhibitor belimumab plus standard therapy compared with placebo plus standard therapy in active systemic lupus erythematosus (SLE).

Methods.—In a phase III, multicenter, randomized, placebo-controlled trial, 819 antinuclear antibody-positive or anti-double-stranded DNA-positive SLE patients with scores ≥ 6 on the Safety of Estrogens in Lupus Erythematosus National Assessment (SELENA) version of the SLE Disease Activity Index (SLEDAI) were randomized in a 1:1:1 ratio to receive 1 mg/kg belimumab, 10 mg/kg belimumab, or placebo intravenously on days 0, 14, and 28 and then every 28 days for 72 weeks. The primary efficacy end point was the SLE Responder Index (SRI) response rate at week 52 (an SRI response was defined as a ≥ 4-point reduction in SELENA-SLEDAI score, no new British Isles Lupus Assessment Group [BILAG] A organ domain score and no more than 1 new BILAG B score, and no worsening in physician's global assessment score versus baseline).

Results.—Belimumab at 10 mg/kg plus standard therapy met the primary efficacy end point, generating a significantly greater SRI response at week 52 compared with placebo (43.2% versus 33.5%; $P = 0.017$). The rate with 1 mg/kg belimumab was 40.6% ($P = 0.089$). Response rates at week 76 were 32.4%, 39.1%, and 38.5% with placebo, 1 mg/kg belimumab, and 10 mg/kg belimumab, respectively. In post hoc sensitivity analyses evaluating higher SELENA-SLEDAI score thresholds, 10 mg/kg belimumab achieved better discrimination at weeks 52 and 76. Risk of severe flares over 76 weeks (based on the modified SLE Flare Index) was reduced with 1 mg/kg belimumab (34%) ($P = 0.023$) and 10 mg/kg belimumab (23%) ($P = 0.13$). Serious and severe adverse events, including infections, laboratory abnormalities, malignancies, and deaths, were comparable across groups.

Conclusion.—Belimumab plus standard therapy significantly improved SRI response rate, reduced SLE disease activity and severe flares, and was generally well tolerated in SLE.

▶ I have commented on belimumab before. It is exciting that we finally have something new for lupus patients. On the other hand, it is disappointing, and perhaps surprising, that its efficacy seems quite modest and limited. I doubt there will be a single critical pathway identified that is amenable for effective therapeutic intervention. I cannot imagine it will be that simple.

R. S. Panush, MD

Depletion of autoreactive plasma cells and treatment of lupus nephritis in mice using CEP-33779, a novel, orally active, selective inhibitor of JAK2

Lu LD, Stump KL, Wallace NH, et al (Cephalon, Inc, West Chester, PA)
J Immunol 187:3840-3853, 2011

Accumulating evidence suggests that autoreactive plasma cells play an important role in systemic lupus erythematosus (SLE). In addition, several proinflammatory cytokines promote autoreactive B cell maturation and autoantibody production. Hence, therapeutic targeting of such cytokine pathways using a selective JAK2 inhibitor, CEP-33779 (JAK2 enzyme IC(50) = 1.3 nM; JAK3 enzyme IC(50)/JAK2 enzyme IC(50) = 65-fold), was tested in two mouse models of SLE. Age-matched, MRL/lpr or BWF1 mice with established SLE or lupus nephritis, respectively, were treated orally with CEP-33779 at 30 mg/kg (MRL/lpr), 55 mg/kg or 100 mg/kg (MRL/lpr and BWF1). Studies included reference standard, dexamethasone (1.5 mg/kg; MRL/lpr), and cyclophosphamide (50 mg/kg; MRL/lpr and BWF1). Treatment with CEP-33779 extended survival and reduced splenomegaly/lymphomegaly. Several serum cytokines were significantly decreased upon treatment including IL-12, IL-17A, IFN-α, IL-1β, and TNF-α. Antinuclear Abs and frequencies of autoantigen-specific, Ab-secreting cells declined upon CEP-33779 treatment. Increased serum complement levels were associated with reduced renal JAK2 activity, histopathology, and spleen CD138(+) plasma cells. The selective JAK2 inhibitor CEP-33779 was able to mitigate several immune parameters associated with SLE advancement, including the protection and treatment of mice with lupus nephritis. These data support the possibility of using potent, orally active, small-molecule inhibitors of JAK2 to treat the debilitative disease SLE.

▶ JAK inhibitors, orally administered antagonists of Janus kinase (interfering with the JAK-STAT signaling pathway, which transmits extracellular signals into gene promotors), are in clinical trials for rheumatoid arthritis and appear promising. These data suggest possible utility for lupus as well.

R. S. Panush, MD

Usefulness of cellular text messaging for improving adherence among adolescents and young adults with systemic lupus erythematosus
Ting TV, Kudalkar D, Nelson S, et al (Cincinnati Children's Hosp Med Ctr, OH)
J Rheumatol 39:174-179, 2012

Objective.—In a cohort of 70 patients with childhood-onset systemic lupus erythematosus (cSLE): to determine the baseline adherence to medications and visits; to investigate the effects of cellular text messaging reminders (CTMR) on adherence to clinic visits; and to study the influence of CTMR on adherence to use of hydroxychloroquine (HCQ).

Methods.—CTMR were sent to 70 patients prior to clinic visits for 14 months. A subgroup of patients were evaluated for medication adherence to HCQ: 19 patients receiving CTMR prior to each scheduled HCQ dose were compared to 22 patients randomized to standard of care education about HCQ. Visit adherence was measured using administrative databases. Pharmacy refill information, self-report of adherence, and HCQ blood levels were utilized to monitor medication adherence to HCQ. Sufficient adherence to visits or HCQ was defined as estimates > 80%. Disease activity was primarily monitored with the Systemic Lupus Erythematosus Disease Activity Index.

Results.—At baseline, 32% of patients were sufficiently adherent to HCQ, and 81% to clinic visits. Visit adherence improved significantly by > 80% among those who were nonadherent to clinic visits at the baseline CTMR ($p = 0.01$). CTMR did not influence adherence to HCQ over time.

Conclusion.—Patients with cSLE were only modestly adherent to HCQ and clinic visits. CTMR may be effective for improving visit adherence among adolescents and young adults with cSLE, but it does not improve adherence to HCQ.

▶ I could have predicted that better education about the implications of having lupus and communication through the technology favored by adolescents would have a salutary impact. I still think we need to imaginatively exploit modern technologies and trends to more effectively reach our patients.

R. S. Panush, MD

3 Vasculitis

2012 Provisional classification criteria for polymyalgia rheumatica: a European League Against Rheumatism/American College of Rheumatology collaborative initiative
Dasgupta B, Cimmino MA, Kremers HM, et al (Southend Univ Hosp, Westcliff-on-Sea, UK)
Arthritis Rheum 64:943-954, 2012

The objective of this study was to develop European League Against Rheumatism/American College of Rheumatology classification criteria for polymyalgia rheumatica (PMR). Candidate criteria were evaluated in a 6-month prospective cohort study of 125 patients with new-onset PMR and 169 non-PMR comparison subjects with conditions mimicking PMR. A scoring algorithm was developed based on morning stiffness > 45 minutes (2 points), hip pain/limited range of motion (1 point), absence of rheumatoid factor and/or anti-citrullinated protein antibody (2 points), and absence of peripheral joint pain (1 point). A score $\geq$ 4 had 68% sensitivity and 78% specificity for discriminating all comparison subjects from PMR. The specificity was higher (88%) for discriminating shoulder conditions from PMR and lower (65%) for discriminating RA from PMR. Adding ultrasound, a score $\geq$ 5 had increased sensitivity to 66% and specificity to 81%. According to these provisional classification criteria, patients $\geq$ 50 years old presenting with bilateral shoulder pain, not better explained by an alternative pathology, can be classified as having PMR in the presence of morning stiffness > 45 minutes, elevated C-reactive protein and/or erythrocyte sedimentation rate, and new hip pain. These criteria are not meant for diagnostic purposes.

▶ I am probably old fashioned, but I prefer the older unofficial criteria (age older than 50 years, limb-girdle symptoms, elevated erythrocyte sedimentation rate, and dramatic, immediate response to steroids). I never liked classification (diagnostic) criteria that required calculations. Complex criteria evolve when we do not really understand pathogenesis, have certain markers of disease, or clear notions of where one syndrome ends and another begins. We do not need diagnostic (classification) criteria for pneumococcal pneumonia. Sadly, we still do for many rheumatic diseases.

R. S. Panush, MD

Adverse events during longterm low-dose glucocorticoid treatment of polymyalgia rheumatica: a retrospective study

Mazzantini M, Torre C, Miccoli M, et al (Univ of Pisa, Italy)
J Rheumatol 39:552-557, 2012

Objective.—To assess the occurrence of adverse events in a cohort of patients with polymyalgia rheumatica (PMR), treated with low-dose glucocorticoids (GC).

Methods.—This was a retrospective study by review of medical records.

Results.—We identified 222 patients who had a mean duration of followup of 60 ± 22 months and a mean duration of GC therapy of 46 ± 22 months. We found that 95 patients (43%) had at least 1 adverse event after a mean duration of GC therapy of 31 ± 22 months and a mean cumulative dose of 3.4 ± 2.4 g. In particular, 55 developed osteoporosis, 31 had fragility fractures; 27 developed arterial hypertension; 11 diabetes mellitus; 9 acute myocardial infarction; 3 stroke; and 2 peripheral arterial disease. Univariate analysis showed that the duration of GC treatment was significantly associated with osteoporosis ($p < 0.0001$), fragility fractures ($p < 0.0001$), arterial hypertension ($p < 0.005$), and acute myocardial infarction ($p < 0.05$). Cumulative GC dose was significantly associated with osteoporosis ($p < 0.0001$), fragility fractures ($p < 0.0001$), and arterial hypertension ($p < 0.01$). The adverse events occurred more frequently after 2 years of treatment. Multivariate analysis showed that GC duration was significantly associated with osteoporosis (adjusted OR 1.02, 95% CI 1.02-1.05) and arterial hypertension (adjusted OR 1.03, 95% CI 1.01-1.06); GC cumulative dose was significantly associated with fragility fractures (adjusted OR 1.4, 95% CI 1.03-1.8).

Conclusion.—Longterm, low-dose GC treatment of PMR is associated with serious adverse events such as osteoporosis, fractures, and arterial hypertension; these adverse events occur mostly after 2 years of treatment.

▶ I would have been surprised if the data were other than as reported. Many of my polymyalgia rheumatica (PMR) patients have unfortunately taken glucocorticoids for years, too often with similarly serious adverse effects. We (still) need a consistently effective, reasonably safe, and well-tolerated alternative to long-term steroids for patients with PMR and GCA. I do not know of one.

R. S. Panush, MD

4 Seronegative Spondyloarthropathies

Combination antibiotics as a treatment for chronic Chlamydia-induced reactive arthritis: a double-blind, placebo-controlled, prospective trial
Carter JD, Espinoza LR, Inman RD, et al (Univ of South Florida College of Medicine, Tampa, FL)
Arthritis Rheum 62:1298-1307, 2010

Objective.—Chlamydia trachomatis and Chlamydophila (Chlamydia) pneumoniae are known triggers of reactive arthritis (ReA) and exist in a persistent metabolically active infection state in the synovium, suggesting that they may be susceptible to antimicrobial agents. The goal of this study was to investigate whether a 6-month course of combination antibiotics is an effective treatment for patients with chronic Chlamydia-induced ReA.

Methods.—This study was a 9-month, prospective, double-blind, triple-placebo trial assessing a 6-month course of combination antibiotics as a treatment for Chlamydia-induced ReA. Eligible patients had to be positive for C trachomatis or C pneumoniae by polymerase chain reaction (PCR). Groups received 1) doxycycline and rifampin plus placebo instead of azithromycin; 2) azithromycin and rifampin plus placebo instead of doxycycline; or 3) placebos instead of azithromycin, doxycycline, and rifampin. The primary end point was the number of patients who improved by 20% or more in at least 4 of 6 variables without worsening in any 1 variable in both combination antibiotic groups combined and in the placebo group at month 6 compared with baseline.

Results.—The primary end point was achieved in 17 of 27 patients (63%) receiving combination antibiotics and in 3 of 15 patients (20%) receiving placebo. Secondary efficacy end points showed similar results. Six of 27 patients (22%) randomized to combination antibiotics believed that their disease went into complete remission during the trial, whereas no patient in the placebo arm achieved remission. Significantly more patients in the active treatment group became negative for C trachomatis or C pneumoniae by PCR at month 6. Adverse events were mild, with no significant differences between the groups.

Conclusion.—These data suggest that a 6-month course of combination antibiotics is an effective treatment for chronic Chlamydia-induced ReA.

▶ Interesting. The change in polymerase chain reaction from positive to negative suggests the effect may have been at least in part antimicrobial; antibiotics have many antiinflammatory effects (ie, tetracyclines for RA). I may consider this in certain patients.

R. S. Panush, MD

5   Osteoarthritis

Statin use is associated with reduced incidence and progression of knee osteoarthritis in the Rotterdam study
Clockaerts S, Van Osch GJ, Bastiaansen-Jenniskens YM, et al (Univ Med Ctr, Rotterdam, The Netherlands)
Ann Rheum Dis 71:642-647, 2012

Background.—Osteoarthritis is the most frequent chronic joint disease causing pain and disability. Besides biomechanical mechanisms, the pathogenesis of osteoarthritis may involve inflammation, vascular alterations and dysregulation of lipid metabolism. As statins are able to modulate many of these processes, this study examines whether statin use is associated with a decreased incidence and/or progression of osteoarthritis.

Methods.—Participants in a prospective population-based cohort study aged 55 years and older (n = 2921) were included. x-Rays of the knee/hip were obtained at baseline and after on average 6.5 years, and scored using the Kellgren and Lawrence score for osteoarthritis. Any increase in score was defined as overall progression (incidence and progression). Data on covariables were collected at baseline. Information on statin use during follow-up was obtained from computerised pharmacy databases. The overall progression of osteoarthritis was compared between users and non-users of statins. Using a multivariate logistic regression model with generalised estimating equation, OR and 95% CI were calculated after adjusting for confounding variables.

Results.—Overall progression of knee and hip osteoarthritis occurred in 6.9% and 4.7% of cases, respectively. The adjusted OR for overall progression of knee osteoarthritis in statin users was 0.43 (95% CI 0.25 to 0.77, $p = 0.01$). The use of statins was not associated with overall progression of hip osteoarthritis.

Conclusions.—Statin use is associated with more than a 50% reduction in overall progression of osteoarthritis of the knee, but not of the hip.

▶ Curious. It will be interesting to see if this is confirmed and validated. Statins do have a wide array of biologic effects, so this is plausible.

R. S. Panush, MD

Teriparatide as a chondroregenerative therapy for injury-induced osteoarthritis

Sampson ER, Hilton MJ, Tian Y, et al (Univ of Rochester Med Ctr, NY)
Sci Transl Med 3:101ra93, 2011

There is no disease-modifying therapy for osteoarthritis, a degenerative joint disease that is projected to afflict more than 67 million individuals in the United States alone by 2030. Because disease pathogenesis is associated with inappropriate articular chondrocyte maturation resembling that seen during normal endochondral ossification, pathways that govern the maturation of articular chondrocytes are candidate therapeutic targets. It is well established that parathyroid hormone (PTH) acting via the type 1 PTH receptor induces matrix synthesis and suppresses maturation of chondrocytes. We report that the PTH receptor is up-regulated in articular chondrocytes after meniscal injury and in osteoarthritis in humans and in a mouse model of injury-induced knee osteoarthritis. To test whether recombinant human PTH(1-34) (teriparatide) would inhibit aberrant chondrocyte maturation and associated articular cartilage degeneration, we administered systemic teriparatide (Forteo), a Food and Drug Administration-approved treatment for osteoporosis, either immediately after or 8 weeks after meniscal/ligamentous injury in mice. Knee joints were harvested at 4, 8, or 12 weeks after injury to examine the effects of teriparatide on cartilage degeneration and articular chondrocyte maturation. Microcomputed tomography revealed increased bone volume within joints from teriparatide-treated mice compared to saline-treated control animals. Immediate systemic administration of teriparatide increased proteoglycan content and inhibited articular cartilage degeneration, whereas delayed treatment beginning 8 weeks after injury induced a regenerative effect. The chondroprotective and chondroregenerative effects of teriparatide correlated with decreased expression of type X collagen, RUNX2 (runt-related transcription factor 2), matrix metalloproteinase 13, and the carboxyl-terminal aggrecan cleavage product NITEGE. These preclinical findings provide proof of concept that Forteo may be useful for decelerating cartilage degeneration and inducing matrix regeneration in patients with osteoarthritis.

▶ Expect more about the possibility that parathormone, with these demonstrated properties of chondroprotection and cartilage regeneration, may have value for treating osteoarthritis. We have nothing (yet) that modifies the course of this, the most common of all arthritis diseases.

R. S. Panush, MD

The impact of knee and hip chondrocalcinosis on disability in older people: the ProVA Study from northeastern Italy

Musacchio E, Ramonda R, Perissinotto E, et al (Univ of Padova, Italy)
Ann Rheum Dis 70:1937-1943, 2011

Objectives.—Chondrocalcinosis is frequently associated with osteoarthritis. The role of osteoarthritis in the onset and progression of disability is well known. The impact of chondrocalcinosis on disability has never been investigated in epidemiological studies.

Methods.—Progetto Veneto Anziani is a survey of 3099 older Italians, focusing on chronic diseases and disability. Assessment was by questionnaires, physical performance tests and clinical evaluations. Chondrocalcinosis was determined by x-ray readings of 1629 consecutive subjects. Knee and hip osteoarthritis severity was evaluated by summing the radiographic features score (RFS) assigned during x-ray reading.

Results.—Subjects with chondrocalcinosis were older and more frequently women (age-adjusted $p < 0.0001$). The gender association disappeared following adjustment for osteoarthritis severity. However, at the knee, the prevalence of osteoarthritis was higher in chondrocalcinosis patients independently of age and sex (age-adjusted $p < 0.0001$). No difference was found between chondrocalcinosis and controls in sociodemographic variables and comorbidity. Knee chondrocalcinosis was strongly associated with clinical features of knee osteoarthritis and with disability assessment parameters in the bivariate analysis. Most associations remained after adjusting for age. After further adjustment for RFS, a significant association remained for knee deformity and pain, the need for a cane, difficulty walking 500 m, using a toilet, shopping and repeatedly rising from a chair.

Conclusions.—Pain and physical function are the outcome measures of choice for assessing disability in osteoarthritis patients. The presence of chondrocalcinosis contributes to both, independently of age and osteoarthritis severity, thus compromising the quality of life and worsening comorbidity.

▶ It has long been thought that calcium pyrophosphate crystals, even when "lanthanic" (asymptomatic), are potentially injurious to cartilage. It is therefore not surprising that the presence of chondrocalcinosis in osteoarthritis was associated with more morbidity.

R. S. Panush, MD

6 Gout and Other Crystal Diseases

Antihypertensive drugs and risk of incident gout among patients with hypertension: population based case-control study
Choi HK, Soriano LC, Zhang Y, et al (Boston Univ School of Medicine, MA)
BMJ 344:d8190, 2012

Objective.—To determine the independent associations of antihypertensive drugs with the risk of incident gout among people with hypertension.

Design.—Nested case-control study.

Setting.—UK general practice database, 2000-7.

Participants.—All incident cases of gout (n = 24,768) among adults aged 20-79 and a random sample of 50,000 matched controls.

Main Outcome Measure.—Relative risk of incident gout associated with use of antihypertensive drugs.

Results.—After adjusting for age, sex, body mass index, visits to the general practitioner, alcohol intake, and pertinent drugs and comorbidities, the multivariate relative risks of incident gout associated with current use of antihypertensive drugs among those with hypertension (n = 29,138) were 0.87 (95% confidence interval 0.82 to 0.93) for calcium channel blockers, 0.81 (0.70 to 0.94) for losartan, 2.36 (2.21 to 2.52) for diuretics, 1.48 (1.40 to 1.57) for β blockers, 1.24 (1.17 to 1.32) for angiotensin converting enzyme inhibitors, and 1.29 (1.16 to 1.43) for non-losartan angiotensin II receptor blockers. Similar results were obtained among those without hypertension. The multivariate relative risks for the duration of use of calcium channel blockers among those with hypertension were 1.02 for less than one year, 0.88 for 1-1.9 years, and 0.75 for two or more years and for use of losartan they were 0.98, 0.87, and 0.71, respectively (both $P < 0.05$ for trend).

Conclusions.—Compatible with their urate lowering properties, calcium channel blockers and losartan are associated with a lower risk of incident gout among people with hypertension. By contrast, diuretics, β blockers, angiotensin converting enzyme inhibitors, and non-losartan angiotensin II receptor blockers are associated with an increased risk of gout.

▶ This report identifies risk for gout for beta-blockers, angiotensin-converting enzyme inhibitors, and nonlosartan angiotensin II receptor blockers. Because hypertension and gout are frequently associated comorbid conditions, these observations have practical implications.

R. S. Panush, MD

7 Fibromyalgia and Other Soft Tissue Musculoskeletal Problems

Does lumbar disc degeneration on magnetic resonance imaging associate with low back symptom severity in young Finnish adults?
Takatalo J, Karppinen J, Niinimäki J, et al (Univ of Oulu, Finland)
Spine (Phila Pa 1976) 36:2180-2189, 2011

Study Design.—A cross-sectional magnetic resonance imaging study with questionnaires on low back pain (LBP) and functional limitations.

Objective.—To investigate the association between lumbar intervertebral disc degeneration (DD) and low back symptom severity among young Finnish adults.

Summary of Background Data.—Both LBP and lumbar DD are common already in adolescence, but very little is known of their association in young adults.

Methods.—Young adults belonging to a birth cohort (n = 874) were invited to lumbar magnetic resonance imaging using a 1.5-T scanner. Data on LBP and functional limitations at the ages of 18, 19, and 21 years were used to cluster the subjects with respect to low back symptoms using latent class analysis. The prevalence and 95% confidence intervals of DD at 21 years and the sum score of DD at all lumbar levels were compared between the clusters. The contribution of DD and other imaging findings (herniations, anular tears, Modic changes, spondylolytic defects) to symptom severity was analyzed with logistic regression analysis.

Results.—Latent class analysis produced five clusters from the 554 subjects, ranging from a cluster where subjects (n = 65) had been painful at all time points to an asymptomatic cluster (n = 168). DD was more prevalent in the three most symptomatic clusters compared to the two least symptomatic ones. Similar findings were obtained for the DD sum scores. Lumbar DD was related to symptom severity independently of other degenerative findings. Moreover, moderately degenerated discs were more likely than mildly degenerated discs to be associated with the most severe low back symptoms.

Conclusion.—Intervertebral DD was associated with low back symptom severity among young adults, suggesting that the symptoms may have a discogenic origin at this age. However, DD was also found in one-third of asymptomatic subjects.

▶ This study illustrates the dilemma about low back pain. Disc degeneration occurred in one-third of asymptomatic young adults.

R. S. Panush, MD

The longitudinal outcome of fibromyalgia: a study of 1555 patients
Walitt B, Fitzcharles MA, Hassett AL, et al (Natl Data Bank for Rheumatic Diseases, Wichita, KS)
J Rheumatol 38:2238-2246, 2011

Objective.—To describe the diagnosis status and outcome of patients diagnosed with fibromyalgia (FM) by US rheumatologists.

Methods.—We assessed 1555 patients with FM with detailed outcome questionnaires during 11,006 semiannual observations for up to 11 years. At entry, all patients satisfied American College of Rheumatology preliminary 2010 FM criteria modified for survey research. We determined diagnosis status, rates of improvement, responder subgroups, and standardized mean differences (effect sizes) between start and study completion scores of global well-being, pain, sleep problems, and health related quality of life (QOL).

Results.—The 5-year improvement rates were pain 0.4 (95% CI 0.2, 0.5), fatigue 0.4 (95% CI 0.2, 0.05), and global 0.0 (95% CI -0.1, 0.1). The standardized mean differences were patient global 0.03 (95% CI -0.02, 0.08), pain 0.22 (95% CI 0.16, 0.28), sleep problems 0.20 (95% CI 0.14, 0.25), physical component summary of the Short-form 36 (SF-36) 0.11 (95% CI -0.14, -0.07), and SF-36 mental component summary 0.03 (95% CI -0.07, 0.02). Patients switched between criteria-positive and criteria-negative states, with 716 patients (44.0%) failing to meet criteria at least once during 4228.5 patient-years (7448 observations). About 10% of patients had substantial improvement and about 15% had moderate improvement of pain. Overall, FM severity worsened in 35.9% and pain in 38.6%.

Conclusion.—Although we found no average clinically meaningful improvement in symptom severity overall, 25% had at least moderate improvement of pain over time. The result that emerged from this longitudinal study was one of generally continuing high levels of self-reported symptoms and distress for most patients, but a slight trend toward improvement.

▶ It is not surprising that most patients did not change much over time, consistent with older data. It will be interesting to see whether there are similar observations for the next decade, now that we approach disease somewhat differently and have some medications that may be genuinely beneficial.

R. S. Panush, MD

8 Miscellaneous Rheumatic Diseases and Therapies

Antibodies targeting the catalytic zinc complex of activated matrix metalloproteinases show therapeutic potential

Sela-Passwell N, Kikkeri R, Dym O, et al (Weizmann Inst of Science, Rehovot, Israel)

Nat Med 18:143-147, 2011

Endogenous tissue inhibitors of metalloproteinases (TIMPs) have key roles in regulating physiological and pathological cellular processes. Imitating the inhibitory molecular mechanisms of TIMPs while increasing selectivity has been a challenging but desired approach for antibody-based therapy. TIMPs use hybrid protein-protein interactions to form an energetic bond with the catalytic metal ion, as well as with enzyme surface residues. We used an innovative immunization strategy that exploits aspects of molecular mimicry to produce inhibitory antibodies that show TIMP-like binding mechanisms toward the activated forms of gelatinases (matrix metalloproteinases 2 and 9). Specifically, we immunized mice with a synthetic molecule that mimics the conserved structure of the metalloenzyme catalytic zinc-histidine complex residing within the enzyme active site. This immunization procedure yielded selective function-blocking monoclonal antibodies directed against the catalytic zinc-protein complex and enzyme surface conformational epitopes of endogenous gelatinases. The therapeutic potential of these antibodies has been demonstrated with relevant mouse models of inflammatory bowel disease. Here we propose a general experimental strategy for generating inhibitory antibodies that effectively target the in vivo activity of dysregulated metalloproteinases by mimicking the mechanism employed by TIMPs.

▶ Expect to see more about metalloproteinase inhibition, as these enzymes participate widely in inflammatory and destructive processes, not only in rheumatic disorders (rheumatoid arthritis, osteoarthritis) but also gastrointestinal and vascular diseases.

R. S. Panush, MD

Combined prednisone and mycophenolate mofetil treatment for retroperitoneal fibrosis: a case series

Scheel PJ Jr, Feeley N, Sozio SM (The Johns Hopkins Univ School of Medicine, Baltimore, MD)
Ann Intern Med 154:31-36, 2011

Background.—Small case series suggest that a combination of mycophenolate mofetil and prednisone may be an effective treatment for patients with retroperitoneal fibrosis.

Objective.—To describe the outcomes of adults with retroperitoneal fibrosis who received a combination of prednisone and mycophenolate mofetil.

Design.—Prospective case series of patients followed between 1 April 2005 and 1 July 2009.

Setting.—Single tertiary care facility.

Patients.—28 patients with retroperitoneal fibrosis.

Intervention.—Prednisone, 40 mg/d, tapered over 6 months, and mycophenolate mofetil, 1000 mg twice daily, for a mean of 24.3 months.

Measurements.—Clinical course, laboratory assessment, and measurement of periaortic mass. Mean follow-up was 1012 days, and no patients were lost to follow-up.

Results.—Systemic symptoms resolved in all patients; 89% had a 25% or greater reduction in periaortic mass. Elevated erythrocyte sedimentation rate and serum creatinine level and decreased hemoglobin level normalized in all patients. Disease recurred in 2 of 28 patients.

Limitation.—This was a small case series.

Conclusion.—Combined prednisone and mycophenolate mofetil therapy is a potentially effective treatment for retroperitoneal fibrosis that warrants evaluation in randomized trials.

▶ I liked this report because I have been asked to see some of these patients in consultation. Most of the literature is anecdotal; some patients' symptoms can be challenging to treat, and there is little robust evidence from which to make recommendations. I was therefore pleased to see a reasonable prospective series of patients with good outcomes.

R. S. Panush, MD

Fumarates improve psoriasis and multiple sclerosis by inducing type II dendritic cells

Ghoreschi K, Brück J, Kellerer C, et al (Eberhard Karls Univ Tübingen, Germany)
J Exp Med 208:2291-2303, 2011

Fumarates improve multiple sclerosis (MS) and psoriasis, two diseases in which both IL-12 and IL-23 promote pathogenic T helper (Th) cell differentiation. However, both diseases show opposing responses to most established therapies. First, we show in humans that fumarate treatment induces IL-4-producing Th2 cells in vivo and generates type II dendritic cells (DCs) that produce IL-10 instead of IL-12 and IL-23. In mice, fumarates also generate type II DCs that induce IL-4-producing Th2 cells in vitro and in vivo and protect mice from experimental autoimmune encephalomyelitis. Type II DCs result from fumarate-induced glutathione (GSH) depletion, followed by increased hemoxygenase-1 (HO-1) expression and impaired STAT1 phosphorylation. Induced HO-1 is cleaved, whereupon the N-terminal fragment of HO-1 translocates into the nucleus and interacts with AP-1 and NF-κB sites of the IL-23p19 promoter. This interaction prevents IL-23p19 transcription without affecting IL-12p35, whereas STAT1 inactivation prevents IL-12p35 transcription without affecting IL-23p19. As a consequence, GSH depletion by small molecules such as fumarates induces type II DCs in mice and in humans that ameliorate inflammatory autoimmune diseases. This therapeutic approach improves Th1- and Th17-mediated autoimmune diseases such as psoriasis and MS by interfering with IL-12 and IL-23 production.

▶ Fumarates improve the immunologically mediated disorders—psoriasis and multiple sclerosis—perhaps by inducing interleukin (IL)-10—producing type II dendritic cells (confounding production of IL-12 and IL-23, which promote pathogenic T helper (Th) cell differentiation). Expect to hear more about these and other therapies that perturb IL-12 and IL-23 in Th1- and Th17-mediated autoimmune diseases.

R. S. Panush, MD

IL-23 is critical for induction of arthritis, osteoclast formation, and maintenance of bone mass

Adamopoulos IE, Tessmer M, Chao CC, et al (Merck Res Laboratories, Palo Alto, CA)
J Immunol 187:951-959, 2011

The role of IL-23 in the development of arthritis and bone metabolism was studied using systemic IL-23 exposure in adult mice via hydrodynamic delivery of IL-23 minicircle DNA in vivo and in mice genetically deficient in IL-23. Systemic IL-23 exposure induced chronic arthritis, severe bone loss, and myelopoiesis in the bone marrow and spleen, which resulted in increased osteoclast differentiation and systemic bone loss. The effect of IL-23 was partly dependent on CD4(+) T cells, IL-17A, and TNF, but could not be reproduced by overexpression of IL-17A in vivo. A key role in the IL-23-induced arthritis was made by the expansion and activity of myeloid cells. Bone marrow macrophages derived from IL-23p19(-/-) mice showed a slower maturation into osteoclasts with reduced tartrate-resistant acid phosphatase-positive cells and dentine resorption capacity in in vitro osteoclastogenesis assays. This correlated with fewer multinucleated osteoclast-like cells and more trabecular bone volume and number in 26-wk-old male IL-23p19(-/-) mice compared with control animals. Collectively, our data suggest that systemic IL-23 exposure induces the expansion of a myeloid lineage osteoclast precursor, and targeting IL-23 pathway may combat inflammation-driven bone destruction as observed in rheumatoid arthritis and other autoimmune arthritides.

▶ Expect to keep seeing interleukin-23 in the literature. It is a critical contributor to inflammatory and autoimmune disease and therefore an attractive potential therapeutic target.

R. S. Panush, MD

Impact of synthetic and biologic disease-modifying antirheumatic drugs on antibody responses to the AS03-adjuvanted pandemic influenza vaccine: a prospective, open-label, parallel-cohort, single-center study
Gabay C, H1N1 Study Group (Univ Hosps of Geneva and Univ of Geneva, Switzerland)
Arthritis Rheum 63:1486-1496, 2011

Objective.—To identify the determinants of antibody responses to adjuvanted split influenza A (H1N1) vaccines in patients with inflammatory rheumatic diseases.

Methods.—One hundred seventy-three patients (82 with rheumatoid arthritis, 45 with spondylarthritis, and 46 with other inflammatory rheumatic diseases) and 138 control subjects were enrolled in this prospective single-center study. Controls received 1 dose of adjuvanted influenza A/09/H1N1 vaccine, and patients received 2 doses of the vaccine. Antibody responses were measured by hemagglutination inhibition assay before and 3-4 weeks after each dose. Geometric mean titers (GMTs) and rates of seroprotection (GMT ≥ 40) were calculated. A comprehensive medical questionnaire was used to identify the determinants of vaccine responses and adverse events.

Results.—Baseline influenza A/09/H1N1 antibody levels were low in patients and controls (seroprotection rates 14.8% and 14.2%, respectively). A significant response to dose 1 was observed in both groups. However, the GMT and the seroprotection rate remained significantly lower in patients (GMT 146 versus 340, seroprotection rate 74.6% versus 87%; both $P < 0.001$). The second dose markedly increased antibody titers in patients, with achievement of a similar GMT and seroprotection rate as elicited with a single dose in healthy controls. By multivariate regression analysis, increasing age, use of disease-modifying antirheumatic drugs (DMARDs) (except hydroxychloroquine and sulfasalazine), and recent (within 3 months) B cell depletion treatment were identified as the main determinants of vaccine responses; tumor necrosis factor α antagonist treatment was not identified as a major determinant. Immunization was well tolerated, without any adverse effect on disease activity.

Conclusion.—DMARDs exert distinct influences on influenza vaccine responses in patients with inflammatory rheumatic diseases. Two doses of adjuvanted vaccine were necessary and sufficient to elicit responses in patients similar to those achieved with 1 dose in healthy controls.

▶ There are several comments to be made about this nice study. (1) Vaccination did not cause flare of disease. (2) Only H1N1 was examined. (3) Prednisone, tumor necrosis factor-alpha inhibitors, hydroxychloroquine, and sulfasalazine did not impair responses. (4) Type of autoimmune disease did not influence vaccine response. (5) Protection from infection was not evaluated. Thus, I think it would be presumptuous to try to generalize from these data. We need to know what level of response to vaccine confers clinical immunity, and we need to know this for each vaccine (eg, pneumonia, shingles) we contemplate using in practice.

R. S. Panush, MD

Retainer medicine: an ethically legitimate form of practice that can improve primary care
Huddle TS, Centor RM (Univ of Alabama at Birmingham)
Ann Intern Med 155:633-635, 2011

Retainer medicine has become an important yet controversial form of primary care practice in the United States, coming under attack for its purported failure to measure up to professional ethics. Critics opine that retainer medicine obstructs professional commitments to health care access and social justice. Some ethicists urge that society should restrict or ban retainer medicine; professional organizations have yet to take a stand. The authors believe that retainer medicine is compatible with professional ethics and will more likely aid in solving the difficulties facing primary care rather than add to them. Although professional ethics should evolve to address new conditions, a condemnation of retainer medicine is warranted neither by traditional ethical precepts nor by contemporary developments in medical ethics. Any move to sanction retainer medicine under the banner of professionalism or professional ethics will be counter-productive. The primary care shortage will only get worse if physicians in retainer practice leave primary care altogether, a likely outcome of legal or professional condemnation of retainer practice.

▶ This article may have changed my thinking. I had considered boutique prac-
tice offensive—unethical and unprofessional. The authors argued in brief that the responsibility for ensuring social justice is societal and that individual responsibilities are to provide the best possible ethical and competent care however they chose to practice. I still worry that this perspective lessens the incentive—indeed, obligation—of all physicians to achieve a more just and equitable health care for all.

R. S. Panush, MD

Rheumatic complaints in women taking aromatase inhibitors for treatment of hormone-dependent breast cancer

Scarpa R, Atteno M, Peluso R, et al (Univ Federico II, Naples, Italy)
J Clin Rheumatol 17:169-172, 2011

Background.—The rheumatic adverse effects accompanying treatment with aromatase inhibitors (AIs) in hormone-dependent breast cancer represent an area of clinical relevance and emerging concern. This report describes these rheumatic complaints detailing their clinical pattern.

Methods.—During 1-year period, 18 consecutive postmenopausal women (mean age, 58.33 years; range, 52-66 years) in treatment with AIs for hormone-dependent breast cancer (mean duration of therapy, 12.0 months; range, 9.1-17.7 months) were referred for evaluation in the outpatient clinic of the rheumatology unit in relation to rheumatic complaints. According to a routine protocol planned with oncologists, patient evaluations consisted of a complete clinical examination with careful assessment of rheumatic complaints and related physical symptoms, followed by laboratory testing and a bone scintiscan. In no cases were rheumatic complaints present before AI therapy.

Results.—On the basis of clinical data and investigations and by applying accepted diagnostic criteria, a diagnosis of an undifferentiated spondyloarthropathy was reached in 10 (55.5%) of the 18 patients studied, and an oligoarthritis was shown in 2 more patients (11.1%), whereas a simple arthralgia was found in the remaining 6 patients (33.3%). In the patients meeting criteria as belonging to a spondyloarthritic subset, a family history positive for psoriasis and celiac disease was shown in 2 and 1 instance, respectively, whereas HLA-CW6 and HLA-B27 were detected in 3 and 1 case. A high serum level of anti-cyclic citrullinated peptide antibodies was shown in 1 patient with oligoarthritis. Most of the patients (16/18) were treated with nonsteroidal antiinflammatory drugs or with corticosteroids. Methotrexate (10 mg weekly) was added in 3 of these patients, nonresponders. Aromatase inhibitor discontinuation was needed in the remaining 2 cases with spontaneous resolution of symptoms over time.

Conclusions.—Data from the present study emphasize a previously unsuspected high prevalence of defined arthritides underlying these rheumatic complaints. Therefore, investigative efforts should be addressed to better clarify the clinical and pathogenetic significance of these important consequences of AI therapy. An accurate monitoring of rheumatic complaints has to be suggested to patients taking AI therapy, with a rapid referral to a rheumatologist in the case of consistent suspicion of an inflammatory arthritis.

▶ Oncologists and rheumatologists recognize this relatively new syndrome, and other physicians should also be aware of it. I have had reasonable success managing this symptomatically, which is really all we can do because patients rarely are prepared to stop the aromatase inhibitor.

R. S. Panush, MD

Singing Intervention for Preoperative Hypertension Prior to Total Joint Replacement: A Case report

Niu NN, Perez MT, Katz JN (Brigham and Women's Hosp and Harvard Univ, Boston, MA)
Arthritis Care Res (Hoboken) 63:630-632, 2011

Background.—The therapy generally instituted for preoperative hypertension includes diuretics, beta blockers, calcium-channel blockers, and angiotensin-converting enzyme (ACE) inhibitors. Even with all these agents and others, some patients do not respond. For refractory cases, clinicians seek alternative methods. Music has the ability to ameliorate anxiety and blood pressure according to a number of randomized controlled trials. A case of preoperative hypertension managed by allowing the patient to make music was reported.

> *Case Report.*—Woman, 76, from the Dominican Republic had hypertension and a 15-year history of bilateral knee osteoarthritis (OA). She also suffered from hyperlipidemia and mild obesity. She was accepted into Operation Walk Boston (Op Walk), a philanthropic program that provides total joint replacement to poor Dominican patients with advanced hip or knee OA. She was admitted to the hospital for bilateral total knee replacement with a blood pressure of 160/90 mm Hg. On the morning of surgery her blood pressure measured 240/120 mm Hg, and surgery was cancelled while she was given additional blood pressure agents. Although this therapy was begun immediately, her systolic pressure stayed at about 200 mm Hg throughout the afternoon. She was concerned, since the Op Walk team could not remain beyond a few more days. She asked if she could sing and was given permission. She sang six religious songs that invoked protection of the poor and the ill in line with her Seventh-Day Adventist beliefs in Jesus, God, and her Savior. She explained that she often sang at home to cheer herself up or to calm herself down. After two songs, her blood pressure was 180/90 mm Hg. After a few more songs, her systolic blood pressure was under 180 mm Hg and remained so for about 20 more minutes of singing and for several hours afterward. She was allowed to sing "ad lib" throughout the night, during which time her blood pressure remained at acceptable levels. She was able to undergo the surgery, had no surgical complications, and had no difficulty managing her blood pressure postoperatively.

Conclusions.—Singing is simple, safe, and free. Music appears to have the power to improve mood, distract from disease, relax people, and enhance the release of natural opiates. These appear to work together to modulate the transmission or perception of pain. Both high blood pressure and chronic arthritic pain have been ameliorated by listening to music. Singing offers patients a form of self-expression for their emotions; allows patients to choose their own songs, which would have the rhythm, pitch, and tempo that provide the most therapeutic effects; and reflects a belief in the power of music, which can provide comfort during times of stress and hardship. Thus singing should be able to reduce anxiety and pain, improve the sense of self-control, provide relief by choosing songs with personal significance, and produce benefits in line with belief that can extend far beyond the effects of just listening to music. Further study is needed to determine if singing can be an alternative or adjuvant therapy for reducing chronic pain and facilitating surgical interventions for patients with arthritis.

▶ Kudos to Jeff Katz and colleagues for their innovative approach to this patient. Although perhaps seeming a strange selection, I perceive several important points here: know your patients; listen to your patients; think outside the box. Remember there's more to medicine than medicine.

R. S. Panush, MD

Suicidal ideation among adults with arthritis: prevalence and subgroups at highest risk. Data from the 2007-2008 National Health and Nutrition Examination Survey
Tektonidou MG, Dasgupta A, Ward MM (Natl Univ of Athens, Greece)
Arthritis Care Res (Hoboken) 63:1322-1333, 2011

Objective.—To evaluate the prevalence, correlates, and subgroups at highest risk for suicidal ideation among adults with arthritis.

Methods.—We used data on US adults with arthritis, ages ≥40 years, participating in the 2007-2008 National Health and Nutrition Examination Survey. Suicidal ideation was assessed by item 9 of the Patient Health Questionnaire 9 (PHQ-9). Sociodemographic factors, health behaviors, and comorbid conditions were examined as potential correlates. Depression was measured by the PHQ-8 score (range 1-24). We used random forests to identify subgroups at highest risk for suicidal ideation. To determine if any correlates were unique to arthritis, we compared results to those for persons with diabetes mellitus and cancer.

Results.—The prevalence ± SEM of suicidal ideation was 5.6% ± 0.8% among persons with arthritis and 2.4% ± 0.4% among those without. The most important correlates for suicidal ideation in adults with arthritis were depression, anxiety, duration of arthritis, age, income:poverty ratio, number of close friends, pain, alcohol, excessive daytime sleepiness, and comorbidities. Eleven of the 16 most important contributors for suicidal ideation among adults with arthritis were also important for people with diabetes mellitus and cancer. Among persons with arthritis, subgroups at highest risk for suicidal ideation were those with a PHQ-8 score between 18 and 24 and less than 4.5 years of arthritis (96.5%), and those with a PHQ-8 score between 7 and 17, ≥1.24 days of binges/month, and either an income of ≥$45,000/year (85.4%) or an income of <$45,000/year and >3 comorbidities (70.8%).

Conclusion.—Depression, short duration of arthritis, binge drinking, income, and >3 comorbidities identified subgroups of adults with arthritis at greatest risk for suicidal ideation.

▶ Suicide ideation is more than twice as common in patients with arthritis than it is in those without. Suicide was also associated with all the expected correlates (depression, poverty, pain, alcohol use, smaller number of close friends). None of this is surprising. We have tended to underestimate (and undertreat) our patients' pain and probably have not fully appreciated the depth and breadth of their suffering. We should be more alert to this.

R. S. Panush, MD

The effect of patch testing on surgical practices and outcomes in orthopedic patients with metal implants

Atanaskova Mesinkovska N, Tellez A, Molina L, et al (Cleveland Clinic, OH)
Arch Dermatol 148:687-693, 2012

Objective.—To determine the effect of patch testing on surgical decision making and outcomes in patients evaluated for suspected metal hypersensitivity related to implants in bones or joints.

Design.—Medical chart review.

Setting.—Tertiary care academic medical center.

Participants.—All patients who had patch testing for allergic contact dermatitis related to orthopedic implants.

Intervention.—Patch testing.

Main Outcome Measures.—The surgeon's preoperative choice of metal implant alloy compared with patch testing results and the presence of hypersensitivity complications related to the metal implant on postsurgical follow-up.

Results.—Patients with potential metal hypersensitivity from implanted devices (N = 72) were divided into 2 groups depending on timing of their patch testing: preimplantation (n = 31) and postimplantation (n = 41). History of hypersensitivity to metals was a predictor of positive patch test results to metals in both groups. Positive patch test results indicating metal hypersensitivity influenced the decision-making process of the referring surgeon in all preimplantation cases (n = 21). Patients with metal hypersensitivity who received an allergen-free implant had surgical outcomes free of hypersensitivity complications (n = 21). In patients who had positive patch test results to a metal in their implant after implantation, removal of the device led to resolution of associated symptoms (6 of 10 patients).

Conclusions.—The findings of this study support a role for patch testing in patients with a clinical history of metal hypersensitivity before prosthetic device implantation. The decision on whether to remove an implanted device after positive patch test results should be made on a case-by-case basis, as decided by the surgeon and patient.

▶ Probably most, if not all, patients with metal implants have at least microscopic reaction to the foreign material. Fortunately, not many have clinically important symptoms. Diagnosis of this complication can be difficult; the distinction of implant-related arthritis from other possibilities must ultimately be made by synovial fluid analysis or histology. A simpler test would be nice. A patch test might be helpful to identify sensitive individuals prior to joint replacement.

R. S. Panush, MD

INFECTIOUS DISEASE

NANCY M. KHARDORI, MD, PHD

PART TWO

INFECTIOUS DISEASE

NANCY M. KHARDORI MD, PHD

Introduction

"A man cannot become a competent surgeon without full knowledge of human anatomy and physiology and the physician without physiology and chemistry flounders along in an aimless fashion, never able to gain any accurate conception of disease, practicing a sort of popgun pharmacy, hitting now the malady and again the patient, he himself not knowing which." This quote from Sir William Oster (1849–1919) is titled "The practice of medicine requires knowledge of basic science." In his time the science of microbiology was in its infancy and antimicrobial agents were yet to become a reality. It is rational to state that this quote is more applicable to the specialty of infectious disease than any others. This year's overview of literature in INFECTIOUS DISEASES continues to provide testament to the fact that common human pathogens continue to cause significant morbidity and mortality by adapting to and surviving challenges they face in the form of antimicrobials. Five selections in the bacteriology section discuss the ongoing epidemic of staphylococcal skin and soft tissue infections driven by the clone USA300 (both MSSA and MRSA), the high incidence of recurrence, clustering within household contacts, and the effectiveness of various decolonization regimens. The blurring of microbiological distinction between community-acquired and nosocomial S aureus infection is clearly documented now along with the higher prevalence rates of MRSA in complicated skin and soft tissue infections.

The multiplicity and diversity of genes associated with toxin production in both MRSA and MSSA allude to the fact that virulence is not determined by any single determinant (eg, PVL toxin) but a multitude of virulence genes. An elegant study on the evolution of biology of S aureus used whole-genome sequencing on isolates from carrier state to disease state and described a clustering of protein-truncating mutations. The role of food processing and chain of the transmission of human pathogens, both bacteria and viruses, is demonstrated in the selections on E coli 0157:H7, Hepatitis A virus, and norovirus. I found the report on safety and efficacy of MVA85A vaccine for tuberculosis in HIV-infected populations with and without latent tuberculosis infection to be of major clinical relevance given that HIV and TB epidemics coexist in sub-Saharan Africa.

Two of the selections in the section on fungal infections describe the role of Candida sp in severe sepsis and the outcome-modifying factors. A cluster of patients with pneumocystic pneumonia and patients colonized by Pneumocystis jirovecii in renal transplant recipients point to the need for enhanced prevention procedures and further define the role of primary prophylaxis in immunocompromised patients. The continued reporting of antimicrobial resistance among human and animal pathogens is reported in a number of selections. However, the only positive step in this regard is the recent FDA recommendation for restriction on the use of antibiotics in animal agriculture, in particular, their addition to the feed for growth promoting effect. Included are 5 selections on major clinical features and routine laboratory tests and early goal-directed strategies in the management of serious infectious diseases. Vaccines continue to be the highlight of advances in infectious disease management as demonstrated by the 4 selections in this edition of the YEAR BOOK OF MEDICINE. This sharply contrasts with the lack of studies on new classes of antimicrobial agents.

I would like to point out the selection on the strong association of Human Papilloma Virus with a subset of oropharyngeal squamous cell carcinoma, 90% of which are related to HPV type 16. The available vaccines for prevention of genital warts and anogenital cancers both contain HPV type 16. Even if we were to get newer classes of antimicrobial agents (not foreseeable in the near future), their short life span and short-term impact on morbidity and mortality and collateral damage will always contrast with the long life span (potentially indefinite), long-term impact on human health, and collateral advantage of herd community offered by the vaccines.

I close with the grateful acknowledgement of assistance provided by Sandy Finch in accomplishing a task that is both daunting and rewarding at the same time.

N. M. Khardori, MD, PhD

9 Bacterial Infections

Efficacy of 5-Day Levofloxacin-Containing Concomitant Therapy in Eradication of *Helicobacter pylori* Infection
Federico A, Nardone G, Gravina AG, et al (Azienda Ospedaliera Universitaria, Napoli, Italy; Universitá Federico II, Napoli, Italy; et al)
Gastroenterology 143:55-61.e1, 2012

Background & Aims.—*Helicobacter pylori* have become resistant to antimicrobial agents, reducing eradication rates. A 10-day sequential regimen that contains levofloxacin was efficient, safe, and cost saving in eradicating *H pylori* infection in an area with high prevalence of clarithromycin resistance. We performed a noninferiority randomized trial to determine whether a 5-day levofloxacin-containing quadruple concomitant regimen was as safe and effective as the 10-day sequential regimen in eradicating *H pylori* in previously untreated patients.

Methods.—We randomly assigned patients with *H pylori* infection to groups that were given 5 days of concomitant therapy (esomeprazole 40 mg twice daily, amoxicillin 1 g twice daily, levofloxacin 500 mg twice daily, and tinidazole 500 mg twice daily; n = 90) or 10 days of sequential therapy (esomeprazole 40 mg twice daily, amoxicillin 1 g twice daily for 5 days followed by esomeprazole 40 mg twice daily, levofloxacin 500 mg twice daily, and tinidazole 500 mg twice daily for 5 more days; n = 90). Antimicrobial resistance was assessed by the E-test. Efficacy, adverse events, and costs were determined.

Results.—Intention-to-treat analysis showed similar eradication rates for concomitant (92.2%; 95% confidence interval [CI], 84.0%−95.8%) and sequential therapies (93.3%; 95% CI, 86.9%−97.3%). Per-protocol eradication results were 96.5% (95% CI, 91%−99%) for concomitant therapy and 95.5% for sequential therapy (95% CI, 89.6%−98.5%). The differences between sequential and concomitant treatments were 1.1% in the intention-to-treat study (95% CI; −7.6% to 9.8%) and −1.0% in the per-protocol analysis (95% CI; −8.0% to 5.9%). The prevalence of antimicrobial resistance and incidence of adverse events were comparable between groups. Concomitant therapy cost $9 less than sequential therapy.

Conclusions.—Five days of levofloxacin-containing quadruple concomitant therapy is as effective and safe, and less expensive, in eradicating

H pylori infection than 10 days of levofloxacin-containing sequential therapy.

▶ Recent decline in the eradication of *Helicobacter pylori* following standard triple-drug therapy has led to a need for alternate approaches.[1] A bismuth-containing quadruple regimen (ie, proton pump inhibitor [PPI] plus bismuth, tetracycline, and metronidazole) has been recommended as the first-line strategy in areas with 15% of *H pylori* resistant to clarithromycin.

A novel 10-day sequential therapy consisting of 5-day dual therapy (PPI plus amoxicillin) followed by 5-day triple therapy (PPI plus clarithromycin plus tinidazole) has shown good results.

An earlier publication from the authors reported that in areas with clarithromycin and clarithromycin plus metronidazole resistance, a levofloxacin-containing regimen achieved eradication rates higher than 95%.[2]

This study was designed to compare the concomitant use of esomeprazole, amoxicillin, levofloxacin, and tinidazole for 5 days to the 10-day sequential regimen of esomeprazole plus amoxicillin for 5 days followed by esomeprazole plus levofloxacin and tinidazole for the next 5 days. This randomized trial in an area of high (>15%) prevalence of clarithromycin-resistant *H pylori* strains showed that the 5-day concomitant regimen is highly effective, with an eradication rate of 92% in the intent-to-treat population. In the sequential therapy group, the eradication rate was 93% and 95% for intent-to-treat and per protocol populations, respectively. The occurrence of adverse events and prevalence of antimicrobial resistance were comparable between the 2 groups. With equal efficacy, reduced cost, and likely improved compliance with a simpler regimen, this regimen represents a safe first-line alternative particularly in areas with low efficacy of triple therapy.

N. M. Khardori, MD, PhD

References

1. Selgrad M, Malfertheiner P. Treatment of Helicobacter pylori. *Curr Opin Gastroenterol.* 2011;27:565-570.
2. Romano M, Cuomo A, Gravina AG, et al. Empirical levofloxacin-containing versus clarithromycin-containing sequential therapy for Helicobacter pylori eradication: a randomised trial. *Gut.* 2010;59:1465-1470.

A Novel Vehicle for Transmission of *Escherichia coli* O157:H7 to Humans: Multistate Outbreak of *E. coli* O157:H7 Infections Associated With Consumption of Ready-to-Bake Commercial Prepackaged Cookie Dough—United States, 2009
Neil KP, Biggerstaff G, MacDonald JK, et al (Ctrs for Disease Control and Prevention, Atlanta, GA; Washington State Dept of Health, Shoreline; et al)
Clin Infect Dis 54:511-518, 2012

Background.—*Escherichia coli* O157:H7 is a Shiga toxin—producing *E. coli* (STEC) associated with numerous foodborne outbreaks in the United States and is an important cause of bacterial gastrointestinal illness.

In May 2009, we investigated a multistate outbreak of *E. coli* O157:H7 infections.

Methods.—Outbreak-associated cases were identified using serotyping and molecular subtyping procedures. Traceback investigation and product testing were performed. A matched case-control study was conducted to identify exposures associated with illness using age-, sex-, and state-matched controls.

Results.—Seventy-seven patients with illnesses during the period 16 March—8 July 2009 were identified from 30 states; 35 were hospitalized, 10 developed hemolytic-uremic syndrome, and none died. Sixty-six percent of patients were <19 years; 71% were female. In the case-control study, 33 of 35 case patients (94%) consumed ready-to-bake commercial prepackaged cookie dough, compared with 4 of 36 controls (11%) (matched odds ratio = 41.3; $P < .001$); no other reported exposures were significantly associated with illness. Among case patients consuming cookie dough, 94% reported brand A. Three nonoutbreak STEC strains were isolated from brand A cookie dough. The investigation led to a recall of 3.6 million packages of brand A cookie dough and a product reformulation.

Conclusions.—This is the first reported STEC outbreak associated with consuming ready-to-bake commercial prepackaged cookie dough. Despite instructions to bake brand A cookie dough before eating, case patients consumed the product uncooked. Manufacturers should consider formulating ready-to-bake commercial prepackaged cookie dough to be as safe as a ready-to-eat product. More effective consumer education about the risks of eating unbaked cookie dough is needed.

▶ *Escherichia coli* O157:H7 has been associated with more than 180 outbreaks of bacterial gastrointestinal illness since the mid-1990s. Uncooked foods, fruit and vegetables, and unpasteurized dairy products have frequently been implicated in outbreaks.[1] The intestinal tract of healthy ruminant animals (eg, cattle, deer, goats, and sheep) is the reservoir for *E coli* O157:H7. Contamination occurs during meat processing, use of contaminated soil, or contaminated irrigation water in produce production, shedding of *E coli* from colonized cattle into milk, or cross-contamination.

Because of the kill steps used in processing, processed foods are less likely to be contaminated. This article adds ready-to-bake commercial prepackaged cookie dough as a novel vehicle for transmission of *E coli* O157:H7. A cluster of 17 cases of *E coli* O157:H7 infection from 13 states in the United States were identified through PulseNet, the national molecular subtyping network for food-borne disease surveillance. The 17 isolates were indistinguishable by pulsed-field gel electrophoresis (PFGE). The cookie dough brand implicated in the outbreak was eaten by case patients uncooked, despite instructions to bake the dough before eating. Three nonoutbreak-related Shiga toxin—producing *E coli* (STEC) strains were isolated from the cookie dough brand used by 94% of case patients. No human isolates had PFGE patterns matching those of food sample STEC isolates. However, the isolation of STEC from the product revealed that STEC can contaminate and survive in these processed products. A large batch of contaminated flour remains a prime suspect for introducing the pathogen to the product based on product contamination occurring over several weeks. The investigators recommend that food processors should consider using pasteurized flour in ready-to-cook or ready-to-bake foods that are likely to be consumed in ways that label statements warn against.

N. M. Khardori, MD, PhD

Reference

1. Rangel JM, Sparling PH, Crowe C, Griffin PM, Swerdlow DL. Epidemiology of *Escherichia coli* O157:H7 outbreaks, United States, 1982–2002. *Emerg Infect Dis.* 2005;11:603-609.

Epidemiology and Outcomes of Complicated Skin and Soft Tissue Infections in Hospitalized Patients

Zervos MJ, Freeman K, Vo L, et al (Henry Ford Health System, Detroit, MI; Albert Einstein College of Medicine, Bronx, NY; Ortho-McNeil Janssen Scientific Affairs, Raritan, NJ)
J Clin Microbiol 50:238-245, 2012

Complicated skin and soft tissue infections (cSSTIs) are among the most rapidly increasing reasons for hospitalization. To describe inpatients with regard to patient characteristics, cSSTI origin, appropriateness of initial antibiotics, and outcomes, we performed a retrospective cohort study in patients hospitalized for cSSTI. To identify independent predictors of outcomes, we performed multivariate analyses. Of 1,096 eligible patients, 48.7% had health care-associated (HCA) cSSTI and 51.3% had community-acquired (CA) cSSTI. After adjustment for baseline variables, hospital length of stay (LOS) was longer for HCA than for CA cSSTI (difference, 2.1 days; 95% confidence interval [CI], 0.8 to 3.5; $P < 0.05$). Other covariates associated with a longer LOS were need for dialysis (regression coefficient ± standard error, 4.5 ± 1.1) and diabetic wound diagnosis (2.6 ± 1.0) (all $P < 0.05$). In the subset with culture-positive cSSTI within 24 h of admission, the most common pathogen was *Staphylococcus aureus* (298/449 [66.4%]), of which 74.8% (223/298) were methicillin-resistant *S. aureus* (MRSA). Eighty-three patients (18.5%) received inappropriate initial antibiotics. After adjustment for other variables, the following were associated with inappropriate initial therapy: direct admission to hospital (not via emergency department), cSSTI caused by MRSA or mixed pathogens, and cSSTI caused by pathogens other than *S. aureus* or streptococci (all $P < 0.05$). We did not find an association between inappropriate therapy and outcomes, except in the subset with ulcers (adjusted odds ratio, 11.8; 95% CI, 1.3 to 111.1; $P = 0.03$). More studies are needed to examine the impact of HCA cSSTI and inappropriate initial therapy on outcomes (Table 2).

▶ The blurring of microbiological distinction between community-acquired and nosocomial infections has prompted the introduction of the category of health

TABLE 2.—Unadjusted and Multivariate Analyses of Outcomes Stratified by Health Care-Associated Infection (HCAI) and Community-Acquired Infection (CAI) ($n = 1,096$)

Outcome	Unadjusted Analysis HCAI ($n = 534$)	CAI ($n = 562$)	P Value	Multivariate Analysis[a]
Hospital length of stay (days)				2.11 (0.75-3.48)[b]
Median (IQR)	5 (1, 73)	4 (1, 103)	<0.0001[c]	
Mean ± SD	8.11 ± 8.46	6.39 ± 9.71	<0.0001[d]	
No. (%) of patients with in-hospital mortality	15 (2.8)	6 (1.1)	<0.05[e]	1.58 (0.58—4.29)[f]
No. (%) of patients with readmission/ death within 30 days	136 (25.5)	67 (11.9)	<0.05[e]	1.08 (0.66—1.76)[f]

[a]Adjusted for variables in Table 1.
[b]Regression mean difference (95% CI); $P < 0.05$; smearing retransformed mean = 2.24 (0.87—3.61).
[c]Wilcoxon rank sum test.
[d]t test on log-transformed length of stay.
[e]Chi-square test.
[f]Adjusted odds ratio (95% CI).

care—associated infections. This category defines infections in community-based patients who have had contact with the health care system with potential for exposure to resistant pathogens.[1]

In patients with pneumonia and bacteremia, the epidemiology, microbiology, and outcomes of health care—associated infections are close to those of nosocomial infection.

This is a retrospective cohort study of hospitalized patients with an admission diagnosis of complicated skin and soft tissue infection (cSSTI). A multivariate analysis showed that 49% of cSSTIs were health care associated. The most common pathogen in both community-acquired and health care—associated cSSTIs was *Staphylococcus aureus* (66%) with 75% of *S aureus* isolates being resistant to methicillin (MRSA).

As shown in Table 2, the length of stay, in-hospital mortality, and readmission/death within 30 days were worse for health care—associated cSSTI compared with those defined as community associated. Inappropriate initial antibiotic therapy was noted in 18.5% of patients. However, the study did not find an association between inappropriate therapy and outcomes except in the subset of patients with ulcers. A striking difference between this and prior studies is in the prevalence rates of MRSA in cSSTIs. The higher rates in this study may be attributed to recent increase in the rates of MRSA in the community.

N. M. Khardori, MD, PhD

Reference

1. Fridkin SK, Hageman JC, Morrison M, et al. Methicillin-resistant Staphylococcus aureus disease in three communities. *N Engl J Med*. 2005;352:1436-1444.

Evolutionary dynamics of *Staphylococcus aureus* during progression from carriage to disease

Young BC, Golubchik T, Batty EM, et al (Univ of Oxford, UK; et al)
Proc Natl Acad Sci U S A 109:4550-4555, 2012

Whole-genome sequencing offers new insights into the evolution of bacterial pathogens and the etiology of bacterial disease. *Staphylococcus aureus* is a major cause of bacteria-associated mortality and invasive disease and is carried asymptomatically by 27% of adults. Eighty percent of bacteremias match the carried strain. However, the role of evolutionary change in the pathogen during the progression from carriage to disease is incompletely understood. Here we use high-throughput genome sequencing to discover the genetic changes that accompany the transition from nasal carriage to fatal bloodstream infection in an individual colonized with methicillin-sensitive *S. aureus*. We found a single, cohesive population exhibiting a repertoire of 30 single-nucleotide polymorphisms and four insertion/deletion variants. Mutations accumulated at a steady rate over a 13-mo period, except for a cluster of mutations preceding the transition to disease. Although bloodstream bacteria differed by just eight mutations from the original nasally carried bacteria, half of those mutations caused truncation of proteins, including a premature stop codon in an *AraC*-family transcriptional regulator that has been implicated in pathogenicity. Comparison with evolution in two asymptomatic carriers supported the conclusion that clusters of protein-truncating mutations are highly unusual. Our results demonstrate that bacterial diversity in vivo is limited but nonetheless detectable by whole-genome sequencing, enabling the study of evolutionary dynamics within the host. Regulatory or structural changes that occur during carriage may be functionally important for pathogenesis; therefore identifying those changes is a crucial step in understanding the biological causes of invasive bacterial disease.

▶ *Staphylococcus aureus* is a common constituent of nasal flora of healthy adults.[1] In bacteremic patients, *S aureus* isolated from the blood could not be distinguished by pulsed field gel electrophoresis from those concomitantly cultured from the nares in 80% of cases.

This study recruited 360 adults with nasal carriage of *S aureus* for regular screening to help them understand the biological factors involved in progression from carriage to disease. Whole-genome sequencing was used to chart the evolution of the bacterial population during carriage and disease using nasal and blood isolates from a participant who developed *S aureus* bloodstream infection during the study. This was compared to ongoing biological evolution of *S aureus* in 2 asymptomatic carriers. The results showed genetic variation evolving over time with dynamic populations of nasal *S aureus*.

Only 8 mutations separated disease-causing *S aureus* from those carried asymptomatically. Half of these mutations caused truncation of proteins. A cluster of protein-truncating mutations preceded disease progression, suggesting a role for loss-of-function mutation in bacterial pathogenesis.

The molecular techniques along with linear study of colonizing and disease causing *S aureus* in this investigation help us understand the role of chance, circumstance, and genetics in invasive bacterial disease.

N. M. Khardori, MD, PhD

Reference

1. von Eiff C, Becker K, Machka K, Stammer H, Peters G. Nasal carriage as a source of Staphylococcus aureus bacteremia. Study Group. *N Engl J Med*. 2001;344: 11-16.

Household Versus Individual Approaches to Eradication of Community-Associated *Staphylococcus aureus* in Children: A Randomized Trial
Fritz SA, Hogan PG, Hayek G, et al (Washington Univ School of Medicine, St Louis, MO)
Clin Infect Dis 54:743-751, 2012

Background.—Community-associated *Staphylococcus aureus* infections often affect multiple members of a household. We compared 2 approaches to *S. aureus* eradication: decolonizing the entire household versus decolonizing the index case alone.

Methods.—An open-label, randomized trial enrolled 183 pediatric patients (cases) with community-onset S. aureus skin abscesses and colonization of anterior nares, axillae, or inguinal folds from 2008 to 2009 at primary and tertiary centers. Participants were randomized to decolonization of the case alone (index group) or of all household members (household group). The 5-day regimen included hygiene education, twice-daily intranasal mupirocin, and daily chlorhexidine body washes. Colonization of cases and subsequent skin and soft tissue infection (SSTI) in cases and household contacts were ascertained at 1, 3, 6, and 12 months.

Results.—Among 147 cases with 1-month colonization data, modified intention-to-treat analysis revealed *S. aureus* eradication in 50% of cases in the index group and 51% in the household group ($P = 1.00$). Among 126 cases completing 12-month follow-up, *S. aureus* was eradicated from 54% of the index group versus 66% of the household group ($P = .28$). Over 12 months, recurrent SSTI was reported in 72% of cases in the index group and 52% in the household group ($P = .02$). SSTI incidence in household contacts was significantly lower in the household versus index group during the first 6 months; this trend continued at 12 months.

Conclusions.—Household decolonization was not more effective than individual decolonization in eradicating community-associated *S. aureus* carriage from cases. However, household decolonization reduced the incidence of subsequent SSTI in cases and their household contacts.

Clinical Trials Registration.—NCT00731783.

▶ The epidemic of staphylococcal skin and soft tissue infection (SSTI) over the past decade has been driven largely by a community-associated *Staphylococcus aureus* clone, designated USA300, which includes methicillin-resistant and methicillin-susceptible strains.[1,2] Recurrence rates of approximately 20% over 3 months have been reported for *S aureus* SSTIs, with clustering within households. It is believed that household contact may serve as a reservoir for *S aureus* transmission, with treated patients reacquiring the organism from colonized household contact. Nasal colonization is a risk factor for developing SSTI.[3] Patients in community settings are often prescribed decolonization measures used to prevent health care–associated MRSA infection.

In this open-label, randomized, controlled trial, the effectiveness of decolonization of all household members was compared with decolonization of the index case alone. In addition to a standardized hygiene curriculum, the 5-day decolonization regimen included twice daily application of 20% mupirocin ointment to anterior nares and daily use of 40% chlorhexidine in the bath or shower. At 1 month, *S aureus* was eradicated from 51% in the household group and 50% in the index patient–only group. Eradication rates between groups did not differ at 6 and 12 months. However, the household decolonization approach resulted in fewer subsequent SSTIs in both cases and their household contacts. It has been proposed that skin-to-skin and skin-to-fomite contact may play a greater role than endogenous colonization in the pathogenesis of *S aureus* infection.[4] In this study, 20% of screened patients with confirmed *S aureus* SSTI were not colonized with *S aureus* in the nares, axillae, or inguinal folds. In a pediatric study with *S aureus* SSTI and nasal colonization, the infecting and colonizing strains were concordant in only 59% of patients, indicating that acquisition of a new strain (from person-to-person contact or from environmental surfaces) led to symptomatic infection.

The significant observation in this study is the reduction in the burden of SSTI with household decolonization, although colonization eradication rate was the same as the group where the index case only was decolonized. There still is a need for optimizing strategies for interrupting staphylococcal transmission including environmental contamination since approximately 50% of the household group in this study reported recurrent SSTI over a 1-year period.

N. M. Khardori, MD, PhD

References

1. McCaskill ML, Mason EO Jr, Kaplan SL, Hammerman W, Lamberth LB, Hultén KG. Increase of the USA300 clone among community-acquired methicillin-susceptible Staphylococcus aureus causing invasive infections. *Pediatr Infect Dis J*. 2007;26:1122-1127.
2. Moran GJ, Krishnadasan A, Gorwitz RJ, et al. Methicillin-resistant *S. aureus* infections among patients in the emergency department. *N Engl J Med*. 2006;355:666-674.
3. Ellis MW, Hospenthal DR, Dooley DP, Gray PJ, Murray CK. Natural history of community-acquired methicillin-resistant Staphylococcus aureus colonization and infection in soldiers. *Clin Infect Dis*. 2004;39:971-979.
4. Miller LG, Diep BA. Colonization, fomites, and virulence: rethinking the pathogenesis of community-associated methicillin-resistant Staphylococcus aureus infection. *Clin Infect Dis*. 2008;46:752-760.

Early goal-directed therapy (EGDT) for severe sepsis/septic shock: which components of treatment are more difficult to implement in a community-based emergency department?
O'Neill R, Morales J, Jule M (Genesys Regional Med Ctr, Grand Blanc, MI)
J Emerg Med 42:503-510, 2012

Background.—Early goal-directed therapy (EGDT) has been shown to reduce mortality in patients with severe sepsis/septic shock, however, implementation of this protocol in the emergency department (ED) is sometimes difficult.

Objectives.—We evaluated our sepsis protocol to determine which EGDT elements were more difficult to implement in our community-based ED.

Methods.—This was a non-concurrent cohort study of adult patients entered into a sepsis protocol at a single community hospital from July 2008 to March 2009. Charts were reviewed for the following process measures: a predefined crystalloid bolus, antibiotic administration, central venous catheter insertion, central venous pressure measurement, arterial line insertion, vasopressor utilization, central venous oxygen saturation measurement, and use of a standardized order set. We also compared the individual component adherence with survival to hospital discharge.

Results.—A total of 98 patients presented over a 9-month period. Measures with the highest adherence were vasopressor administration (79%; 95% confidence interval [CI] 69–89%) and antibiotic use (78%; 95% CI 68–85%). Measures with the lowest adherence included arterial line placement (42%; 95% CI 32–52%), central venous pressure measurement (27%; 95% CI 18–36%), and central venous oxygen saturation measurement (15%; 95% CI 7–23%). Fifty-seven patients survived to hospital discharge (Mortality: 33%). The only element of EDGT to demonstrate a statistical significance in patients surviving to hospital discharge was the crystalloid bolus (79% vs. 46%) (respiratory rate [RR] = 1.76, 95% CI 1.11–2.58).

Conclusion.—In our community hospital, arterial line placement, central venous pressure measurement, and central venous oxygen saturation measurement were the most difficult elements of EGDT to implement. Patients who survived to hospital discharge were more likely to receive the crystalloid bolus.

▶ In spite of advances in critical care and antimicrobial therapy, severe sepsis continues to have a mortality rate of around 30%. A mortality benefit has been demonstrated with Early Goal-Directed Therapy (EGDT).[1,2] The integration of this approach in day-to-day clinical practice has been difficult and slow, especially in the community hospitals.

This study is done at a 410-bed community hospital with a 35-bed emergency department. It evaluates the difficulty involved in adhering to specific elements of the EGDT and their impact on survival to hospital discharge. The highest adherence was shown with vasopressor administration (79%) and antibiotic use (78%). The adherence rate with arterial line placement, central venous pressure measurement, and central venous oxygen saturation measurement was 42%, 27%, and 15%, respectively. Mortality rate for severe sepsis in this study was 33%. A statistically significant difference in patients surviving to hospital discharge was demonstrated with a 2-L crystalloid bolus within 1 hour of identification of severe sepsis/septic shock. The study suggests that early fluid administration may be the most important element of EGDT.

N. M. Khardori, MD, PhD

References

1. Angus DC, Linde-Zwirble WT, Lidicker J, Clermont G, Carcillo J, Pinsky MR. Epidemiology of severe sepsis in the United States: analysis of incidence, outcome, and associated costs of care. *Crit Care Med.* 2001;29:1303-1310.
2. Otero RM, Nguyen HB, Huang DT, et al. Early goal-directed therapy in severe sepsis and septic shock revisited: concepts, controversies, and contemporary findings. *Chest.* 2006;130:1579-1595.

Illness Severity in Community-Onset Invasive *Staphylococcus aureus* Infection and the Presence of Virulence Genes

Wehrhahn MC, Robinson JO, Pascoe EM, et al (Royal Perth Hosp and PathWest Laboratory Medicine, WA; Princess Margaret Hosp, Toronto, Ontario, Canada; et al)
J Infect Dis 205:1840-1848, 2012

Background.—It is uncertain whether particular clones causing invasive community-onset methicillin-resistant and methicillin-sensitive *Staphylococcus aureus* (cMRSA/cMSSA) infection differ in virulence.

Methods.—Invasive cMRSA and cMSSA cases were prospectively identified. Principal component analysis was used to derive an illness severity score (ISS) from clinical data, including 30-day mortality, requirement for intensive hospital support, the presence of bloodstream infection, and hospital length of stay. The mean ISS for each *S. aureus* clone (based on MLST) was compared with its DNA microarray-based genotype.

Results.—Fifty-seven cMRSA and 50 cMSSA infections were analyzed. Ten clones caused 82 (77%) of these infections and had an ISS calculated. The enterotoxin gene cluster (*egc*) and the collagen adhesin (*cna*) gene were found in 4 of the 5 highest-ranked clones (ST47-MSSA, ST30-MRSA-IV [2B], ST45-MSSA, and ST22-MRSA-IV[2B]) compared with none and 1 of the lowest 5 ranked clones, respectively. cMSSA clones caused more severe infection than cMRSA clones. The *lukF/lukS* Panton–Valentine leukocidin (PVL) genes did not directly correlate with the ISS, being present in the second, fourth, and 10th most virulent clones.

Conclusions.—The clinical severity of invasive cMRSA and cMSSA infection is likely to be attributable to the isolates' entire genotype rather than a single putative virulence determinant such as PVL (Figs 1 and 2, Table 4).

▶ Invasive infection caused by community-onset methicillin-resistant *Staphylococcus aureus* (cMRSA) has been reported worldwide over the last decade.[1]

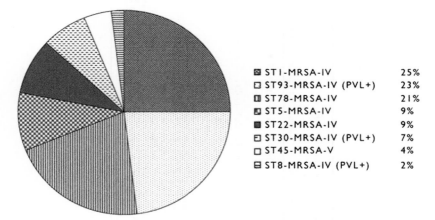

⊠ ST1-MRSA-IV	25%
☐ ST93-MRSA-IV (PVL+)	23%
⊞ ST78-MRSA-IV	21%
◪ ST5-MRSA-IV	9%
■ ST22-MRSA-IV	9%
⊟ ST30-MRSA-IV (PVL+)	7%
☐ ST45-MRSA-V	4%
⊟ ST8-MRSA-IV (PVL+)	2%

FIGURE 1.—cMRSA clones. (Reprinted from Wehrhahn MC, Robinson JO, Pascoe EM, et al. Illness severity in community-onset invasive *Staphylococcus aureus* infection and the presence of virulence genes. *J Infect Dis*. 2012;205:1840-1848, by permission of Oxford University Press.)

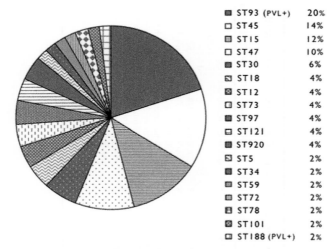

■ ST93 (PVL+)	20%
☐ ST45	14%
⊟ ST15	12%
☐ ST47	10%
■ ST30	6%
⊠ ST18	4%
⊠ ST12	4%
☐ ST73	4%
■ ST97	4%
☐ ST121	4%
■ ST920	4%
⊠ ST5	2%
■ ST34	2%
⊞ ST59	2%
⊡ ST72	2%
⊟ ST78	2%
⊠ ST101	2%
⊡ ST188 (PVL+)	2%

FIGURE 2.—cMSSA clones. (Reprinted from Wehrhahn MC, Robinson JO, Pascoe EM, et al. Illness severity in community-onset invasive *Staphylococcus aureus* infection and the presence of virulence genes. *J Infect Dis*. 2012;205:1840-1848, by permission of Oxford University Press.)

The virulence factors in *S aureus* include Panton-Valentine leukocidin (PVL), the superantigen (SAg) family including toxic shock syndrome toxin-1, and the Staphylococcal enterotoxins and adhesion proteins like collagen adhesion protein (cna). It remains unclear if MRSA is inherently more virulent than methicillin-sensitive *S aureus* (MSSA). The authors of this study have recently published data that demonstrate no difference in 30-day mortality between patients with invasive Panton—Valentine leukocidin (PVL)-positive and negative

TABLE 4.—*S. aureus* Clones Ranked by Illness Severity Score (ISS) and Their Associated Virulence Profiles

Rank	Clone (n)	ISS	agr	Capsule	Adhesion	Enterotoxins	lukF/lukS PVL Genes	Haemolysins and Leukocidins
1	ST47-MSSA (5)	1.114	I	8	clfA/B fib fnbA/B cna	egc (all), c + l (3/5), d + j + r (1/5)	No	hla/hlg/hld (all), hlb (1/5)
2	ST30-MRSA-IV[2B] (4)	0.481	III	8	clfA/B fib fnbA/B cna	egc (all)	Yes	hla/hlb/hlg/hld (all)
3	ST45-MSSA (7)	0.394	I	8	clfA/B fib fnbA/B cna	egc (all)	No	hla/hlg/hld (all)
4	ST93-MSSA (10)	0.345	III	8	clfA/B fib fnbA/B	egc (all), b (1/7), c + l (4/7)	Yes	hla/hlb/hlg/hld (all), lukD (all)
5	ST22-MRSA-IV[2B] (5)	0.269	I	5	clfA/B fib fnbA cna	egc (all), b (3/5), c + l (3/5)	No	hla/hlb/hlg/hld (all)
6	ST78-MRSA-IV[2B] (12)	0.188	III	8	clfA/B fib fnbA/B	b (1/12), c + l (11/12)	No	hla/hlb/hlg/hld (all), lukD/E (all)
7	ST1-MRSA-IV[2B] (15)	−0.281	III	8	clfA/B fib fnbA/B	a (14/15), h (all), k + q (13/15)	No	hla/hlb/hlg/hld (all), lukD/E (all)
8	ST15-MSSA (6)	−0.411	II	8	clfA/B fib fnbA/B	0	No	hla/hlg/hld (all), lukD/E (all)
9	ST5-MRSA-IV[2B] (5)	−0.528	II	5	clfA/B fib fnbA/B	a (4/5), egc (all)	No	hlb/hlg/hld (all), hla (4/5)
10	ST93-MRSA-IV[2B] (13)	−0.655	III	8	clfA/B fib fnbA/B	0	Yes	hla/hlb/hld (all), lukD (all), lukE (6/13)

Abbreviations: agr, accessory gene regulator; clfA/B, clumping factor A/B; cna, collagen adhesion protein; *egc*, enterotoxin gene cluster; fib, fibrinogen binding protein; fnbA/B, fibronectin binding protein A/B; ISS, illness severity score; PVL Panton—Valentine leukocidin.

cMRSA and cMSSA infection. Invasive infection was noted from both cMRSA and cMSSA by isolates lacking the PVL genes, including patients without obvious risk factors for poor outcome.[2]

This prospective study examines markers of illness severity (illness severity score [ISS]) associated with invasive community-onset *S aureus* infection and the presence of known virulence genes in *S aureus*. As shown in Table 4, the clones ST30-MRSA and ST45-MSSA caused the most severe invasive infections based on their mean illness severity. cMSSA clones caused more severe illness than cMRSA clones.

The mean ISS for all MSSA clones was higher than that of MRSA clones. ST93-MSSA ranked higher (4th highest ISS) compared with ST93-MRSA (10th). This finding lends support to the hypothesis that β-lactam resistance in *S aureus* may result in a fitness cost. The expression of enterotoxin gene cluster (*egc*) gene may also explain the difference between MSSA (45%) and MRSA (17%) isolates.

The distribution of various virulence genes among cMSSA and cMRSA clones is shown in Figs 1 and 2. PVL gene was demonstrated in 20% of cMSSA clones compared with 23% of cMRSA clones. The adhesion, *cna* gene was found in all but one of the top 5 ISS clones compared with none of the lower 5 clones. No clear association was found between a clone's mean ISS and the presence of gene-encoding PVL.

The apparent association with genes such as *cna* and *egc* and the diversity of ISS values for *S aureus* clones support the evidence that virulence is not determined by any single determinant (eg, PVL) but a multitude of interacting virulence determinants. Virulence profile data may influence treatment of patients with invasive *S aureus* infection, for example, the use of ribosomal-active agents for toxin producers, use of intravenous immunoglobulin as an adjunct, and specific anti-SAg agents. These data will also be useful in refining infection control practices and guiding *S aureus* vaccine development.

N. M. Khardori, MD, PhD

References

1. Robinson JO, Pearson JC, Christiansen KJ, Coombs GW, Murray RJ. Community-associated versus healthcare-associated methicillin-resistant Staphylococcus aureus bacteraemia: a 10-year retrospective review. *Eur J Clin Microbiol Infect Dis.* 2009;28:353-361.
2. Wehrhahn MC, Robinson JO, Pearson JC, et al. Clinical and laboratory features of invasive community-onset methicillin-resistant *Staphylococcus aureus* infection: a prospective-case control study. *Eur J Clin Microbiol Infect Dis.* 2010;29:1025-1033.

In-feed antibiotic effects on the swine intestinal microbiome

Looft T, Johnson TA, Allen HK, et al (Natl Animal Disease Ctr, Ames, IA; Michigan State Univ, East Lansing)
Proc Natl Acad Sci U S A 109:1691-1696, 2012

Antibiotics have been administered to agricultural animals for disease treatment, disease prevention, and growth promotion for over 50 y. The impact of such antibiotic use on the treatment of human diseases is hotly debated. We raised pigs in a highly controlled environment, with one portion of the littermates receiving a diet containing performance-enhancing antibiotics [chlortetracycline, sulfamethazine, and penicillin (known as ASP250)] and the other portion receiving the same diet but without the antibiotics. We used phylogenetic, metagenomic, and quantitative PCR-based approaches to address the impact of antibiotics on the swine gut microbiota. Bacterial phylotypes shifted after 14 d of antibiotic treatment, with the medicated pigs showing an increase in *Proteobacteria* (1−11%) compared with nonmedicated pigs at the same time point. This shift was driven by an increase in *Escherichia coli* populations. Analysis of the metagenomes showed that microbial functional genes relating to energy production and conversion were increased in the antibiotic-fed pigs. The results also indicate that antibiotic resistance genes increased in abundance and diversity in the medicated swine microbiome despite a high background of resistance genes in nonmedicated swine. Some enriched genes, such as aminoglycoside O-phosphotransferases, confer resistance to antibiotics that were not administered in this study, demonstrating the potential for indirect selection of resistance to classes of antibiotics not fed. The collateral effects of feeding subtherapeutic doses of antibiotics to agricultural animals are apparent and must be considered in cost-benefit analyses.

▶ The Food and Drug Administration has recently recommended restrictions on the use of antibiotics in animal agriculture.[1] The Infectious Disease Society of America supported this recommendation and testified before a congressional subcommittee. The impact of antibiotic use for growth promotion over a 50-year period has led to widespread emergence of multiple antibiotic resistance in both animal and human pathogens. The selective pressure caused by the addition of antibiotics to feed may lead to lasting changes in livestock commensal bacteria. Even in the absence of continued antibiotics, the recovery of antibiotic resistance genes in bacterial communities may remain stable.

This article reports on the comprehensive effects of daily feeding of subtherapeutic doses of antibiotics on livestock macrobiotas. Piglets born to sows not exposed to antibiotics before the study were raised in a highly controlled environment. ASP250 is an antibiotic (medicated) supplemental feed containing chlortetracycline, sulfamethazine, and penicillin commonly given to swine for the treatment of bacterial enteritis and enhanced food efficiency. At week 18 after birth, 1 group received the medicated feed and the other the same feed without antibiotics for 3 weeks. The effect of ASP250 on the swine antibiotic resistome was assessed using phenotype, metagenomic, and quantitative polymerase chain reaction approaches. Diverse resistant genes (5 genes in particular) were detected at high frequency in the stool microbiomes of both unmedicated and medicated piglets. This finding suggests that the constant selective pressure after 50 years of in-feed antibiotics has established a high background level of resistance in the swine microbiome. A detectable increase above the high background of resistance occurred because of direct interaction with the antibiotics in ASP250. Some enriched genes conferred resistance to antibiotics that were not present in the feed used in this study, demonstrating the potential for indirect in addition to direct collateral effects of antibiotic supplemented feed. These effects should be considered seriously in cost-benefit analyses, in spite of the data to suggest numerous possibilities for how the swine gut microbiota might be involved in improved feed efficiency, which parallels a growth-promoting effect afforded by certain in-feed antibiotics.[2]

N. M. Khardori, MD, PhD

References

1. US Department of Health and Human Services, Food and Drug Administration, and Center for Veterinary Medicine (2010) Draft guidance #209. http://www.fda.gov/downloads/animalveterinary/guidancecomplianceenforcement/guidanceforindustry/ucm216936.pdf. Accessed October 12, 2010.
2. Santacruz A, Collado MC, García-Valdés L, et al. Gut microbiota composition is associated with body weight, weight gain and biochemical parameters in pregnant women. *Br J Nutr.* 2010;104:83-92.

Linezolid in Methicillin-Resistant *Staphylococcus aureus* Nosocomial Pneumonia: A Randomized, Controlled Study

Wunderink RG, Niederman MS, Kollef MH, et al (Northwestern Univ Feinberg School of Medicine, Chicago, IL; Winthrop-Univ Hosp, Mineola, NY; Washington Univ School of Medicine, St Louis, MO; et al)

Clin Infect Dis 54:621-629, 2012

Background.—Post hoc analyses of clinical trial data suggested that linezolid may be more effective than vancomycin for treatment of methicillin-resistant *Staphylococcus aureus* (MRSA) nosocomial pneumonia. This study prospectively assessed efficacy and safety of linezolid, compared with a dose-optimized vancomycin regimen, for treatment of MRSA nosocomial pneumonia.

Methods.—This was a prospective, double-blind, controlled, multicenter trial involving hospitalized adult patients with hospital-acquired or health-care—associated MRSA pneumonia. Patients were randomized to receive intravenous linezolid (600 mg every 12 hours) or vancomycin (15 mg/kg every 12 hours) for 7—14 days. Vancomycin dose was adjusted on the basis of trough levels. The primary end point was clinical outcome at end of study (EOS) in evaluable per-protocol (PP) patients. Prespecified secondary end points included response in the modified intent-to-treat (mITT) population at end of treatment (EOT) and EOS and microbiologic response in the PP and mITT populations at EOT and EOS. Survival and safety were also evaluated.

Results.—Of 1184 patients treated, 448 (linezolid, n = 224; vancomycin, n = 224) were included in the mITT and 348 (linezolid, n = 172; vancomycin, n = 176) in the PP population. In the PP population, 95 (57.6%) of 165 linezolid-treated patients and 81 (46.6%) of 174 vancomycin-treated patients achieved clinical success at EOS (95% confidence interval for difference, 0.5%—21.6%; P = .042). All-cause 60-day mortality was similar (linezolid,

15.7%; vancomycin, 17.0%), as was incidence of adverse events. Nephrotoxicity occurred more frequently with vancomycin (18.2%; linezolid, 8.4%).

Conclusions.—For the treatment of MRSA nosocomial pneumonia, clinical response at EOS in the PP population was significantly higher with linezolid than with vancomycin, although 60-day mortality was similar (Fig 2).

▶ Pneumonia, especially that associated with mechanical ventilation, is the second most common hospital-associated infection in the United States.[1]

Methicillin-resistant *Staphylococcus aureus* (MRSA) as an etiologic agent accounts for 10% to 40% of cases of health care—associated (HCAP), hospital acquired (HAP), and ventilation-associated pneumonia.

Vancomycin and linezolid were found to be statistically equally effective for treatment of nosocomial pneumonia in 2 prospective, randomized, double-blind trials. A combined post hoc analysis of these trials found that in the MRSA pneumonia subgroup, survival (80% vs 63.5%) and clinical cure (59.0% vs 35.5%) were significantly improved in patients treated with linezolid compared with vancomycin.[2]

Vancomycin in those trials was used at a fixed dose of 1 gm twice a day. Therefore, the lower efficacy and higher mortality in the vancomycin group may have been because of a lack of dose optimization. Current guidelines recommend a body weight—based initial dose of vancomycin followed by adjustment based on trough levels.

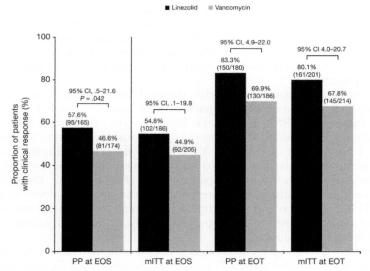

FIGURE 2.—Clinical response rates in per-protocol (PP) and modified intent-to-treat (mITT) patients at end-of-study (EOS) and end of therapy (EOT). *P* values and 95% confidence intervals (CI) are included for the differences between treatment groups in the primary end point. (Reprinted from Wunderink RG, Niederman MS, Kollef MH, et al. Linezolid in methicillin-resistant staphylococcus aureus nosocomial pneumonia: a randomized, controlled study. *Clin Infect Dis.* 2012;54:621-629, by permission of the Infectious Diseases Society of America.)

This prospective, double-blind, controlled, multicenter trial was conducted in hospitalized adult patients with HCAP and HAP. The efficacy, safety, and tolerability of fixed-dose linezolid was compared with that of dose-optimized vancomycin for 7 to 14 days in the treatment of documented MRSA pneumonia. As shown in Fig 2, clinical efficacy (primary endpoint) was greater for linezolid compared with vancomycin. Microbiologic response, as demonstrated by MRSA clearance at the end of treatment, paralleled clinical outcomes. Linezolid was better tolerated than vancomycin. The higher rate of nephrotoxicity in the vancomycin group may reflect the higher (adjusted) doses of vancomycin based on current guidelines.

Compared with previous studies, hematologic abnormalities (including thrombocytopenia) were not more frequent in the linezolid group, likely because of the short duration of therapy. All-cause 60-day mortality in linezolid treated groups (15.7%) was similar to that in the previous post hoc analyses. However, mortality among vancomycin-treated (35%) observed patients was lower (17%) in the current trial compared with previous results. This difference may reflect the positive aspect of optimized vancomycin dosing in this trial. The treatment of colonization only as a variable in the difference in efficacy was equally likely in both groups. Clinical success rates were equal in nonquantitative and quantitative culture-diagnosed cases. The overall tolerability profile of both agents was equivalent.

N. M. Khardori, MD, PhD

References

1. Emori TG, Gaynes RP. An overview of nosocomial infections, including the role of the microbiology laboratory. *Clin Micrbiol Rev.* 1993;6:428-442.
2. Wunderink RG, Rello J, Cammarata SK, Croos-Dabrera RV, Kollef MH. Linezolid vs vancomycin: analysis of two double-blind studies of patients with amethicillin-resistant Staphylococcus aureus nosocomial pneumonia. *Chest.* 2003;124: 1789-1797.

Rapid Whole-Genome Sequencing for Investigation of a Neonatal MRSA Outbreak

Köser CU, Holden MTG, Ellington MJ, et al (Univ of Cambridge, UK; Wellcome Trust Sanger Inst, Hinxton, UK; Health Protection Agency, Cambridge, UK; et al)
N Engl J Med 366:2267-2275, 2012

Background.—Isolates of methicillin-resistant *Staphylococcus aureus* (MRSA) belonging to a single lineage are often indistinguishable by means of current typing techniques. Whole-genome sequencing may provide improved resolution to define transmission pathways and characterize outbreaks.

Methods.—We investigated a putative MRSA outbreak in a neonatal intensive care unit. By using rapid high-throughput sequencing technology with a clinically relevant turnaround time, we retrospectively sequenced the DNA from seven isolates associated with the outbreak and another seven MRSA isolates associated with carriage of MRSA or bacteremia in the same hospital.

Results.—We constructed a phylogenetic tree by comparing single-nucleotide polymorphisms (SNPs) in the core genome to a reference genome (an epidemic MRSA clone, EMRSA-15 [sequence type 22]). This revealed a distinct cluster of outbreak isolates and clear separation between these and the nonoutbreak isolates. A previously missed transmission event was detected between two patients with bacteremia who were not part of the outbreak. We created an artificial "resistome" of antibiotic-resistance genes and demonstrated concordance between it and the results of phenotypic susceptibility testing; we also created a "toxome" consisting of toxin genes. One outbreak isolate had a hypermutator phenotype with a higher number of SNPs than the other outbreak isolates, highlighting the difficulty of imposing a simple threshold for the number of SNPs between isolates to decide whether they are part of a recent transmission chain.

Conclusions.—Whole-genome sequencing can provide clinically relevant data within a time frame that can influence patient care. The need for automated data interpretation and the provision of clinically meaningful reports represent hurdles to clinical implementation. (Funded by the U.K. Clinical Research Collaboration Translational Infection Research Initiative and others.)

▶ Whole-genome sequencing for microbes has been shown to have excellent discriminatory power in a number of recent outbreaks including cholera, tuberculosis, and *Escherichia coli* 0104:H4. Availability of this tool in the routine diagnostic setting within a clinically relevant turnaround time would be distinctly superior to currently available phenotypic and genotypic methods for infection control and outbreak investigation.

The authors of this study have previously shown that whole-genome sequencing can be used to describe the intercontinental and local transmission of methicillin-resistant *Staphylococcus aureus* (MRSA).[1] In this investigation, they improve on the methodology by using a rapid-sequencing platform. A retrospective study was done on DNA from 7 isolates associated with a MRSA outbreak in a neonatal unit at a university hospital.

Another 7 MRSA isolates associated with carriage or bacteremia in the same hospital were used for comparison. The rapid whole-genome sequencing was able to show a clear distinction between isolates in the outbreak and non-outbreak groups.

The genotypes using artificial antibiotic-resistant genes and antimicrobial phenotypes showed concordance, which is useful for guiding therapy. The technique also represents a powerful tool for the study of antibiotic resistance mechanisms. A "toxome," consisting of toxin genes from the study isolated, was created that would allow immediate identification of the toxin genes. Currently this takes multiple polymerase chain reactions at reference laboratories. The genetic defect for a small-colony variant isolate in the study was rapidly identified. Such isolates are known to be associated with persistence and treatment failure.

The authors predict that once data interpretation is fully automated, whole-genome sequencing will become a standard tool for infection control and aid in monitoring the spread and evolution of major pathogens in the health care and community settings in real time.

N. M. Khardori, MD, PhD

Reference

1. Harris SR, Feil EJ, Holden MT, et al. Evolution of MRSA during hospital transmission and intercontinental spread. *Science.* 2010;327:469-474.

Rising rates of macrolide-resistant *Mycoplasma pneumoniae* in the central United States
Yamada M, Buller R, Bledsoe S, et al (Washington Univ School of Medicine, St Louis, MO; St Louis Children's Hosp, MO)
Pediatr Infect Dis J 31:409-411, 2012

Macrolide-resistant *Mycoplasma pneumoniae* is widespread in Asia, and severe cases of pneumonia have been described in children. Little information is available about the resistance pattern in the United States. We collected respiratory samples from 49 patients with *Mycoplasma* infection in the central United States between 2007 and 2010. We found a macrolide resistance rate of 8.2%. Resistance should be considered when patients with *M. pneumoniae* infection do not have a satisfactory response to macrolides. Alternative antibiotics include tetracyclines or fluoroquinolones.

▶ The emergence of resistance of *Mycoplasma pneumoniae* to macrolide class of antimicrobial agents has had a significant clinical impact in Asia and Europe. Resistance rates are 10% to 26% in Europe and 30% to 90% in Asia, the highest being in China.

Resistance to macrolides in *M pneumoniae* has been associated with single-base mutations in the peptidyl transferase region (domain V) of the 23SrRNA gene, also called the macrolide binding site.[1]

M pneumoniae remains one of the leading causes of community-acquired pneumonia among children and young adults.[2]

Using a polymerase chain reaction assay, this study found *M pneumoniae* DNA in 2.4% of 2251 upper respiratory samples submitted to the virology laboratory at a children's hospital between 2007 and 2010. Of these, 8.2% harbored a mutation associated with macrolide resistance. The mutation rate was 3.3% in samples collected between 2007 and 2008 and 15.8% for samples from 2009 to 2010. The mutation A2063G transition found in this study is also the most common mutation reported from Asia and Europe. The same mutation has been reported in *Mycoplasma genitalium* in Denmark and can be selected in vitro by exposure to subinhibitory concentrations of azithromycin.

The upward trend in resistance of *M pneumoniae* to macrolides in the United States is of concern. Alternate classes of antimicrobial agents that have been used for refractory cases include tetracyclines and fluoroquinolones.

N. M. Khardori, MD, PhD

References

1. Morozumi M, Takahashi T, Ubukata K. Macrolide-resistant Mycoplasma pneumoniae: characteristics of isolates and clinical aspects of community-acquired pneumonia. *J Infect Chemother.* 2010;16:78-86.
2. Block S, Hedrick J, Hammerschlag MR, et al. Mycoplasma pneumoniae and Chlamydia pneumoniae in pediatric community-acquired pneumonia: comparative efficacy and safety of clarithromycin vs. erythromycin ethylsuccinate. *Pediatr Infect Dis J.* 1995;14:471-477.

Vancomycin for Surgical Prophylaxis?

Crawford T, Rodvold KA, Solomkin JS (Univ of Illinois at Chicago; Univ of Cincinnati College of Medicine, OH)
Clin Infect Dis 54:1474-1479, 2012

The increasing prevalence of methicillin-resistant *Staphylococcus aureus* (MRSA) has resulted in a reevaluation of the role of vancomycin for surgical prophylaxis. Two systematic reviews of randomized control studies have concluded that cephalosporins are as effective as vancomycin for the prevention of surgical site infections (SSIs). However, most of these studies were conducted more than 10 years ago and cannot be generalized to the current rates of MRSA. Several time-series analyses have recently evaluated the effectiveness of vancomycin for surgical prophylaxis in institutions with a high prevalence of MRSA. Decision analysis models have also been used to estimate thresholds of MRSA prevalence for which vancomycin would minimize the incidence and cost of SSIs. Combination therapy and the emergence of resistant pathogens following vancomycin prophylaxis are reviewed. Vancomycin is not recommended for routine use in surgical prophylaxis but may be considered as a component of a MRSA prevention bundle for SSIs in selective circumstances.

▶ Surgical site infection (SSI) is the second most common health care—associated infection in the United States.[1]

Staphylococcus aureus resistant to methicillin (MRSA) and coagulase-negative *staphylococci* (often resistant to methicillin) are now the primary pathogens associated with SSIs in cardiothoracic, vascular, orthopedic, and neurosurgical procedures involving sternotomy and insertion of vascular grafts and other devices, particularly prosthetic joints that have significant consequences if patients develop SSIs. Based on earlier studies,[2] first- or second-generation cephalosporins are preferred for perioperative surgical prophylaxis. Vancomycin is recommended as an alternative agent for patients with a life-threatening β lactam allergy and in situations in which a high prevalence of MRSA exists.

This study analyzes 2 systemic reviews that compare the rate of SSIs in patients receiving antibiotic prophylaxis with either vancomycin or Teicoplanin versus β lactam agents; 2 randomized, prospective studies that evaluated antibiotic prophylaxis in hospitals with a high prevalence of MRSA; 3 clinical studies that used pre- and postintervention periods to assess the effect of switching to vancomycin for surgical prophylaxis in cardiothoracic surgery patients; and a recent time-series analysis evaluating the use of vancomycin and a MRSA bundle program.[3]

The bundle program resulted in a significant reduction in SSI rate and a 93% reduction in postoperative MRSA wound infections. It is not clear if vancomycin is a critical component in bundled approaches for most types of surgical prophylaxis.

N. M. Khardori, MD, PhD

References

1. Alexander JW, Solomkin JS, Edwards MJ. Updated recommendations for control of surgical site infections. *Ann Surg.* 2011;253:1082-1093.
2. Chambers D, Worthy G, Myers L, et al. Glycopeptide vs. non-glycopeptide antibiotics for prophylaxis of surgical site infections: a systematic review. *Surg Infect.* 2010;11:455-462.
3. Walsh EE, Greene L, Kirshner R. Sustained reduction in methicillin-resistant Staphylococcus aureaus wound infections after cardiothoracic surgery. *Arch Intern Med.* 2011;171:68-73.

10 Fungal Infections

A Cluster of *Pneumocystis* Infections Among Renal Transplant Recipients: Molecular Evidence of Colonized Patients as Potential Infectious Sources of *Pneumocystis jirovecii*

Le Gal S, Damiani C, Rouillé A, et al (Univ of Brest, France; Amiens Univ Hosp, France; et al)

Clin Infect Dis 54:e62-e71, 2012

Background.—Eighteen renal transplant recipients (RTRs) developed *Pneumocystis jirovecii* infections at the renal transplantation unit of Brest University Hospital (Brest, Brittany, France) from May 2008 through April 2010, whereas no cases of *P. jirovecii* infection had been diagnosed in this unit since 2002. This outbreak was investigated by identifying *P. jirovecii* types and analyzing patient encounters.

Methods.—The identification of *P. jirovecii* internal transcribed spacer (ITS) types was performed on *P. jirovecii* isolates from the 18 RTRs (12 patients with *Pneumocystis* pneumonia [PCP], 6 colonized patients), 22 unlinked control patients (18 patients with PCP, 4 colonized patients), and 69 patients (34 patients with PCP, 35 colonized patients) with contemporaneously diagnosed *P. jirovecii* infections in the Brest geographic area. A transmission map was drawn up. Its analysis was combined with the results of *P. jirovecii* typing.

Results.—*P. jirovecii* ITS type identification was successful in 14 of 18 RTRs, 15 of 22 control patients, and 48 of the 69 patients. Type Eg was the most frequent type in the 3 patient groups. However, its frequency was significantly higher in the first patient group than in the 2 other groups ($P < .05$ and $P < .01$, respectively). Fourteen encounters between RTRs who harbored an identical type were observed. Ten patients were considered as possible index patients, of whom 3 were colonized by the fungus, and 7 presented PCP.

Conclusions.—The results provide to our knowledge the first data on the role of colonized patients as potential sources of *P. jirovecii* in a context of nosocomial acquisition of the fungus.

▶ *Pneumocystis* pneumonia (PCP) is currently considered to result from acquisition of the fungus rather than reactivation of latent infection with *Pneumocystis jirovecii* in the lung.[1] There is no animal reservoir for *P jirovecii* because organisms infecting each mammalian species are host-specific. The potential human sources of *P jirovecii* may be all infected patients, including those with mild symptoms and respiratory colonization. Host-to-host transmission has been reported through animal models and suspected nosocomial transmission in renal transplant recipients.[2]

This study reports a cluster of *Pneumocystis* infections in renal transplant recipients at a university hospital in France. Of the 18 patients in the cluster, 16 developed PCP and 6 were colonized. In the prior 6 years, no cases of *P jirovecii* had been diagnosed in this unit. The patients in the clusters (renal transplant recipients [RTRs]) were compared with 22 unlinked control patients (18 with PCP and 4 colonized) and 69 patients (34 patients with PCP and 35 colonized patients) with *P jirovecii* infections in the same geographic area. Internal transcribed spacer typing was performed on all *P jirovecii* isolates. In all 3 patient groups, type Eg was the most frequent. The frequency of type Eg was significantly higher in the RTR group. Of a total of 25 encounters involving 16 patients among RTRs, 14 were considered to be the cause of *P jirovecii* transmission. These 14 RTRs harbored an identical type of *P jirovecii*. Of the 10 considered to be index patients, 3 were colonized by the fungus and 7 presented with PCP.

The authors suggest further discussion of the current recommendation of 4 to 6 months of PCP prophylaxis in RTRs and the consideration of extending the isolation policy to patients in whom pulmonary colonization with *P jirovecii* is documented.[3]

N. M. Khardori, MD, PhD

References

1. Keely SP, Stringer JR. Sequences of Pneumocystis carinii f. sp. hominis strains associated with recurrent pneumonia vary at multiple loci. *J Clin Microbiol.* 1997;35: 2745-2747.
2. Schmoldt S, Schuhegger R, Wendler T, et al. Molecular evidence of nosocomial *Pneumocystis jirovecii* transmission among 16 patients after kidney transplantation. *J Clin Microbiol.* 2008;46:966-971.
3. Siegel JD, Rhinehart E, Jackson M, Chiarello L. 2007 guideline for isolation precautions: preventing transmission of infectious agents in health care settings. *Am J Infect Control.* 2007;35:S65-S164.

Impact of Treatment Strategy on Outcomes in Patients with Candidemia and Other Forms of Invasive Candidiasis: A Patient-Level Quantitative Review of Randomized Trials
Andes DR, for the Mycoses Study Group (Univ of Wisconsin, Madison; et al)
Clin Infect Dis 54:1110-1122, 2012

Background.—Invasive candidiasis (IC) is an important healthcare-related infection, with increasing incidence and a crude mortality exceeding 50%. Numerous treatment options are available yet comparative studies have not identified optimal therapy.

Methods.—We conducted an individual patient-level quantitative review of randomized trials for treatment of IC and to assess the impact of host-, organism-, and treatment-related factors on mortality and clinical cure. Studies were identified by searching computerized databases and queries of experts in the field for randomized trials comparing the effect of ≥2 antifungals for treatment of IC. Univariate and multivariable analyses were performed to determine factors associated with patient outcomes.

Results.—Data from 1915 patients were obtained from 7 trials. Overall mortality among patients in the entire data set was 31.4%, and the rate of treatment success was 67.4%. Logistic regression analysis for the aggregate data set identified increasing age (odds ratio [OR], 1.01; 95% confidence interval [CI], 1.00–1.02; *P* = .02), the Acute Physiology and Chronic Health Evaluation II score (OR, 1.11; 95% CI, 1.08–1.14; *P* = .0001), use of immunosuppressive therapy (OR, 1.69; 95% CI, 1.18–2.44; *P* = .001), and infection with *Candida tropicalis* (OR, 1.64; 95% CI, 1.11–2.39; *P* = .01) as predictors of mortality. Conversely, removal of a central venous catheter (CVC) (OR, 0.50; 95% CI, .35–.72; *P* = .0001) and treatment with an echinocandin antifungal (OR, 0.65; 95% CI, .45–.94; *P* = .02) were associated with decreased mortality. Similar findings were observed for the clinical success end point.

Conclusions.—Two treatment-related factors were associated with improved survival and greater clinical success: use of an echinocandin and removal of the CVC (Fig 1, Table 4).

▶ In the past 2 decades, epidemiologic studies have identified *Candida* species as the fourth-most common cause of nosocomial bloodstream infection. *Candida* spp—related hospitalizations and mortality have continued to rise.[1] Invasive

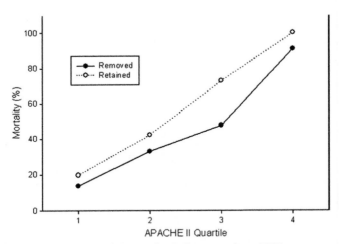

FIGURE 1.—Impact of severity of illness and central venous catheter (CVC) management on patient mortality. Each symbol represents the mortality rate as a percentage for patients in 1 of 4 Acute Physiology and Chronic Health Evaluation (APACHE) II score quartiles: quartile 1, 0–11; 2, 12–23; 3, 24–35; and 4, 36–47. Closed symbols represent patients with CVC removal; open symbols, patients with CVC retention. Differences in mortality were statistically significant for quartiles 1, 2, and 3 (quartile 1, *P* = .05; 2, *P* = .01; 3, *P* = .002; and 4, *P* = .41). (Reprinted from Andes DR, for the Mycoses Study Group. Impact of treatment strategy on outcomes in patients with candidemia and other forms of invasive candidiasis: a patient-level quantitative review of randomized trials. *Clin Infect Dis.* 2012;54:1110-1122, by permission of the Infectious Diseases Society of America.)

TABLE 4.—Multivariate Analysis of Host, Disease, and Treatment Factors and Outcome in Patients With Invasive Candidiasis

Organisms[a]	Factor	Mortality OR	P	95% CI	Factor	Success OR	P	95% CI
All organisms (n = 978)	Age	1.01	.02	1.00–1.02	APACHE II	0.94	.0001	.93–.96
	APACHE II score	1.11	.0001	1.08–1.14	Echinocandin	2.33	.01	1.27–4.35
	Immunosuppressive therapy	1.69	.001	1.18–2.44	CVC removed	1.69	.001	1.23–2.33
	Candida tropicalis	1.64	.01	1.11–2.39	Study		NS	
	Echinocandin	0.65	.02	.45–.94				
	CVC removed	0.50	.0001	.35–.72				
	Study		NS					
Candida albicans (n = 408)	APACHE II score	1.09	.0001	1.05–1.13	APACHE II score	0.92	.005	.92–99
	Immunosuppressive therapy	2.22	.002	1.30–3.70	Echinocandin	3.70	.005	1.49–9.09
	Surgery	0.58	.05	.34–98	Study		NS	
	Malignancy	1.89	.03	1.05–3.45				
	Echinocandin	0.55	.03	.32–95				
	CVC removed	0.52	.01	.31–90				
	Study		NS					
Non-albicans species (n = 570)	APACHE II score	1.14	.0001	1.1–1.17	Age	1.02	.004	1.01–1.03
	Echinocandin	0.52	.04	.36–78	APACHE II score	0.93	.0001	.91–96
	CVC removed	0.69	.05	.48–98	CVC removed	1.74	.007	1.16–2.61
	Study		NS		Study		NS	
Candida glabrata (n = 104)	CVC removed	0.13	.001	.04–.45	APACHE II score	0.95	.05	.90–99
	Study		NS		Echinocandin	2.63	.05	1.10–625
					Study		NS	
Candida tropicalis[b]	APACHE II score	1.13	.0001	1.08–1.18	Age	0.98	.04	.96–99
	Study		NS		APACHE II score	0.93	.0001	.89–96
					CVC removed	1.97	.02	1.10–3.52
					Study		NS	
Candida parapsilosis[c]	APACHE II score	1.11	.001	1.04–1.19	APACHE II score	0.95	.01	.90–99
	ICU admission	2.63	.02	1.12–6.25	Study		NS	
	Study		NS					

Abbreviations: APACHE, Acute Physiology and Chronic Health Evaluation; CI, confidence interval; CVC, central venous catheter; ICU, intensive care unit; NS, not significant ($P > .05$); OR, odds ratio; Study = individual study publication.

[a]Parenthetical numbers represent number of individuals available for each model.

[b]For *Candida tropicalis*, n = 262 for analysis of mortality and 261 for analysis of success.

[c]For *Candida parapsilosis*, n = 158 for analysis of mortality and 212 for analysis of success.

candidiasis is associated with mortality rates of 50%. There has been a global shift in epidemiology toward nonalbicans species, particularly *Candida glabrata.*[2] The variable susceptibility of nonalbicans *Candida* species to antifungal agents further adds to the complexity of choosing initial antifungal therapy.

This study reviewed 7 randomized treatment trials of invasive candidiasis. This is currently the largest patient-level quantitative review to have been done to help optimize management strategy for an important clinical issue with high mortality. Table 4 shows differences in treatment success and mortality in relationship to host and microbiologic factors. The study identified 2 modifiable management strategies. First, the use of an echinocandin antifungal was associated with reduced mortality compared with use of agents from triazole or polyene classes. Second, the findings further support the previous retrospective analysis demonstrating that central venous catheter (CVC) removal can shorten the duration of candidemia and enhance the likelihood of survival. The reduced mortality in the patients in whom the CVC was removed is clearly shown in Fig 1. Based on findings presented, the authors suggest that the choice of echinocandin drug class should be considered as initial therapy for most patient groups in contrast to the current guidelines.

N. M. Khardori, MD, PhD

References

1. Zilberberg MD, Shorr AF, Kollef MH. Secular trends in candidemia-related hospitalization in the United States, 2000—2005. *Infect Control Hosp Epidemiol.* 2008; 29:978-980.
2. Chow JK, Golan Y, Ruthazer R, et al. Factors associated with candidemia caused by non-albicans Candida species versus Candida albicans in the intensive care unit. *Clin Infect Dis.* 2008;46:1206-1213.

Septic Shock Attributed to *Candida* Infection: Importance of Empiric Therapy and Source Control
Kollef M, Micek S, Hampton N, et al (Washington Univ School of Medicine; Barnes-Jewish Hosp, St Louis, MO; Hosp Informatics Group, St Louis, MO; et al)
Clin Infect Dis 54:1739-1746, 2012

Background.—Delayed treatment of candidemia has previously been shown to be an important determinant of patient outcome. However, septic shock attributed to *Candida* infection and its determinants of outcome have not been previously evaluated in a large patient population.

Methods.—A retrospective cohort study of hospitalized patients with septic shock and blood cultures positive for *Candida* species was conducted at Barnes-Jewish Hospital, a 1250-bed urban teaching hospital (January 2002—December 2010).

Results.—Two hundred twenty-four consecutive patients with septic shock and a positive blood culture for *Candida* species were identified. Death during hospitalization occurred among 155 (63.5%) patients. The hospital mortality rate for patients having adequate source control and antifungal therapy administered within 24 hours of the onset of shock was 52.8% (n = 142), compared to a mortality rate of 97.6% (n = 82) in patients who did not have these goals attained (*P* < .001). Multivariate logistic regression analysis demonstrated that delayed antifungal treatment (adjusted odds ratio [AOR], 33.75; 95% confidence interval [CI], 9.65−118.04; *P* = .005) and failure to achieve timely source control (AOR, 77.40; 95% CI, 21.52−278.38; *P* = .001) were independently associated with a greater risk of hospital mortality.

Conclusions.—The risk of death is exceptionally high among patients with septic shock attributed to *Candida* infection. Efforts aimed at timely source control and antifungal treatment are likely to be associated with improved clinical outcomes (Table 3).

▶ A recent point-prevalence study of severe sepsis with 13 796 adult patients reported that 51% of patients were classified as infected on the day of the study.[1] Of these, 30% were culture negative. Among the 70%, the organism cultures were gram-positive (47%), gram-negative (62%), and fungal (19%).

The hospital mortality of severe sepsis and septic shock remains at 30% to 50%. The outcomes are further negatively impacted by inappropriate initial antimicrobial therapy.[2]

This is a retrospective cohort study of patients with septic shock from *Candida* bloodstream infection (BSI) at a large urban teaching hospital. The study examines the appropriateness of antimicrobial therapy and its influence on the outcome in patients with septic shock and *Candida* BSI.

Of the 224 patients with septic shock attributed to monomicrobial infection with *Candida* spp as documented by a positive blood culture, 155 (69.2%) died during hospitalization. No antifungal therapy was given to 18.3% of patients prior to their death because of delayed recognition of the fungal infection.

Table 3 shows that delayed administration of appropriate antifungal therapy (≤24 hours) and inadequate source control were the most important determinants of outcome in patients with septic shock and microbiologically documented *Candida* BSI.

TABLE 3.—Multivariate Analysis of Risk Factors for Hospital Mortality[a]

	AOR	95% CI	*P* Value
Solid cell tumor with metastases	6.01	2.98−12.10	.010
Class IV congestive heart failure	4.95	2.53−9.68	.017
APACHE II Score (1-point increments)	1.37	1.26−1.48	<.001
Inadequate source control	77.40	21.52−278.38	.001
Red blood cell transfusion	6.49	4.06−10.38	<.001
Serum albumin (1 g/dL increments)	0.42	0.30−0.59	.012
Delayed antifungal treatment[b]	33.75	9.65−118.04	.005

Hosmer-Lemeshow goodness-of-fit test, *P* = .920.

Abbreviations: AOR, adjusted odds ratio; APACHE, Acute Physiology and Chronic Health Evaluation; CI, confidence interval.

[a]Other covariates not in the table had a *P* value >.05, including age, corticosteroids, granulocyte colony−stimulating factor, and total crystalloid fluid administered within 24 hours of shock.

[b]Defined as patients who received no antifungal therapy within 24 hours of the onset of shock.

Severity of illness, red blood cell transfusion, and comorbidities were also associated with mortality in multivariate analysis.

In the absence of more rapid and accurate microbiologic techniques, the high index of suspicion for *Candida* BSI in patients with risk factors is needed to start prescription antifungal therapy.

N. M. Khardori, MD, PhD

References

1. Vincent JL, Rello J, Marshall J, et al. International study of the prevalence and outcomes of infection in intensive care units. *JAMA*. 2009;302:2323-2329.
2. Kollef MH. Broad-spectrum antimicrobials and the treatment of serious bacterial infections: getting it right up front. *Clin Infect Dis*. 2008;47:S3-S13.

11 Miscellaneous

A Randomized Trial of the Efficacy of Hand Disinfection for Prevention of Rhinovirus Infection

Turner RB, Fuls JL, Rodgers ND, et al (Univ of Virginia, Charlottesville; Henkel, Scottsdale, AZ; et al)
Clin Infect Dis 54:1422-1426, 2012

Background.—Hand disinfection is frequently recommended for prevention of rhinovirus (RV) infection and RV-associated common colds. The effectiveness of this intervention has not been established in a natural setting. The purpose of this study was to determine the effect of hand disinfection on RV infection and RV-associated common cold illness in a natural setting.

Methods.—A controlled clinical trial was done in young adult volunteers during 9 weeks of the fall 2009 RV season. Volunteers were randomized to either an antiviral hand treatment containing 2% citric acid and 2% malic acid in 62% ethanol (n = 116) or to a no-treatment control group (n = 96). The hand treatment was applied every 3 hours while the subjects were awake. All volunteers kept a daily diary of symptoms and had a nasal lavage for polymerase chain reaction once each week and 2 additional lavages around the time of each common cold illness. The primary endpoint was the number of RV-associated illnesses. The incidence of RV infection and of common cold illnesses were evaluated as secondary endpoints.

Results.—The hand treatment did not significantly reduce RV infection or RV-related common cold illnesses. The total number of common cold illnesses was significantly reduced in the intent-to-treat analysis, but this effect was not seen in the per protocol analysis.

Conclusions.—In this study, hand disinfection did not reduce RV infection or RV-related common cold illnesses.

Clinical Trials Registration.—NCT00993759 (Table 1).

▶ Hand-to-hand transfer of rhinovirus (RV) has been identified as a likely mechanism of transmission of the infection.[1] The addition of organic acids to ethanol hand sanitizers in an experimental setting provides an additional antiviral effect lasting for up to 4 hours.[2]

This controlled clinical trial reports on the efficacy of hand disinfection on transmission of RV infection in the natural setting. Healthy adult volunteers recruited from the University of Virginia community were randomly assigned to treatment and no-treatment group. Study treatment consisted of a lotion containing 62% ethanol, 2% citric acid, and 2% malic acid applied every 3 hours while

TABLE 1.—Comparison of the Antiviral Hand Sanitizer Treatment Group and the No-Treatment (Control) Group

Type of Analysis	Antiviral Treatment	No Treatment
Intent-to-treat analysis	(n = 116)	(n = 96)
Common cold illnesses	56 (48; 39–57)	72 (75; 65–83)[a]
Rhinovirus infections	49 (42; 34–51)	49 (51; 41–61)
Rhinovirus-associated illnesses	26 (22; 16–31)	24 (25; 17–35)
Per protocol analysis	(n = 91)	(n = 95)
Common cold illnesses	50 (55; 45–65)	71 (75; 65–82)
Rhinovirus infections	45 (50; 39–60)	49 (52; 42–61)
Rhinovirus-associated illnesses	25 (28; 19–37)	24 (25; 18–35)

Data are presented as no. (no. per 100 subjects; 95% confidence interval).
[a] $P = .01$ for comparison to active treatment.

awake and after hand washing for the 9 weeks of the fall 2009 RV season. The intervention was evaluated through a daily diary of symptoms, detection of RV by polymerase chain reaction in the nasal lavage once a week and 2 additional lavages around the time of each common cold illness.

As shown in Table 1, the total number of common cold illnesses was significantly reduced in the intent-to-treat analysis. This effect did not extend to per protocol analysis or to the RV infections and RV-associated illnesses in the intent-to-treat analysis. No treatment effect was demonstrated on coronavirus and influenza A and B viruses as detected by polymerase chain reaction assay done on RV-negative specimens from volunteers with common cold illnesses. An earlier study of RV transmission in the natural setting done using an iodine hand treatment focused on preventing infection in mothers in contact with children in the household setting. The results of that study, along with experimental studies, led to the opinion that RV is transmitted by direct contact. This study calls into question this commonly held assumption and suggests that the route of RV spread in different populations in the natural setting needs to be better defined.

N. M. Khardori, MD, PhD

References

1. Hendley JO, Gwaltney JM Jr. Mechanisms of transmission of rhinovirus infections. *Epidemiol Rev.* 1988;10:243-258.
2. Turner RB, Fuls JL, Rodgers ND. Effectiveness of hand sanitizers with and without organic acids for removal of rhinovirus from hands. *Antimicrob Agents Chemother.* 2010;54:1363-1364.

Early peak temperature and mortality in critically ill patients with or without infection

Young PJ, Saxena M, Beasley R, et al (Wellington Regional Hosp, New Zealand; Univ of New South Wales, Sydney, Australia; Med Res Inst of New Zealand, Wellington; et al)
Intensive Care Med 38:437-444, 2012

Purpose.—To determine whether fever is associated with an increased or decreased risk of death in patients admitted to an intensive care unit (ICU) with infection.

Methods.—We evaluated the independent association between peak temperature in the first 24 h after ICU admission and in-hospital mortality according to whether there was an admission diagnosis of infection using a database of admissions to 129 ICUs in Australia and New Zealand (ANZ) ($n = 269,078$). Subsequently, we sought to confirm or refute the ANZ database findings using a validation cohort of admissions to 201 ICUs in the UK ($n = 366,973$).

Results.—A total of 29,083/269,078 (10.8%) ANZ patients and 103,191/366,973 (28.1%) of UK patients were categorised as having an infection. In the ANZ cohort, adjusted in-hospital mortality risk progressively decreased with increasing peak temperature in patients with infection. Relative to the risk at 36.5—36.9°C, the lowest risk was at 39—39.4°C (adjusted OR 0.56; 95% CI 0.48—0.66). In patients without infection, the adjusted mortality risk progressively increased above 39.0°C (adjusted OR 2.07 at 40.0°C or above; 95% CI 1.68—2.55). In the UK cohort, findings were similar with adjusted odds ratios at corresponding temperatures of 0.77 (95% CI 0.71—0.85) and 1.94 (95% CI 1.60—2.34) for infection and noninfection groups, respectively.

Conclusions.—Elevated peak temperature in the first 24 h in ICU is associated with decreased in-hospital mortality in critically ill patients with an infection; randomised trials are needed to determine whether controlling fever increases mortality in such patients (Figs 1 and 2).

▶ Fever as a marker of illness and severity of illness is common in critical patients. On one hand, it may be part of a protective response and may result in survival benefit during infection.[1] This may be related to enhanced production of pyrogenic cytokines linked to a robust immunologic response or because temperatures in the febrile range can cause direct inhibition of microbial growth.[2,3] In addition, the in vitro activity of antibiotics has been shown to increase at temperatures within the physiologic febrile range.

Using a large database, this study from Australia and New Zealand evaluated the independent association between peak temperatures in the first 24 hours after intensive care unit (ICU) admission and outcome. The findings were verified by using a validation cohort of admissions to ICUs in the United Kingdom.

Patients from both databases were categorized into infection and noninfection groups. Illness severity—adjusted in-hospital mortality associated with peak documented temperature in the first 24 hours following admission to ICU was

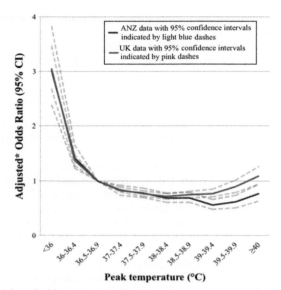

FIGURE 1.—Adjusted odds ratios (see Tables 2, 3 in the original article) for in-hospital mortality versus peak temperature in the first 24 h in ICU for patients in the infection group. (With kind permission from Springer Science+Business Media: Young PJ, Saxena M, Beasley R, et al. Early peak temperature and mortality in critically ill patients with or without infection. *Intensive Care Med*. 2012;38:437-444, with permission from Springer and ESICM.)

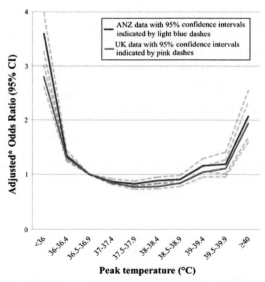

FIGURE 2.—Adjusted odds ratios (see Tables 2, 3 in the original article) for in-hospital mortality versus peak temperature in the first 24 h in ICU for patients in the non-infection group. (With kind permission from Springer Science+Business Media: Young PJ, Saxena M, Beasley R, et al. Early peak temperature and mortality in critically ill patients with or without infection. *Intensive Care Med*. 2012;38:437-444, with permission from Springer and ESICM.)

used as the primary outcome. As shown in Fig 1, in both cohorts, adjusted in-hospital mortality risk progressively decreased with increasing peak temperature in patients with infection. The lowest risk was at the temperature of 39°C to 39.4°C.

These findings were in contrast to those of the patients categorized as non-infection. As shown in Fig 2, in the noninfection group, the adjusted mortality progressively increased to greater than 39.0°C. Fever is known to be associated with a marked metabolic cost, increasing metabolic rate, minute ventilation, and cardiac output. Critically ill patients with fever in the absence of infection are exposed to deleterious effects without the beneficial effect of suppression of the infectious agent. Hypothermia puts both infection and noninfection patients at an increased risk of mortality. In spite of the limitations in the study that the authors discuss, the differential association of fever with outcome in the infection and noninfection groups is statistically significant.

N. M. Khardori, MD, PhD

References

1. Laupland KB, Shahpori R, Kirkpatrick AW, Ross T, Gregson DB, Stelfox HT. Occurrence and outcome of fever in critically ill adults. *Crit Care Med*. 2008; 36:1531-1535.
2. Enders JF, Shaffer MF. Studies on natural immunity to Pneumococcus type III: I. The capacity of strains of Pneumococcus type III to grow at 40 degrees C. and their virulence for rabbits. *J Exp Med*. 1936;64:7-18.
3. Chu CM, Tian SF, Ren GF, Zhang YM, Zhang LX, Liu GQ. Occurrence of temperature-sensitive influenza A viruses in nature. *J Virol*. 1982;41:353-359.

Hydroxyethyl Starch 130/0.42 versus Ringer's Acetate in Severe Sepsis

Perner A, for the 6S Trial Group and the Scandinavian Critical Care Trials Group (Copenhagen Univ Hosp, Denmark; et al)
N Engl J Med 367:124-134, 2012

Background.—Hydroxyethyl starch (HES) 130/0.42 is widely used for fluid resuscitation in intensive care units (ICUs), but its safety and efficacy have not been established in patients with severe sepsis.

Methods.—In this multicenter, parallel-group, blinded trial, we randomly assigned patients with severe sepsis to fluid resuscitation in the ICU with either 6% HES 130/0.42 (Tetraspan) or Ringer's acetate at a dose of up to 33 ml per kilogram of ideal body weight per day. The primary outcome measure was either death or end-stage kidney failure (dependence on dialysis) at 90 days after randomization.

Results.—Of the 804 patients who underwent randomization, 798 were included in the modified intention-to-treat population. The two intervention groups had similar baseline characteristics. At 90 days after randomization, 201 of 398 patients (51%) assigned to HES 130/0.42 had died, as compared with 172 of 400 patients (43%) assigned to Ringer's acetate (relative risk, 1.17; 95% confidence interval [CI], 1.01 to 1.36; $P = 0.03$); 1 patient in each group had end-stage kidney failure. In the 90-day period,

87 patients (22%) assigned to HES 130/0.42 were treated with renal-replacement therapy versus 65 patients (16%) assigned to Ringer's acetate (relative risk, 1.35; 95% CI, 1.01 to 1.80; $P = 0.04$), and 38 patients (10%) and 25 patients (6%), respectively, had severe bleeding (relative risk, 1.52; 95% CI, 0.94 to 2.48; $P = 0.09$). The results were supported by multivariate analyses, with adjustment for known risk factors for death or acute kidney injury at baseline.

Conclusions.—Patients with severe sepsis assigned to fluid resuscitation with HES 130/0.42 had an increased risk of death at day 90 and were more likely to require renal-replacement therapy, as compared with those receiving Ringer's acetate. (Funded by the Danish Research Council and others; 6S ClinicalTrials.gov number, NCT00962156.)

▶ International guidelines for management of severe sepsis and septic shock in The Surviving Sepsis Campaign recommend the use either of colloids or crystalloids for volume replacement in severe sepsis.[1] As observed in 2 randomized trials, high-molecular-weight hydroxyethyl starch (HES) may cause kidney failure in patients with severe sepsis.[2]

The HES solutions used in these studies have 200KD hydroxyethyl groups per glucose molecule (substitution ratio) of more than 0.4%. These have now largely been replaced by lower molecular weight and lower substitution ratio (ie, HES 130/0.42).

This study reports on the Scandinavian Starch for Severe Sepsis/Septic Shock trial to compare HES 130/0.42 with Ringer's acetate. The primary outcomes measured are death or end-stage kidney failure in patients with severe sepsis. Patients were randomly assigned to the HES or Ringer's acetate group. Baseline characteristics in the 2 groups were similar. Compared with Ringer's lactate, HES 130/0.42 significantly increased the risk of death or dependence on dialysis at day 90. The increased risk of death with HES 130/0.42 observed in this trial is similar to that observed in the severe sepsis trial that used HES 200/0.52. The survival curves separated around day 20 in both trials indicating late deaths induced by HES. HES was associated with kidney failure and increased use of renal-replacement therapy in both trials. There was no significant difference in trial fluid volumes between the 2 groups even though colloids like HES are considered to be more potent plasma volume expanders than crystalloids. Routine practice was maintained in this protocol except for fluid resuscitation. Overall, outcomes rates in this trial were similar to those in previous trials.

N. M. Khardori, MD, PhD

References

1. Dellinger RP, Levy MM, Carlet JM, et al. Surviving Sepsis Campaign: international guidelines for management of severe sepsis and septic shock: 2008. *Intensive Care Med.* 2008;34:17-60.
2. Brunkhorst FM, Engel C, Bloos F, et al. Intensive insulin therapy and pentastarch resuscitation in severe sepsis. *N Engl J Med.* 2008;358:125-139.

Inadequacy of temperature and white blood cell count in predicting bacteremia in patients with suspected infection

Seigel TA, Cocchi MN, Salciccioli J, et al (Beth Israel Deaconess Med Ctr, Boston, MA; et al)
J Emerg Med 42:254-259, 2012

Background.—Early treatment of sepsis in Emergency Department (ED) patients has lead to improved outcomes, making early identification of the disease essential. The presence of systemic inflammatory response criteria aids in recognition of infection, although the reliability of these markers is variable.

Study Objective.—This study aims to quantify the ability of abnormal temperature, white blood cell (WBC) count, and bandemia to identify bacteremia in ED patients with suspected infection.

Methods.—This was a post hoc analysis of data collected for a prospective, observational, cohort study. Consecutive adult (age ≥18 years) patients who presented to the ED of a tertiary care center between February 1, 2000 and February 1, 2001 and had blood cultures obtained in the ED or within 3 h of admission were enrolled. Patients with bacteremia were identified and charts were reviewed for presence of normal temperature (36.1−38°C/97−100.4°F), normal WBC (4−12 K/μL), and presence of bandemia (>5% of WBC differential).

Results.—There were 3563 patients enrolled; 289 patients (8.1%) had positive blood cultures. Among patients with positive blood cultures, 33% had a normal body temperature and 52% had a normal WBC count. Bandemia was present in 80% of culture-positive patients with a normal temperature and 79% of culture-positive patients with a normal WBC count. Fifty-two (17.4%) patients with positive blood cultures had neither an abnormal temperature nor an abnormal WBC.

Conclusion.—A significant percentage of ED patients with blood culture-proven bacteremia have a normal temperature and WBC count upon presentation. Bandemia may be a useful clue for identifying occult bacteremia.

▶ As part of criteria that define systemic inflammatory response syndrome (SIRS), abnormal body temperature and white blood cell (WBC) count are often used as markers for infection, even though their accuracy has not been documented. The role of abnormal body temperature and WBC count in predicting bacteremia in patients presenting to emergency departments has not been defined.

This publication presents a post hoc secondary analysis of data collected for a prospective, observational cohort study.[1] The patients included in this analysis presented to the emergency department with suspected infection (based on symptom report or physical examination findings) and ultimately had positive blood culture results. Of these patients with proven bacteremia, 17.4% had normal temperature, normal WBC count, or both on initial evaluation in the ED. Normal body temperature was noted in 33% and normal WBC count in 52% of patients with positive blood cultures. However, bandemia (75% of WBC differential) was present in 80% of culture positive patients with a normal temperature and 79% of culture positive patients with a normal WBC count. Even in bacteremia patients with hypotension or septic shock, 33% had a normal temperature and 21% had normal WBC count on initial evaluation suggesting the insensitivity of these parameters even in the presence of severe physiologic derangement. These results are similar to those demonstrated in other cohorts of patients (eg, patients with community-acquired pneumonia, infected surgical patients, critically ill patients, geriatric patients). Significant infectious diseases including bacteremia may be present in patients without the traditionally associated findings of fever or hypothermia and leukocytosis or leukopenia.

N. M. Khardori, MD, PhD

Reference

1. Shapiro NI, Wolfe RE, Moore RB, et al. Mortality in Emergency Department Sepsis (MEDS) score: a prospectively derived and validated clinical prediction rule. *Crit Care Med.* 2003;31:670-675.

What's new in respiratory infections and tuberculosis 2008–2010
Brown JS, Lipman MCI, Zar HJ (Rayne Inst, London, UK; Univ College Med School, London, UK; Univ of Cape Town, South Africa)
Thorax 67:350-354, 2012

Over the past few years there have been an increasing number of research articles published in *Thorax* on respiratory tract infections (including tuberculosis) affecting children and adults. Although these articles cover a wide variety of areas, several broad themes can be discerned. These include greater interest in viral respiratory infections (partially stimulated by the recent influenza A pandemic), improved characterisation of who is at risk of community-acquired pneumonia and mycobacterial infection, research into better diagnostics and attempts to develop new or improved scoring scales for a range of respiratory infection syndromes. There have also been a limited number of articles on how to manage patients with respiratory infection, including describing the efficacy of prevention by vaccination. Overall, there has been a discernible emphasis on transferring advances in clinical science to actual clinical practice, with several papers using molecular methodologies or measuring levels of cytokines or other potential biomarkers to improve diagnostic accuracy in patients with lung infection. There have also been manuscripts linking specific pathogen genotypes to infection phenotype, an area that is likely to be increasingly important in explaining some of the variations in severity between patients with respiratory infection. However, many questions remain on the optimum strategies for the management and prevention of pneumonia, bronchiectasis and tuberculosis, and there remains a strong need for further clinical research in

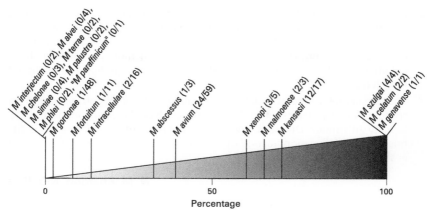

FIGURE 1.—Clinical relevance of pulmonary non-tuberculous mycobacteria isolates, per species. (x/y), number of patients who met the American Thoracic Society diagnostic criteria/total number of patients per species (reproduced from van Ingen *et al*[22]). *Editor's Note:* Please refer to original journal article for full references. (Reproduced from Thorax, Brown JS, Lipman MCI, Zar HJ. What's new in respiratory infections and tuberculosis 2008–2010. *Thorax.* 2012;67:350-354. Copyright 2012 with permission from BMJ Publishing Group Ltd.)

order to make substantial improvements in the management of patients with lung infection (Fig 1).

▶ This is a well-written and highly clinically relevant summary of more than 75 major research articles on respiratory infection published in *Thorax* between 2008 and 2010. The highlights include the following.

1. The H1N1 pandemic of 2009 started in Mexico from triple reassortment of porcine H1N1, resulting in transmission from pigs to humans of a strain with human pandemic potential. The pandemic affected younger rather than age groups older than 45 years probably because of preexisting immunity from exposure in earlier outbreaks. Preexisting comorbidities, especially obesity and asthma, were associated with higher mortality. Poor outcomes were also associated with abnormal chest radiographs or raised C-reactive protein on admission. In contrast with seasonal influenza, 50% of patients who died were previously healthy, with pregnancy as one of the strongest risk factors. Like the previous influenza pandemics, there was a second and third wave, with the third wave leading to 411 deaths in the United Kingdom compared with a combined total of 474 deaths during the first 2 waves.

2. Association of bacterial pneumonia with viral respiratory infection and its impact on mortality was again demonstrated in a comprehensive survey of the patients presenting with community-acquired pneumonia. Twenty-nine percent had viral infection with influenza virus, rhinovirus, adenovirus, and respiratory syncytial virus. Bacterial pathogen coinfection mainly by *Streptococcus pneumoniae* was seen in 46% of patients with viral infection.

3. Diabetes was estimated to be a population-attributable risk in 11% of cases of tuberculosis in the United Kingdom, similar to that of HIV co-infection. The proportion of nonpulmonary tuberculosis cases in United Kingdom has increased between 1999 and 2006 and is seen mostly in foreign born patients who develop disease several years after immigration to the United Kingdom.

4. The clinical relevance of isolation of nontuberculosis mycobacterium from sputum was demonstrated in 1 of 4 subjects based on American Thoracic Society/Infectious Diseases Society of America criteria for disease diagnosis. The relative significance of various nontuberculosis mycobacterium is shown in Fig 1.

N. M. Khardori, MD, PhD

12 Vaccines

A Cell Culture–Derived Influenza Vaccine Provides Consistent Protection Against Infection and Reduces the Duration and Severity of Disease in Infected Individuals

Ehrlich HJ, Singer J, Berezuk G, et al (Global R&D, Vienna, Austria; Vaccine R&D, Beltsville, MD; et al)

Clin Infect Dis 54:946-954, 2012

Background.—Current knowledge of the consistency of protection induced by seasonal influenza vaccines over the duration of a full influenza season is limited, and little is known about the clinical course of disease in individuals who become infected despite vaccination.

Methods.—Data from a randomized double-blind placebo-controlled clinical trial undertaken in healthy young adults in the 2008–2009 influenza season were used to investigate the weekly cumulative efficacy of a Vero cell culture–derived influenza vaccine. In addition, the duration and severity of disease in vaccine and placebo recipients with cell culture–confirmed influenza infection were compared.

Results.—Vaccine efficacy against matching strains was consistently high (73%–82%) throughout the study, including the entire period of the influenza season during which influenza activity was above the epidemic threshold. Vaccine efficacy was also consistent (68%–83%) when calculated for all strains, irrespective of antigenic match. Vaccination also ameliorated disease symptoms when infection was not prevented. Bivariate analysis of duration and severity showed a significant amelioration of myalgia ($P = .003$), headache ($P = .025$), and fatigue ($P = .013$) in infected vaccinated subjects compared with placebo. Cough ($P = .143$) and oropharyngeal pain ($P = .083$) were also reduced in infected vaccinated subjects.

Conclusions.—A Vero cell culture–derived influenza vaccine provides consistently high levels of protection against cell culture–confirmed infection by seasonal influenza virus and significantly reduces the duration and severity of disease in those individuals in which infection is not prevented.

Clinical Trials Registration.—ClinicalTrials.gov NCT00566345 (Fig 2).

▶ Annual influenza vaccination is now recommended for all individuals older than 6 months in the United States.[1] The aim of the US Healthy People 2020 initiative is to achieve 80% to 90% influenza vaccine coverage. This will require improvements in influenza vaccine supply through novel and more efficient technologies.[2]

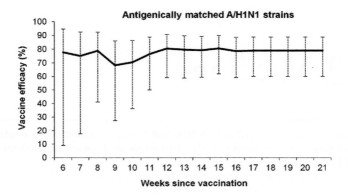

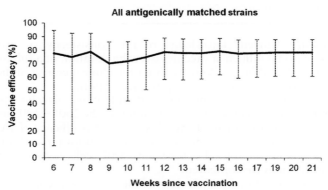

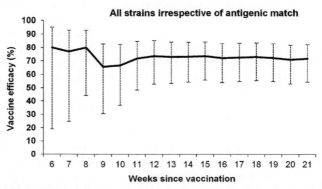

FIGURE 2.—Weekly cumulative vaccine efficacy against cell culture–confirmed influenza infection. Vaccine efficacy could be calculated from 24 January 2009, ~6 weeks after vaccination of the last subject on 15 December. Analysis of specimens from influenzalike illness visits continued until 15 May; the last laboratory-confirmed influenza infection was recorded in the week ending 9 May 2009. (Reprinted from Ehrlich HJ, Singer J, Berezuk G, et al. A cell culture–derived influenza vaccine provides consistent protection against infection and reduces the duration and severity of disease in infected individuals. *Clin Infect Dis*. 2012;54:946-954, by permission of the Infectious Diseases Society of America.)

A recent phase III placebo-controlled trial using a novel Vero cell culture—derived seasonal influenza vaccine demonstrated a 78.5% efficacy against cell culture—confirmed influenza infection with antigenically matched virus strains.[3]

This article presents additional analyses of the data from this trial to assess the vaccine efficacy over a complete influenza season and to determine the duration and severity of disease in infected individuals. The efficacy against matching strains (73% to 82%) was consistently high throughout the entire period of the influenza season. Vaccine efficacy against all strains (irrespective of antigenic match) was 68% to 83% (Fig 2). The benefit of the vaccination extended beyond the prevention of infection. The majority of the influenza like illness symptoms in patients who were infected despite vaccination were milder and of shorter duration compared with placebo recipients. The high efficacy with no reduction up to 5 months after vaccination would allow earlier vaccination to offer season-long protection. This, in conjunction with reduction in the severity and duration of symptoms in infected patients, would further enhance the overall medical and socioeconomic benefits of the seasonal influenza vaccination.

N. M. Khardori, MD, PhD

References

1. Fiore AE, Uyeki TM, Broder K, et al. Prevention and control of influenza with vaccines: recommendations of the Advisory Committee on Immunization Practices (ACIP), 2010. *MMWR Recomm Rep.* 2010;59:1-62.
2. Glezen WP. Cell-culture-derived influenza vaccine production. *Lancet.* 2011;377: 698-700.
3. Barrett PN, Berezuk G, Fritsch S, et al. Efficacy, safety, and immunogenicity of a Vero-cell-culture-derived trivalent influenza vaccine: a multicentre, double-blind, randomised, placebo-controlled trial. *Lancet.* 2011;377:751-759.

A Comparison of 2 Strategies to Prevent Infection Following Pertussis Exposure in Vaccinated Healthcare Personnel

Goins WP, Edwards KM, Vnencak-Jones CL, et al (Baylor College of Medicine, Houston, TX; Vanderbilt Univ School of Medicine, Nashville, TN)
Clin Infect Dis 54:938-945, 2012

Background.—Antibiotic postexposure prophylaxis (PEP) following pertussis exposure is recommended but has never been evaluated in healthcare personnel (HCP) vaccinated with acellular pertussis vaccine (Tdap).

Methods.—Tdap-vaccinated HCP were randomized to receive azithromycin PEP or no PEP following pertussis exposure. Acute and convalescent nasopharyngeal swabs and sera were obtained for pertussis testing by polymerase chain reaction (PCR) and anti—pertussis toxin (PT) immunoglobulin G, respectively. A nasopharyngeal aspirate was also collected for PCR and culture from subjects who reported respiratory symptoms within 21 days following identification of the exposure. Pertussis infection was defined as a positive culture or PCR, a 2-fold rise in anti-PT titer, or a single anti-PT titer of ≥94 enzyme-linked immunosorbent assay units/mL. Daily symptom monitoring without PEP was considered noninferior to PEP after pertussis exposure if the lower limit of the 1-sided 95% confidence interval (CI) for the reduction in pertussis was greater than −7%.

Results.—During 30 months of study, 86 subjects were randomized following a pertussis exposure. Using the predefined definition of infection, pertussis infection did not develop in 41 (97.6%) of 42 subjects who received azithromycin PEP and 38 (86.4%) of 44 subjects who did not receive PEP (absolute risk difference, −11.3%; lower bound of the 1-sided 95% CI, −20.6%; $P = .81$). However, no subject developed symptomatic pertussis confirmed with culture or a specific PCR assay, and possibly no subject developed subclinical pertussis infection based upon additional serologic testing.

Conclusions.—Using the predefined definition of pertussis infection, noninferiority for preventing pertussis following exposure was not demonstrated for daily symptom monitoring of Tdap-vaccinated HCP without PEP when compared with antibiotic PEP. However, the small number of exposed HCP warrants further study of this approach.

Clinical Trial Registration.—NCT00469274.

▶ Health care personnel (HCP) are an important link in the transmission chain of pertussis. They are at increased risk for acquiring infection from infected patients and likely to transmit the infection to susceptible patients and other HCP.[1] Prior to 2005, the only method to reduce the transmission after pertussis exposure was postexposure prophylaxis (PEP) with an antibiotic. In 2005, a vaccine containing tetanus toxoid and acellular pertussis vaccine was licensed for use in those aged 11 to 64 years old.

The Centers for Disease Control and Prevention (CDC) in 2006 recommended that all HCP with direct patient contact receive a single dose of Tdap (tetanus, diphtheria, pertussis) vaccine to reduce transmission of pertussis within health care facilities.[2] The CDC also recommended that exposed vaccinated HCP receive PEP with either antibiotic or daily symptom monitoring only with prompt evaluation, treatment, and furlough if symptoms develop.

This is a randomized, open-label trial to compare the 2 CDC recommended strategies following pertussis exposure in vaccinated HCP. Tdap was given to most subjects at enrollment, but some had received it previously. Postexposure (86 subjects during 30 months of study) Tdap-vaccinated HCP were randomized to receive azithromycin PEP or no PEP. A predefined definition of pertussis infection in HCP was used for further evaluation. Pertussis infection did not develop in 97.6% of 42 subjects who received azithromycin PEP and in 86.4% of 44 subjects who did not receive azithromycin. Based on confirmed culture or a specific polymerase chain reaction, no subject developed subclinical pertussis infection.

The Advisory Committee on Immunization Practices recently recommended antibiotic PEP for all exposed HCP who are likely to expose high-risk patients (eg neonates, pregnant women) to pertussis.[3]

N. M. Khardori, MD, PhD

References

1. Baggett HC, Duchin JS, Shelton W, et al. Two nosocomial pertussis outbreaks and their associated costs-King County, Washington, 2004. *Infect Control Hosp Epidemiol.* 2007;28:537-543.
2. Kretsinger K, Broder KR, Cortese MM, et al. Preventing tetanus, diphtheria, and pertussis among adults: use of tetanus toxoid, reduced diphtheria toxoid and acellular pertussis vaccine recommendations of the Advisory Committee on Immunization Practices (ACIP) and recommendation of ACIP, supported by the Healthcare Infection Control Practices Advisory Committee (HICPAC), for use of Tdap among health-care personnel. *MMWR Recomm Rep.* 2006;55:1-37.
3. Advisory Committee on Immunization Practices, Centers for Disease Control and Prevention (CDC). Immunization of health-care personnel: recommendations of the Advisory Committee on Immunization Practices (ACIP). *MMWR Recomm Rep.* 2011;60:1-45.

A Phase IIa Trial of the New Tuberculosis Vaccine, MVA85A, in HIV- and/or *Mycobacterium tuberculosis*–infected Adults

Scriba TJ, Tameris M, Smit E, et al (Univ of Cape Town, South Africa; et al)
Am J Respir Crit Care Med 185:769-778, 2012

Rationale.—Novel tuberculosis (TB) vaccines should be safe and effective in populations infected with *Mycobacterium tuberculosis* (*M.tb*) and/or HIV for effective TB control.

Objective.—To determine the safety and immunogenicity of MVA85A, a novel TB vaccine, among *M.tb*- and/or HIV-infected persons in a setting where TB and HIV are endemic.

Methods.—An open-label, phase IIa trial was conducted in 48 adults with *M.tb* and/or HIV infection. Safety and immunogenicity were analyzed up to 52 weeks after intradermal vaccination with 5×10^7 plaque-forming units of MVA85A. Specific T-cell responses were characterized by IFN-γ enzyme-linked immunospot and whole blood intracellular cytokine staining assays.

Measurements and Main Results.—MVA85A was well tolerated and no vaccine-related serious adverse events were recorded. MVA85A induced robust and durable response of mostly polyfunctional CD4$^+$T cells, coexpressing IFN-γ, tumor necrosis factor-α, and IL-2. Magnitudes of pre- and postvaccination T-cell responses were lower in HIV-infected, compared with HIV-uninfected, vaccinees. No significant effect of antiretroviral therapy on immunogenicity of MVA85A was observed.

Conclusions.—MVA85A was safe and immunogenic in persons with HIV and/or *M.tb* infection. These results support further evaluation of safety and efficacy of this vaccine for prevention of TB in these target populations.

▶ Past experience with tuberculosis (TB) clearly suggests that an effective TB vaccine will be critical for TB elimination.[1] The currently available BCG vaccine is used routinely for infants in settings where TB is endemic. Although BCG confers reliable protection against severe forms of TB in infancy, protection against pulmonary disease in all age groups is poor. This is further complicated by the fact that human immunodeficiency virus (HIV) and TB epidemics coexist in sub-Saharan Africa.

Epidemiological modeling suggests that a 92% reduction in TB incidence can be achieved by 2050 with a mass preexposure and postexposure vaccination of uninfected and latent infected individuals (LTBI), respectively. Therefore, new TB vaccines should be safe and effective in population infection with *Mycobacterium tuberculosis* (*Mtb*) with or without HIV.

Human clinical trials are being conducted with 14 new TB candidate vaccines.[2] MVA85A was the first to be used in safety and immunogenicity studies in LTBI patients. This article reports on the safety and efficacy of MVA85A in populations infected with Mtb with or without HIV in Worcester, South Africa. The 4 study groups were (1) healthy HIV-infected volunteers with no evidence of LTBI, not receiving antiretroviral (ARV) therapy; (2) HIV-infected volunteers with no evidence of LTBI; (3) HIV-infected volunteers with LTBI not receiving ARV therapy; and (4) healthy HIV-infected volunteers who had been stable on ARV therapy for more than 1 year irrespective of LTBI status. The vaccine was well tolerated by all groups and no serious adverse events related to the vaccine were noted. It induced a robust and durable response involving polyfunctional CD4-positive T cells, interferon-γ, interleukin-2, and tumor necrosis factor-α.

ARV therapy had no significant effect on the immunogenicity of MVA85A. Overall, the prevaccination and postvaccination T-cell responses were lower in HIV-infected compared with HIV-uninfected vaccines.

N. M. Khardori, MD, PhD

References

1. Abu-Raddad LJ, Sabatelli L, Achterberg JT, et al. Epidemiological benefits of more-effective tuberculosis vaccines, drugs, and diagnostics. *Proc Natl Acad Sci U S A*. 2009;106:13980-13985.
2. Stop TB Partnership. *Working Group on New TB Vaccines*. Geneva, Switzerland: Stop TB Partnership; 2009. http://www.stoptb.org/wg/new_vaccines/2009. Accessed October 1, 2012.

Early Impact of the US Tdap Vaccination Program on Pertussis Trends

Skoff TH, Cohn AC, Clark TA, et al (US Ctrs for Disease Control and Prevention, Atlanta, GA)
Arch Pediatr Adolesc Med 166:344-349, 2012

Objective.—To evaluate the impact of the adolescent Tdap (tetanus toxoid, reduced diphtheria toxoid, and acellular pertussis vaccine) vaccination program on pertussis trends in the United States.

Design.—Retrospective analysis of nationally reported pertussis cases, January 1, 1990, through December 31, 2009.

Setting.—United States.

Participants.—Confirmed and probable pertussis cases.

Intervention.—The US Tdap vaccination program.

Main Outcome Measure.—Rate ratios of reported pertussis incidence (defined as incidence among 11- to 18-year-olds divided by the combined incidence in all other age groups) modeled through segmented regression analysis and age-specific trends in reported pertussis incidence over time.

Results.—A total of 200 401 pertussis cases were reported in the United States from 1990 to 2009. Overall incidence ranged from 1.0 to 8.8 per 100 000 persons (1991 and 2004, respectively). Slope coefficients (estimated annual rate of change in rate ratios) from segmented regression showed a steady increase in pertussis incidence among adolescents 11 to 18 years old compared with all other age groups before Tdap introduction (slope = 0.22; $P < .001$), and a steep decreasing trend post introduction (slope = -0.48; $P < .001$), suggesting a direct impact of vaccination among adolescents. Indirect effects of adolescent vaccination were not observed among infants younger than 1 year.

Conclusions.—Changes in pertussis incidence in the United States from 2005 to 2009 revealed a divergence between 11- to 18-year-olds and other age groups, suggesting that targeted use of Tdap among adolescents reduced disease preferentially in this age group. Increased Tdap coverage in adolescents and adults is needed to realize the full direct and indirect benefits of vaccination.

► Effective childhood vaccines against pertussis have been used in the United States since the late 1940s. Dtap (tetanus, diphtheria, pertussis) vaccine coverage is high, at 83.9% in 2009, although pertussis has remained endemic in the United States. An increase in cases occurs every 3 to 5 years, with the highest incidence among infants younger than 1 year old. Increased rates have also been reported since 1980 among adolescents and adults. Pertussis is difficult to diagnose in older age groups because of a lack of classic symptoms, and they serve as an important reservoir of infection for the infant prior to being fully vaccinated.

A reduced-dose acellular pertussis vaccine in Tdap was licensed in 2005 as a booster for adolescents and adults in the United States. The Advisory Committee on Immunization Practices recommended routine use of a single-dose Tdap in adolescents 11 to 18 years old. Among adults 19 to 64 years old, a single dose of Tdap was recommended to replace a single dose of Td (tetanus, diphtheria). The coverage offered by this recommendation among adolescents 13 to 17 years of age increased from 10.8% to 55.6%. However, coverage among adults has remained low at 6.6%.[1]

This retrospective analysis of nationally reported pertussis cases (January 1, 1990, through December 31, 2000) revealed a divergence between those aged 11 to 18 years old and other age groups. A steep decreasing trend in the incidence of pertussis in this age group was noted after the introduction of Tdap, suggesting a direct impact of booster vaccination among adolescents. This, however, did not have an indirect effect on infants younger than 1 year old. It will take increased Tdap coverage in both adolescents and adults to realize the full direct and indirect beneficial impacts of Tdap vaccine.

N. M. Khardori, MD, PhD

Reference

1. Centers for Disease Control and Prevention. National Health Interview Survey, 2008–2009: Self-Reported Tetanus, Diphtheria, and Acellular Pertussis (Tdap) Vaccination Coverage Among Adults 19–64 Years in the United States. (Table 2). http://www.cdc.gov/vaccines/stats-surv/nhis/2009-nhis.htm#8. Accessed August 25, 2011.

Efficacy, Safety, and Tolerability of Herpes Zoster Vaccine in Persons Aged 50–59 Years
Schmader KE, Levin MJ, Gnann JW Jr, et al (Duke Univ, NC; Univ of Colorado School of Medicine, Aurora; Univ of Alabama at Birmingham; et al)
Clin Infect Dis 54:922-928, 2012

Background.—Herpes zoster (HZ) adversely affects individuals aged 50–59, but vaccine efficacy has not been assessed in this population. This study was designed to determine the efficacy, safety, and tolerability of zoster vaccine for preventing HZ in persons aged 50–59 years.

Methods.—This was a randomized, double-blind, placebo-controlled study of 22 439 subjects aged 50–59 years conducted in North America and Europe. Subjects were given 1 dose of licensed zoster vaccine (ZV) (Zostavax; Merck) and followed for occurrence of HZ for ≥1 year (mean, 1.3 years) postvaccination until accrual of ≥96 confirmed HZ cases (as determined by testing lesions swabs for varicella zoster virus DNA by polymerase chain reaction). Subjects were followed for all adverse events (AEs) from day 1 to day 42 postvaccination and for serious AEs (SAEs) through day 182 postvaccination.

Results.—The ZV reduced the incidence of HZ (30 cases in vaccine group, 1.99/1000 person-years vs 99 cases in placebo group, 6.57/1000 person-years). Vaccine efficacy for preventing HZ was 69.8% (95% confidence interval, 54.1–80.6). AEs were reported by 72.8% of subjects in the ZV group and 41.5% in the placebo group, with the difference primarily due to higher rates of injection-site AEs and headache. The proportion of subjects reporting SAEs occurring within 42 days postvaccination (ZV,

0.6%; placebo, 0.5%) and 182 days postvaccination (ZV, 2.1%; placebo, 1.9%) was similar between groups.

Conclusions.—In subjects aged 50—59 years, the ZV significantly reduced the incidence of HZ and was well tolerated.

Clinical Trials Registration.—NCT00534248.

▶ Live, attenuated zoster vaccine was shown to reduce the burden of illness due to herpes zoster virus by 61%, the incidence of postherpetic neuralgia by 66%, and the incidence of herpes zoster by 51% in persons aged 60 years or older.[1] The efficacy decreased with increasing age (64%) in those aged 60 to 69 years compared to 41% in those aged 70 to 79 years and 18% in those aged 80 or older. Pain and postherpetic neuralgia related to herpes zoster increase with increasing age. The incidence of herpes zoster among individuals aged 50 to 59 years in the United States is 4.2 to 5.3 per 1000 person-years. A population-based study showed that about 20% of cases of herpes zoster occur in those aged 50 to 59 years.[2]

This randomized, double-blind, placebo-controlled study demonstrates a 70% vaccine efficacy in this age group. The higher efficacy of the vaccine in this age group than previously reported for those aged 60 to 69 and those aged 70 or older is likely a result of a more robust booster effect on the V2V-specific cell-mediated immune response in the younger age groups. The total burden of acute pain in all patients receiving zoster vaccine was significantly lower than in the placebo group. However, among patients who developed herpes zoster, there was no difference in acute pain between the vaccinated and placebo groups, indicating that the effect on pain is due to prevention of herpes zoster rather than decreasing the severity of illness. Since individuals aged 50 to 59 are regularly employed, prevention of herpes zoster by vaccination would decrease lost productivity at work. The vaccine effect was stable over the average of 1.3 years of follow-up. The duration of efficacy would be expected to be at least as long as that observed in the older age groups. The vaccine was well tolerated in this age group. The incidence of severe adverse events within 42 days of vaccination was lower than that reported in older age groups.

N. M. Khardori, MD, PhD

References

1. Oxman MN, Levin MJ, Johnson GR, et al. A vaccine to prevent herpes zoster and postherpetic neuralgia in older adults. *N Engl J Med.* 2005;352:2271-2284.
2. Yawn BP, Saddier P, Wollan PC, St Sauver JL, Kurland MJ, Sy LS. A population-based study of the incidence and complication rates of herpes zoster before zoster vaccine introduction. *Mayo Clin Proc.* 2007;82:1341-1349.

Risk of Intussusception Following Administration of a Pentavalent Rotavirus Vaccine in US Infants

Shui IM, Baggs J, Patel M, et al (Harvard Med School and Harvard Pilgrim Health Care Inst, Boston, MA; Ctrs for Disease Control and Prevention, Atlanta, GA; et al)
JAMA 307:598-604, 2012

Context.—Current rotavirus vaccines were not associated with intussusception in large prelicensure trials. However, recent postlicensure data from international settings suggest the possibility of a low-level elevated risk, primarily in the first week after the first vaccine dose.

Objective.—To examine the risk of intussusception following pentavalent rotavirus vaccine (RV5) in US infants.

Design, Setting, and Patients.—This cohort study included infants 4 to 34 weeks of age, enrolled in the Vaccine Safety Datalink (VSD) who received RV5 from May 2006-February 2010. We calculated standardized incidence ratios (SIRs), relative risks (RRs), and 95% confidence intervals for the association between intussusception and RV5 by comparing the rates of intussusception in infants who had received RV5 with the rates of intussusception in infants who received other recommended vaccines without concomitant RV5 during the concurrent period and with the expected number of intussusception visits based on background rates assessed prior to US licensure of the RV5 (2001-2005).

Main Outcome Measure.—Intussusception occurring in the 1- to 7-day and 1- to 30-day risk windows following RV5 vaccination.

Results.—During the study period, 786 725 total RV5 doses, which included 309 844 first doses, were administered. We did not observe a statistically significant increased risk of intussusception with RV5 for either comparison group following any dose in either the 1- to 7-day or 1- to 30-day risk window. For the 1- to 30-day window following all RV5 doses, we observed 21 cases of intussusception compared with 20.9 expected cases (SIR, 1.01; 95% CI, 0.62-1.54); following dose 1, we observed 7 cases compared with 5.7 expected cases (SIR, 1.23; 95% CI, 0.5-2.54). For the 1- to 7-day window following all RV5 doses, we observed 4 cases compared with 4.3 expected cases (SIR, 0.92; 95% CI, 0.25-2.36); for dose 1, we observed 1 case compared with 0.8 expected case (SIR, 1.21; 95% CI, 0.03-6.75). The upper 95% CI limit of the SIR (6.75) from the historical comparison translates to an upper limit for the attributable risk of 1 intussusception case per 65 287 RV5 dose-1 recipients.

Conclusion.—Among US infants aged 4 to 34 weeks who received RV5, the risk of intussusception was not increased compared with infants who did not receive the rotavirus vaccine.

▶ Since the withdrawal of Rhesus tetravalent rotavirus vaccine in 1999, 2 vaccines have been licensed for use in the United States. The pentavalent rotavirus vaccine (RV5), given at ages 2, 4, and 6 months, was licensed in 2006. The monovalent rotavirus vaccine (RV1), given at ages 2 and 4 months, was licensed in 2008.

This is the largest prospective study to assess the association of RV5 vaccination and intussusception. Compared with the cohort who did not receive RV5, no increased risk of intussusception was found after RV5 vaccination in either the 1-day to 30-day risk window or the 1-day to 7-day risk window. Based on analysis of 800 000 doses (300 000 first doses) of RV5 vaccine administered, an excess risk of 1 intussusception event per 65 287 RV5 vaccinees following dose 1 can be reliably excluded. At the same time, the reintroduction of rotavirus vaccine in 2006 caused an estimated reduction of 55 000 rotavirus hospitalizations in 2008. The rotavirus vaccine coverage in the United States is increasing steadily, averaging 72% in June 2009 among 5-month-olds from 8 different sentinel sites across the country. Earlier analysis from the same cohort did not find an association of intussusception and RV5 in the 30 days following vaccination.[1]

The benefits of rotavirus vaccination in the United States outweigh any potential low-level risk for intussusception that might not have been detected yet.

N. M. Khardori, MD, PhD

Reference

1. Belongia EA, Irving SA, Shui IM, et al; Vaccine Safety Datalink Investigation Group. Real-time surveillance to assess risk of intussusception and other adverse events after pentavalent, bovine-derived rotavirus vaccine. *Pediatr Infect Dis J*. 2010;29:1-5.

13 Viral Infections

A Multistate Outbreak of Hepatitis A Associated With Semidried Tomatoes in Australia, 2009
Donnan EJ, Fielding JE, Gregory JE, et al (The Australian Natl Univ, Melbourne, Australia; et al)
Clin Infect Dis 54:775-781, 2012

Background.—A large outbreak of hepatitis A affected individuals in several Australian states in 2009, resulting in a 2-fold increase in cases reported to state health departments compared with 2008. Two peaks of infection occurred (April—May and September—November), with surveillance data suggesting locally acquired infections from a widely distributed food product.

Methods.—Two case-control studies were completed. Intensive product trace-back and food sampling was undertaken. Genotyping was conducted on virus isolates from patient serum and food samples. Control measures included prophylaxis for close contacts, public health warnings, an order by the chief health officer under the Victorian Food Act 1984, and trade-level recalls on implicated batches of semidried tomatoes.

Results.—A multijurisdictional case-control study in April—May found an association between illness and consumption of semidried tomatoes (odds ratio [OR], 3.0; 95% CI 1.4—6.7). A second case-control study conducted in Victoria in October—November also implicated semidried tomatoes as being associated with illness (OR, 10.3; 95% CI, 4.7—22.7). Hepatitis A RNA was detected in 22 samples of semidried tomatoes. Hepatitis A virus genotype IB was identified in 144 of 153 (94%) patients tested from 2009, and partial sequence analysis showed complete identity with an isolate found in a sample of semidried tomatoes.

Conclusions.—The results of both case-control studies and food testing implicated the novel vehicle of semidried tomatoes as the cause of this hepatitis A outbreak. The outbreak was extensive and sustained despite public health interventions, the design and implementation of which were complicated by limitations in food testing capability and complex supply chains.

▶ Common source outbreaks of hepatitis A virus (HAV) infection in industrialized countries are usually related to food contaminated by infected handlers or contamination of food at the primary production stage.[1] During 2009, 562 cases of HAV were reported across several states in Australia, representing a 2-fold increase in the number of cases reported in 2004 to 2008 annually.

This article reports the results of 2 case-control studies, intensive product trace back, and food sampling. Both studies associated semidried tomatoes with the illness. HAV-1B genotype was found by polymerase chain reaction in serum samples of 144 of 153 cases (94%) tested across the states; all were identical. A multijurisdictional case-control questionnaire was used for both studies. The foods used in the questionnaire were identified through an earlier hypothesis-generating questionnaire and through an earlier cluster investigation. Semidried and sundried tomatoes were found to be significantly associated with the illness in both case-control studies. HAV RNA was detected in 21 of 67 samples of semidried tomatoes. One positive semidried tomato sample had enough RNA to allow sequencing that was found to be identical to that obtained from 7 of the infected serum samples. Notification of the World Health Organization International Food Safety Authorities Network and the European Center for Disease Control was followed by identification of HAV clusters in the Netherlands and France. Case-control studies revealed semidried tomatoes as the source of infection in both of these outbreaks.

The HAV samples from the Netherlands and Australian outbreaks were identical. The HAV sample in France was of a similar but nonidentical strain. Semidried tomatoes have previously been reported as a potential vehicle for *Salmonella* spp. The public health lessons learned from these investigations are difficulty of product traceability, limitation in food testing capability, complexity of food chains, and most importantly, the risks associated with uncooked ready-to-eat food products.

N. M. Khardori, MD, PhD

Reference

1. Heyman DL, ed. *Control of Communicable Disease Manual*. 19th ed. Washington DC: American Public Health Association; 2008.

A Point-Source Norovirus Outbreak Caused by Exposure to Fomites
Repp KK, Keene WE (Oregon Health and Science Univ, Portland; Oregon Public Health Division, Portland)
J Infect Dis 205:1639-1641, 2012

We investigated a norovirus outbreak (genotype GII.2) affecting 9 members of a soccer team. Illness was associated with touching a reusable grocery bag or consuming its packaged food contents (risk difference, 0.636; $P < .01$). By polymerase chain reaction, GII norovirus was recovered from the bag, which had been stored in a bathroom used before the outbreak by a person with norovirus-like illness. Airborne contamination of fomites can lead to subsequent point-source outbreaks. When feasible, we recommend dedicated bathrooms for sick persons and informing cleaning staff (professional or otherwise) about the need for adequate environmental sanitation of surfaces and fomites to prevent spread.

▶ Noroviruses are the most common cause of foodborne outbreaks in the United States and a leading cause of gastroenteritis worldwide.[1,2] Efficient transmission occurs through fecal-oral route, airborne spread, and environmental contamination by fomites. Outbreaks linked to fomites have been reported on cruise ships, hotels, and in institutional settings.

This study reports on a point-source norovirus outbreak caused by exposure to fomites using real-time reverse transcriptase polymerase chain reaction. The index case spent the night in a chaperone's hotel room and was away from the group 2 days prior to symptoms being reported by other subjects. However, cookies, packaged chips, and fresh grapes had been stored in a reusable, open-top grocery bag in the hotel bathroom of the chaperone who had shared the room with the index case.

The food items in this bag were passed around at a group lunch hours after the index case had departed and reported having used the bathroom with the stored bag but never touching or handling the bag.

Genogroup GII norovirus was detected in 2 of 10 swabs from the grocery bag 2 weeks after the group lunch and from 3 stool specimens from ill people. No food items were available for virus detection. The results indicate that norovirus settled on the grocery bag and its contents by fomite aerosolization in the chaperone's hotel bathroom. Both handling the grocery bag and consumption of food contained in it were strongly associated with illness. The authors recommend dedicated bathrooms for sick people and the need for adequate environmental sanitation of surfaces and fomites to prevent spread.

N. M. Khardori, MD, PhD

References

1. Patel MM, Hall AJ, Vinjé J, Parashar UD. Noroviruses: a comprehensive review. *J Clin Virol.* 2009;44:1-8.
2. Gould LH, Nisler AL, Herman KM, et al. Surveillance for foodborne disease outbreaks—United States, 2008. *MMWR Morb Mortal Wkly Rep.* 2011;60:1197-1202.

HIV-1 Dual Infection Is Associated With Faster CD4+ T-Cell Decline in a Cohort of Men With Primary HIV Infection
Cornelissen M, Pasternak AO, Grijsen ML, et al (Univ of Amsterdam, Netherlands)
Clin Infect Dis 54:539-547, 2012

Background.—In vitro, animal, and mathematical models suggest that human immunodeficiency virus (HIV) co- or superinfection would result in increased fitness of the pathogen and, possibly, increased virulence. However, in patients, the impact of dual HIV type 1 (HIV-1) infection on disease progression is unclear, because parameters relevant for disease progression have not been strictly analyzed. The objective of the present study is to analyze the effect of dual HIV-1 infections on disease progression in a well-defined cohort of men who have sex with men.

Methods.—Between 2000 and 2009, 37 men who had primary infection with HIV-1 subtype B, no indication for immediate need of combination antiretroviral therapy (cART), and sufficient follow-up were characterized with regard to dual infection or single infection and to coreceptor use.

Patients were followed to estimate the effect of these parameters on clinical disease progression, as defined by the rate of CD4$^+$ T-cell decline and the time to initiation of cART.

Results.—Four patients presented with HIV-1 coinfection; 6 patients acquired HIV-1 superinfection, on average 8.5 months from their primary infection; and 27 patients remained infected with a single strain. Slopes of longitudinal CD4$^+$ T-cell counts and time-weighted changes from baseline were significantly steeper for patients with dual infection compared with patients with single infection. Multivariate analysis showed that the most important parameter associated with CD4$^+$ T-cell decline over time was dual infection ($P = .001$). Additionally, patients with HIV-1 coinfection had a significantly earlier start of cART ($P < .0001$).

Conclusions.—Dual HIV-1 infection is the main factor associated with CD4$^+$ T-cell decline in men who have untreated primary infection with HIV-1 subtype B.

▶ Dual human immunodeficiency virus (HIV) infections can be a coinfection with both virus strains infecting before HIV seroconversion or superinfection with a second virus strain infecting after seroconversion from infection with the first strain. Dual infection of cats with feline immunodeficiency virus led to rapid outgrowth of viruses, with increased replication capability and virulence. Superinfection in humans was first reported in 2002 and cases of serial superinfections were reported in 2005.[1]

In vitro, superinfection with different HIV-1 strains causes an increase in virus production and T-cell line mortality. In human infection, the second strain of HIV-1 can have greater replicative fitness, leading to greater virulence, and superinfection could potentiate immune escape with compromise of the patient's immune system. Both replicative fitness and immune escape as well as drug resistance could be acquired by the virus through recombination between 2 strains of virus following dual infection. Evolutionary expansion following recombination can affect the individual patient as well as the epidemic at large.

This prospective study provides an assessment of disease progression involving 37 well-characterized patients with primary HIV-1 subtype B infection (PHI). The patients were selected from a multicenter cohort in the Netherlands between 2000 and 2009, did not need immediate antiretroviral therapy, and were followed for at least 2 years. HIV-1 coinfection (4 patients) was defined as having 2 different *env* sequence clusters in the first sample obtained during PHI. HIV-1 superinfection (6 patients) was defined as infection with a second strain demonstrated at a point after initial PHI. Superinfection was demonstrated on an average of 8.5 months from their primary infection. These results demonstrate that recent dual HIV-1 infection is an independent factor associated with disease progression shown by a faster decline in CD4-positive T-cell counts. Patients with HIV-1 coinfection needed combination antiretroviral therapy earlier.

The best practice for clinical management of acute HIV infection remains unknown because of lack of randomized data.[2] However, an additional advantage of temporary antiretroviral therapy could be prevention of early HIV-1 superinfection.

The findings from this study suggest that the practice of unsafe sex with partners with HIV-1 positive serostatus should be discouraged.

N. M. Khardori, MD, PhD

References

1. van der Kuyl AC, Kozaczynska K, van den Burg R, et al. Triple HIV-1 infection. *N Engl J Med.* 2005;352:2557-2559.
2. Bell SK, Little SJ, Rosenberg ES. Clinical management of acute HIV infection: best practice remains unknown. *J Infect Dis.* 2010;202:S278-S288.

Prevalence of Oral HPV Infection in the United States, 2009-2010

Gillison ML, Broutian T, Pickard RKL, et al (Ohio State Univ, Columbus; et al)
JAMA 307:693-703, 2012

Context.—Human papillomavirus (HPV) infection is the principal cause of a distinct form of oropharyngeal squamous cell carcinoma that is increasing in incidence among men in the United States. However, little is known about the epidemiology of oral HPV infection.

Objective.—To determine the prevalence of oral HPV infection in the United States.

Design, Setting, and Participants.—A cross-sectional study was conducted as part of the National Health and Nutrition Examination Survey (NHANES) 2009-2010, a statistically representative sample of the civilian noninstitutionalized US population. Men and women aged 14 to 69 years examined at mobile examination centers were eligible. Participants (N = 5579) provided a 30-second oral rinse and gargle with mouthwash. For detection of HPV types, DNA purified from oral exfoliated cells was evaluated by polymerase chain reaction and type-specific hybridization. Demographic and behavioral data were obtained by standardized interview. Statistical analyses used NHANES sample weights to provide weighted prevalence estimates for the US population.

Main Outcome Measures.— Prevalence of oral HPV infection.

Results.—The prevalence of oral HPV infection among men and women aged 14 to 69 years was 6.9% (95% CI, 5.7%-8.3%) and of HPV type 16 was 1.0% (95% CI, 0.7%-1.3%). Oral HPV infection followed a bimodal pattern with respect to age, with peak prevalence among individuals aged 30 to 34 years (7.3%; 95% CI, 4.6%-11.4%) and 60 to 64 years (11.4%; 95% CI, 8.5%-15.1%). Men had a significantly higher prevalence than women for any oral HPV infection (10.1% [95% CI, 8.3%-12.3%] vs 3.6% [95% CI, 2.6%-5.0%], $P < .001$; unadjusted prevalence ratio [PR], 2.80 [95% CI, 2.02-3.88]). Infection was less common among those without vs those with a history of any type of sexual contact (0.9% [95% CI, 0.4%-1.8%] vs 7.5% [95% CI, 6.1%-9.1%], $P < .001$; PR, 8.69 [95% CI, 3.91-19.31]) and increased with number of sexual partners ($P < .001$ for trend) and cigarettes smoked per day ($P < .001$ for trend). Associations with age, sex, number of sexual partners, and current number of cigarettes smoked per day were independently associated with oral HPV infection in multivariable models.

Conclusion.—Among men and women aged 14 to 69 years in the United States, the overall prevalence of oral HPV infection was 6.9%, and the prevalence was higher among men than among women.

▶ Human papilloma virus (HPV) infection causes a subset of oropharyngeal squamous cell carcinomas (OSCCs). Oral HPV infection confers about a 50-fold increase in risk for OSCC, and 90% of HPV-positive OSCCs are associated with the oncogenic HPV-16 type.[1]

HPV-negative OSCCs are associated with chronic tobacco and alcohol use. HPV has been directly implicated as the underlying cause for the significant increase in OSCC over the past 3 decades. In the United States, the incidence of HPV-negative OSCC declined by 50% from 1999 to 2004 (2 to 1 case per 100 000 population). During that same time, the incidence of HPV-positive OSCC increased by 225% (0.8 to 2.6 per 100 000). The increase has been predominantly among young individuals, which is consistent with sexual behavior changes since the 1950s. Male predominance in the increase in HPV-positive OSCC is more difficult to explain.

This article reports on the first population-based study of oral HPV prevalence conducted within the US National Health and Nutrition Examination Survey. The overall prevalence of oral HPV infection was 6.9%, comprising high-risk HPV infection (3.7%) and low-risk HPV infection (3.1%). HPV-16 was the most prevalent type detected. A significantly higher prevalence (10.1%) was seen in men compared with women (3.6%).

The prevalence among black participants (10.5%) was higher but not statistically different from among white participants (6.5%). Age-related prevalence showed a bimodal pattern (ie, first peak [7.3%] at 30 to 34 years and second higher peak [11.4%] at 60 to 64 years). Sexual behavior and current smoking were identified to be potentially modifiable risk factors for oral HPV infection. The epidemiology of oral HPV infection is consistent with differences in incidence of HPV-positive OSCC across subgroups. Quadrivalent HPV vaccine, which includes the HPV-16 type, is currently recommended for females 9 to 21 years and males 9 to 21 years for prevention of genital warts and anogenital cancers. The vaccine efficacy against oral HPV infection is not known at this point. Given the fact that the number of HPV-positive oropharyngeal cancers are projected to surpass that of invasive cervical cancers by 2020, such trials are warranted.

N. M. Khardori, MD, PhD

Reference

1. Gillison ML, D'Souza G, Westra W, et al. Distinct risk factor profiles for human papillomavirus type 16-positive and human papillomavirus type 16-negative head and neck cancers. *J Natl Cancer Inst.* 2008;100:407-420.

HEMATOLOGY AND ONCOLOGY

JAMES TATE THIGPEN, MD

14 Breast Cancer

Axillary Dissection vs No Axillary Dissection in Women With Invasive Breast Cancer and Sentinel Node Metastasis: A Randomized Clinical Trial
Giuliano AE, Hunt KK, Ballman KV, et al (John Wayne Cancer Inst at Saint John's Health Ctr, Santa Monica, CA; M D Anderson Cancer Ctr, Houston, TX; Mayo Clinic Rochester, MN; et al)
JAMA 305:569-575, 2011

Context.—Sentinel lymph node dissection (SLND) accurately identifies nodal metastasis of early breast cancer, but it is not clear whether further nodal dissection affects survival.

Objective.—To determine the effects of complete axillary lymph node dissection (ALND) on survival of patients with sentinel lymph node (SLN) metastasis of breast cancer.

Design, Setting, and Patients.—The American College of Surgeons Oncology Group Z0011 trial, a phase 3 noninferiority trial conducted at 115 sites and enrolling patients from May 1999 to December 2004. Patients were women with clinical T1-T2 invasive breast cancer, no palpable adenopathy, and 1 to 2 SLNs containing metastases identified by frozen section, touch preparation, or hematoxylin-eosin staining on permanent section. Targeted enrollment was 1900 women with final analysis after 500 deaths, but the trial closed early because mortality rate was lower than expected.

Interventions.—All patients underwent lumpectomy and tangential whole-breast irradiation. Those with SLN metastases identified by SLND were randomized to undergo ALND or no further axillary treatment. Those randomized to ALND underwent dissection of 10 or more nodes. Systemic therapy was at the discretion of the treating physician.

Main Outcome Measures.—Overall survival was the primary end point, with a noninferiority margin of a 1-sided hazard ratio of less than 1.3 indicating that SLND alone is noninferior to ALND. Disease-free survival was a secondary end point.

Results.—Clinical and tumor characteristics were similar between 445 patients randomized to ALND and 446 randomized to SLND alone. However, the median number of nodes removed was 17 with ALND and 2 with SLND alone. At a median follow-up of 6.3 years (last follow-up, March 4, 2010), 5-year overall survival was 91.8% (95% confidence interval [CI], 89.1%-94.5%)with ALND and 92.5% (95% CI, 90.0%-95.1%) with SLND alone; 5-year disease-free survival was 82.2% (95% CI, 78.3%-86.3%) with ALND and 83.9% (95% CI, 80.2%-87.9%) with SLND alone. The hazard ratio for treatment-related overall survival was 0.79 (90% CI, 0.56-1.11) without adjustment and 0.87 (90% CI, 0.62-1.23) after adjusting for age and adjuvant therapy.

Conclusion.—Among patients with limited SLN metastatic breast cancer treated with breast conservation and systemic therapy, the use of SLND alone compared with ALND did not result in inferior survival.

Trial Registration.—clinicaltrials.gov Identifier: NCT00003855.

▶ The development of sentinel lymph node dissection and its use in identifying women with breast cancer who do not need an axillary lymph node dissection has saved thousands of women the significant toxicities of axillary lymph node dissection. It is well documented that axillary lymph node dissection results in a significant risk of complications from seroma and infection to lymphedema. Thus, the use of axillary lymph node dissection needs to be justified given the potential debilitating toxicities.

Although patients with negative sentinel lymph node dissection clearly do not need axillary lymph node dissection, it has been the standard of care to perform axillary lymph node dissection on patients with positive sentinel lymph nodes. These authors have performed a phase III randomized trial to question whether these positive sentinel lymph node patients in fact need the axillary lymph node dissection. Their results have shown no benefit to the axillary lymph node dissection over sentinel lymph node dissection alone at 5 years. Yet it is important to realize that these results only apply to patients who receive lumpectomy and postoperative irradiation to the whole breast (supine position), which usually will result in radiation to the low axilla. Patients who had mastectomy, prone radiation after lumpectomy, or partial breast irradiation were not part of this trial. Applying these results to the appropriate breast cancer population is critical in its correct usage.

C. Lawton, MD

Adjuvant Therapy in Stage I Carcinoma of the Breast: The Influence of Multigene Analyses and Molecular Phenotyping
Schwartz GF, Bartelink H, Burstein HJ, et al (Jefferson Med College, Philadelphia, PA; The Netherlands Cancer Inst, Amsterdam; Harvard Med School, Boston, MA; et al)
Breast J 18:303-311, 2012

A consensus conference was held in order to provide guidelines for the use of adjuvant therapy in patients with Stage I carcinoma of the breast, using traditional information, such as tumor size, microscopic character, Nottingham index, patient age and co-morbidities, but also incorporating steroid hormone and Her-2-neu data as well as other immunohistochemical markers. The role of the genetic analysis of breast cancer and proprietary gene prognostic signatures was discussed, along with the molecular profiling of breast cancers into several groups that may predict prognosis. These molecular data are not currently sufficiently mature to make them part of decision making algorithms of recommendations for the treatment of individual patients.

▶ This article summarizes the deliberations of a consensus conference on the use of molecular profiling as a basis for determining adjuvant treatment. The panel focused primarily on stage I cancers but also discussed briefly some node-positive patients. There are several noteworthy recommendations. First, the panel concluded that current molecular profiling (OncotypeDx and Mammaprint) should not be used as a substitute for clinical judgment in determining adjuvant therapy for stage I breast cancers. Second, they felt that assigning breast cancer type (basal, luminal A, luminal B) on the basis of molecular profiling was not sufficiently consistent among the various tests to routinely serve as a basis for clinical decision making. Third, they recommended that molecular profiling, if ordered, should be ordered from 1 source per patient because the various tests can give discordant answers and lead to confusion. Fourth, they felt that molecular profiling, at its current state, should be adjunct to other factors in clinical decision making. Finally, they recommended that molecular profiling not be used in node-positive patients because this is already a major adverse prognostic factor. The panel also encouraged further clinical studies to validate the clinical utility of these tests. The article is worth reading in detail if one plans to use these tests in the clinical management of patients.

J. T. Thigpen, MD

Comparisons between different polychemotherapy regimens for early breast cancer: meta-analyses of long-term outcome among 100 000 women in 123 randomised trials
Early Breast Cancer Trialists' Collaborative Group (EBCTCG) (Clinical Trial Service Unit (CTSU), Oxford, UK)
Lancet 379:432-444, 2012

Background.—Moderate differences in efficacy between adjuvant chemotherapy regimens for breast cancer are plausible, and could affect treatment choices. We sought any such differences.

Methods.—We undertook individual-patient-data meta-analyses of the randomised trials comparing: any taxane-plus-anthracycline-based regimen versus the same, or more, non-taxane chemotherapy (n = 44 000); one anthracycline-based regimen versus another (n = 7000) or versus cyclophosphamide, methotrexate, and fluorouracil (CMF; n=18 000); and polychemotherapy versus no chemotherapy (n = 32 000). The scheduled dosages of these three drugs and of the anthracyclines doxorubicin (A) and epirubicin (E) were used to define standard CMF, standard 4AC, and CAF and CEF. Log-rank breast cancer mortality rate ratios (RRs) are reported.

Findings.—In trials adding four separate cycles of a taxane to a fixed anthracycline-based control regimen, extending treatment duration, breast cancer mortality was reduced (RR $0\cdot86$, SE $0\cdot04$, two-sided significance [2p] = $0\cdot0005$). In trials with four such extra cycles of a taxane counterbalanced in controls by extra cycles of other cytotoxic drugs, roughly doubling non-taxane dosage, there was no significant difference (RR 0·94, SE 0·06, 2p = 0·33). Trials with CMF-treated controls showed that standard 4AC and standard CMF were equivalent (RR 0·98, SE 0·05, 2p = 0·67), but that anthracycline-based regimens with substantially higher cumulative dosage than standard 4AC (eg, CAF or CEF) were superior to standard CMF (RR 0·78, SE 0·06, 2p = 0·0004). Trials versus no chemotherapy also suggested greater mortality reductions with CAF (RR 0·64, SE 0·09, 2p < 0·0001) than with standard 4AC (RR 0·78, SE 0·09, 2p = 0·01) or standard CMF (RR 0·76, SE 0·05, 2p < 0·0001). In all meta-analyses involving taxane-based or anthracycline-based regimens, proportional risk reductions were little affected by age, nodal status, tumour diameter or differentiation (moderate or poor; few were well differentiated), oestrogen receptor status, or tamoxifen use. Hence, largely independently of age (up to at least 70 years) or the tumour characteristics currently available to us for the patients selected to be in these trials, some taxane-plus-anthracycline-based or higher-cumulative-dosage anthracycline-based regimens (not requiring stem cells) reduced breast cancer mortality by, on average, about one-third. 10-year overall mortality differences paralleled breast cancer mortality differences, despite taxane, anthracycline, and other toxicities.

Interpretation.—10-year gains from a one-third breast cancer mortality reduction depend on absolute risks without chemotherapy (which, for oestrogen-receptor-positive disease, are the risks remaining with appropriate endocrine therapy). Low absolute risk implies low absolute benefit, but information was lacking about tumour gene expression markers or quantitative immunohistochemistry that might help to predict risk, chemosensitivity, or both.

▶ It should always be remembered that meta-analyses do not represent the highest form of evidence, although we are often impressed by the massive numbers. This meta-analysis does provide some interesting information concerning adjuvant therapy for early stage breast cancer. It confirms an observation in an earlier meta-analysis that cyclophosphamide, methotrexate, and fluorouracil (CMF) and anthracycline (AC) yield essentially the same efficacy and that CAF appears to have a slight advantage over either CMF or AC. A regimen containing a taxane and an AC appears to offer some advantage. Unfortunately, data regarding gene expression markers were insufficient to allow these markers to be factored into the equation. Two thoughts represent a reasonable bottom line: First, current approaches to adjuvant therapy for breast cancer clearly reduce mortality. What we lack is solid information about the very best approach to use in each individual situation. Second, we need improved information about the assessment of risk so we can properly evaluate whether benefit outweighs risk in a given situation. These needs should be met as our knowledge of the biology of the disease continues to grow.

J. T. Thigpen, MD

Effect of Obesity on Prognosis After Early-Stage Breast Cancer

Ewertz M, Jensen M-B, Gunnarsdóttir KÁ, et al (Univ of Southern Denmark, Odense, Denmark; Aarhus Univ Hosp, Denmark; Vejle Hosp, Denmark; et al)
J Clin Oncol 29:25-31, 2011

Purpose.—This study was performed to characterize the impact of obesity on the risk of breast cancer recurrence and death as a result of breast cancer or other causes in relation to adjuvant treatment.

Patients and Methods.—Information on body mass index (BMI) at diagnosis was available for 18,967 (35%) of 53,816 women treated for early-stage breast cancer in Denmark between 1977 and 2006 with complete follow-up for first events (locoregional recurrences and distant metastases) up to 10 years and for death up to 30 years. Information was available on prognostic factors and adjuvant treatment for all patients. Univariate analyses were used to compare the associations of known prognostic factors and risks of recurrence or death according to BMI categories. Cox proportional hazards regression models were used to assess the influence of BMI after adjusting for other factors.

Results.—Patients with a BMI of 30 kg/m^2 or more were older and had more advanced disease at diagnosis compared with patients with a BMI below 25 kg/m^2 ($P < .001$). When data were adjusted for disease characteristics, the risk of developing distant metastases after 10 years was significantly increased by 46%, and the risk of dying as a result of breast cancer after 30 years was significantly increased by 38% for patients with a BMI of 30 kg/m^2 or more. BMI had no influence on the risk of locoregional recurrences. Both chemotherapy and endocrine therapy seemed to be less effective after 10 or more years for patients with BMIs greater than 30 kg/m^2.

Conclusion.—Obesity is an independent prognostic factor for developing distant metastases and for death as a result of breast cancer; the effects of adjuvant therapy seem to be lost more rapidly in patients with breast cancer and obesity.

▶ Obesity for men and women is a huge health concern in the United States. Increased risk of heart disease, diabetes, and cancer all relate to our obesity epidemic. The extra fat that exists in obese patients is known to increase estrogen levels and is thought to play a role in the incidence of both breast and prostate cancer in our country.

What has not been well studied is the role of obesity and overall outcome of patients with breast cancer. It has been shown that obesity can negatively affect outcomes in breast cancer patients, but exactly why has not been well elucidated.

These data confirm the finding of an association between obesity and an increased risk of breast cancer deaths in patients with early stage breast cancer. The interesting fact that the breast cancer deaths are related to an increase in distant metastasis and not related to an increase in local regional recurrences should be an aid to oncologists. It should prompt us to work on more effective systemic agents for this population of breast cancer patients.

C. Lawton, MD

Adjuvant Tamoxifen Reduces Subsequent Breast Cancer in Women With Estrogen Receptor–Positive Ductal Carcinoma in Situ: A Study Based on NSABP Protocol B-24

Allred DC, Anderson SJ, Paik S, et al (Natl Surgical Adjuvant Breast and Bowel Project (NSABP), St Louis, MO; et al)
J Clin Oncol 30:1268-1273, 2012

Purpose.—The NSABP (National Surgical Adjuvant Breast and Bowel Project) B-24 study demonstrated significant benefit with adjuvant tamoxifen in patients with ductal carcinoma in situ (DCIS) after lumpectomy and radiation. Patients were enrolled without knowledge of hormone receptor status. The current study retrospectively evaluated the relationship between receptors and response to tamoxifen.

Patients and Methods.—Estrogen (ER) and progesterone receptors (PgR) were evaluated in 732 patients with DCIS (41% of original study population). An experienced central laboratory determined receptor status in all patient cases with available paraffin blocks (n = 449) by immunohistochemistry (IHC) using comprehensively validated assays. Results for additional patients (n = 283) determined by various methods (primarily IHC) were available from enrolling institutions. Combined results were evaluated for benefit of tamoxifen by receptor status at 10 years and overall follow-up (median, 14.5 years).

Results.—ER was positive in 76% of patients. Patients with ER-positive DCIS treated with tamoxifen (*v* placebo) showed significant decreases in subsequent breast cancer at 10 years (hazard ratio [HR], 0.49; $P < .001$) and overall follow-up (HR, 0.60; $P = .003$), which remained significant in multivariable analysis (overall HR, 0.64; $P = .003$). Results were similar, but less significant, when subsequent ipsilateral and contralateral, invasive and noninvasive, breast cancers were considered separately. No significant benefit was observed in ER-negative DCIS. PgR and either receptor were positive in 66% and 79% of patients, respectively, and in general, neither was more predictive than ER alone.

Conclusion.—Patients in NSABP B-24 with ER-positive DCIS receiving adjuvant tamoxifen after standard therapy showed significant reductions in subsequent breast cancer. The use of adjuvant tamoxifen should be considered for patients with DCIS.

▶ The National Surgical Adjuvant Breast and Bowel Project (NSABP) B24 study randomized patients with ductal carcinoma in situ (DCIS) treated with lumpectomy plus radiation to either tamoxifen or placebo. Prior reports of NSABP B24 showed an advantage for the use of tamoxifen in these patients. This article reports subset analyses of those patients according to estrogen receptor status. These analyses show a clear reduction in the incidence of both ipsilateral and contralateral subsequent breast cancers in those patients with estrogen receptor (ER)—positive DCIS. The results are not so clear for patients with ER-negative DCIS. Trends show no difference between tamoxifen and placebo in regard to ipsilateral subsequent breast cancers, but trends also suggest there may be a reduction in the incidence of subsequent contralateral breast cancers. In evaluating these observations, the reader must remember two facts: First, these are unplanned subset analyses and thus cannot be regarded as definitive observations. Second, the number of contralateral breast cancers is extremely small and thus does not permit definitive conclusions. It would seem, however, that it would be reasonable to continue to use tamoxifen in all these patients until it is clear that patients with ER-negative DCIS do not benefit from a reduction in subsequent contralateral breast cancers.

J. T. Thigpen, MD

Management of hot flashes in patients who have breast cancer with venlafaxine and clonidine: a randomized, double-blind, placebo-controlled trial

Boekhout AH, Vincent AD, Dalesio OB, et al (The Netherlands Cancer Inst-Antoni van Leeuwenhoek Hosp, Amsterdam)

J Clin Oncol 29:3862-3868, 2011

Purpose.—Therapies for breast cancer may induce hot flashes that can affect quality of life. We undertook a double-blind, placebo-controlled trial with the primary objective of comparing the average daily hot flash scores in the twelfth week among patients treated with venlafaxine, clonidine, and placebo. Additional analyses of the hot flash score over the full 12 weeks of treatment were performed.

Patients and Methods.—In all, 102 patients with a history of breast cancer were randomly assigned (2:2:1) to venlafaxine 75 mg, clonidine 0.1 mg, or placebo daily for 12 weeks. Questionnaires at baseline and during treatment assessed daily hot flash scores, sexual function, sleep quality, anxiety, and depression.

Results.—After 12 weeks, a total of 80 patients were evaluable for the primary end point. During week 12, hot flash scores were significantly lower in the clonidine group versus placebo $(P = .03)$; for venlafaxine versus placebo, the difference was borderline not significant $(P = .07)$. However, hot flash scores were equal in the clonidine and venlafaxine groups. Over the course of 12 weeks, the differences between both treatments and placebo were significant $(P < .001$ for venlafaxine v placebo; $P = .045$ for clonidine v placebo). Frequencies of treatment-related adverse effects of nausea $(P = .02)$, constipation $(P = .04)$, and severe appetite loss were higher in the venlafaxine group.

Conclusion.—Venlafaxine and clonidine are effective treatments in the management of hot flashes in patients with breast cancer. Venlafaxine resulted in a more immediate reduction of hot flash scores when compared with clonidine; however, hot flash scores at week 12 were lower in the clonidine group than in the venlafaxine group.

▶ Hot flashes as a result of treatment for women with breast cancer and men with prostate cancer are a debilitating complication. Methods to mitigate this toxicity are important.

These authors report a significant randomized, placebo-controlled trial of 2 agents frequently used to treat hot flashes, venlafaxine and clonidine. Their results are somewhat mixed in that venlafaxine caused a more immediate reduction in hot flash scores, yet the clonidine had better hot flash scores at 12 weeks (the endpoint of the study).

So there are 2 important messages regarding this research: The first is that while the effects of hot flash scores were mixed for these drugs, both cause significant reduction in hot flash scores overall. The second message is that we need more data in larger trials (there were only 102 patients on this study) to validate these data and to consider other medications to help treat this challenging toxicity for some breast and prostate cancer patients.

C. Lawton, MD

Nodal status and clinical outcomes in a large cohort of patients with triple-negative breast cancer

Hernandez-Aya LF, Chavez-Macgregor M, Lei X, et al (The Univ of Texas MD Anderson Cancer Ctr, Houston)
J Clin Oncol 29:2628-2634, 2011

Purpose.—To evaluate the clinical outcomes and relationship between tumor size, lymph node status, and prognosis in a large cohort of patients with confirmed triple receptor-negative breast cancer (TNBC).

Patients and Methods.—We reviewed 1,711 patients with TNBC diagnosed between 1980 and 2009. Patients were categorized by tumor size and nodal status. Kaplan-Meier product limit method was used to calculate overall survival (OS) and relapse-free survival (RFS). A Sidak adjustment was used for multiple group comparisons. Cox proportional hazards models were fit to determine the association of tumor size and nodal status with survival outcomes after adjustment for other patient and disease characteristics.

Results.—Median age was 48 years (range, 21 to 87 years). At a median follow-up of 53 months (range, 0.7 to 317 months), there were 614 deaths and 747 recurrences. The 5-year OS was 80% for node-negative patients (N0), 65% for one to three positive lymph nodes (N1), 48% for four to nine positive lymph nodes (N2), and 44% for ≥10 positive lymph nodes (N3; $P < .0001$). The 5-year RFS rates were 67% for N0, 52% for N1, 36% for N2, and 33% for N3 ($P < .0001$). Pairwise comparison by nodal status showed that when comparing N0 with node-positive disease, there was a significant difference in OS and RFS ($P < .001$ all comparisons). However, when comparing N1 with N2 and N3 disease regardless of tumor size, there were no significant differences in OS or RFS.

Conclusion.—In patients with TNBC, once there is evidence of lymph node metastasis, the prognosis may not be affected by the number of positive lymph nodes.

▶ Breast cancer remains a serious problem in our country, despite years of research and encouraging results. It has long been understood that increasing tumor size and number of positive lymph nodes in patients with this diagnosis portends for poorer outcomes. Yet many other factors have been shown to play prognostic roles in this disease, with receptor status being just one of them.

The development of targeted therapy such as trastuzumab for human epidermal growth factor receptor 2 (HER2)—positive patients has lead to markedly improved outcomes for these patients. This is in addition to the previously well-documented benefit of tamoxifen for estrogen receptor—positive breast cancer patients. Yet for patients who are estrogen receptor-, progesterone receptor-, and HER2—negative (ie, triple negative), the results are unquestionably poorer. The clear relationship between tumor size and number of lymph nodes involved and outcomes may not be well correlated in patients with triple-negative tumors.

These authors have evaluated the question of lymph node status and outcome for over 1000 patients in the MD Anderson Cancer Center database. Their results support the well-known effect of lymph node positivity on outcomes, but the increasing number of lymph nodes involved did not appear to worsen the outcome.

These data support the need for significant research for triple-negative breast cancer patients, as they appear to have a uniquely separate biology from nontriple-negative breast cancer tumors.

C. Lawton, MD

15 Cancer Prevention

Effect of daily aspirin on risk of cancer metastasis: a study of incident cancers during randomised controlled trials
Rothwell PM, Wilson M, Price JF, et al (Univ of Oxford, UK; Univ of Edinburgh, UK; et al)
Lancet 379:1591-1601, 2012

Background.—Daily aspirin reduces the long-term incidence of some adenocarcinomas, but effects on mortality due to some cancers appear after only a few years, suggesting that it might also reduce growth or metastasis. We established the frequency of distant metastasis in patients who developed cancer during trials of daily aspirin versus control.

Methods.—Our analysis included all five large randomised trials of daily aspirin (≥ 75 mg daily) versus control for the prevention of vascular events in the UK. Electronic and paper records were reviewed for all patients with incident cancer. The effect of aspirin on risk of metastases at presentation or on subsequent follow-up (including post-trial follow-up of in-trial cancers) was stratified by tumour histology (adenocarcinoma vs other) and clinical characteristics.

Findings.—Of 17 285 trial participants, 987 had a new solid cancer diagnosed during mean in-trial follow-up of $6 \cdot 5$ years (SD $2 \cdot 0$). Allocation to aspirin reduced risk of cancer with distant metastasis (all cancers, hazard ratio [HR] $0 \cdot 64$, 95% CI $0 \cdot 48 - 0 \cdot 84$, $p = 0 \cdot 001$; adenocarcinoma, HR $0 \cdot 54$, 95% CI $0 \cdot 38 - 0 \cdot 77$, $p = 0 \cdot 0007$; other solid cancers, HR $0 \cdot 82$, 95% CI $0 \cdot 53 - 1 \cdot 28$, $p = 0 \cdot 39$), due mainly to a reduction in proportion of adenocarcinomas that had metastatic versus local disease (odds ratio $0 \cdot 52$, 95% CI $0 \cdot 35 - 0 \cdot 75$, $p = 0 \cdot 0006$). Aspirin reduced risk of adenocarcinoma with metastasis at initial diagnosis (HR $0 \cdot 69$, 95% CI $0 \cdot 50 - 0 \cdot 95$, $p = 0 \cdot 02$) and risk of metastasis on subsequent follow-up in patients without metastasis initially (HR $0 \cdot 45$, 95% CI $0 \cdot 28 - 0 \cdot 72$, $p = 0 \cdot 0009$), particularly in patients with colorectal cancer (HR $0 \cdot 26$, 95% CI $0 \cdot 11 - 0 \cdot 57$, $p = 0 \cdot 0008$) and in patients who remained on trial treatment up to or after diagnosis (HR $0 \cdot 31$, 95% CI $0 \cdot 15 - 0 \cdot 62$, $p = 0 \cdot 0009$). Allocation to aspirin reduced death due to cancer in patients who developed adenocarcinoma, particularly in those without metastasis at diagnosis (HR $0 \cdot 50$, 95% CI $0 \cdot 34 - 0 \cdot 74$, $p = 0 \cdot 0006$). Consequently, aspirin reduced the overall risk of fatal adenocarcinoma in the trial populations (HR $0 \cdot 65$, 95% CI $0 \cdot 53 - 0 \cdot 82$, $p = 0 \cdot 0002$), but not the risk of other fatal cancers (HR $1 \cdot 06$, 95% CI $0 \cdot 84 - 1 \cdot 32$, $p = 0 \cdot 64$; difference, $p = 0 \cdot 003$). Effects were independent of age and sex, but absolute benefit was greatest in smokers. A low-dose, slow-release formulation of aspirin designed to inhibit platelets but to have little systemic bioavailability was as effective as higher doses.

Interpretation.—That aspirin prevents distant metastasis could account for the early reduction in cancer deaths in trials of daily aspirin versus control. This finding suggests that aspirin might help in treatment of some cancers and provides proof of principle for pharmacological intervention specifically to prevent distant metastasis.

▶ This article looks at 5 randomized trials of aspirin versus no therapy to prevent vascular events in the United Kingdom. A total 17 285 individuals participated in these 5 studies. The objective of the study was to determine whether aspirin could reduce or prevent the diagnosis of cancers with metastases at initial diagnosis. Among the participants, 987 cancers were diagnosed. In the individuals on aspirin, the risk of a new solid cancer with metastases at diagnosis was reduced by 36% (hazard ratio [HR] = 0.64; P = .001). The likelihood of adenocarcinomas was impacted more (HR = 0.54; P = .0007) than other histologies. In particular, there was a major reduction in metastatic adenocarcinoma of the colon. In addition, the risk of fatal adenocarcinoma was reduced substantially (HR = 0.65; P = .0002). Low-dose, slow release formulations were as effective as higher doses of aspirin. These data suggest that the beneficial effects of daily aspirin extend beyond vascular disease and include a reduction in the likelihood of developing metastatic adenocarcinomas particularly of the colon. Aspirin, anyone?

J. T. Thigpen, MD

16 Chemotherapy: Mechanisms and Side Effects

Appropriate Chemotherapy Dosing for Obese Adult Patients With Cancer:
American Society of Clinical Oncology Clinical Practice Guideline
Griggs JJ, Mangu PB, Anderson H, et al (Univ of Michigan, Ann Arbor; American
Society of Clinical Oncology, Alexandria, VA; Breast Cancer Coalition of
Rochester, NY; et al)
J Clin Oncol 30:1553-1561, 2012

Purpose.—To provide recommendations for appropriate cytotoxic che-motherapy dosing for obese adult patients with cancer.

Methods.—The American Society of Clinical Oncology convened a Panel of experts in medical and gynecologic oncology, clinical pharmacology, pharmacokinetics and pharmacogenetics, and biostatistics and a patient representative. MEDLINE searches identified studies published in English between 1996 and 2010, and a systematic review of the literature was con-ducted. A majority of studies involved breast, ovarian, colon, and lung cancers. This guideline does not address dosing for novel targeted agents.

Results.—Practice pattern studies demonstrate that up to 40% of obese patients receive limited chemotherapy doses that are not based on actual body weight. Concerns about toxicity or overdosing in obese patients with cancer, based on the use of actual body weight, are unfounded.

Recommendations.—The Panel recommends that full weight–based cytotoxic chemotherapy doses be used to treat obese patients with cancer, particularly when the goal of treatment is cure. There is no evidence that short- or long-term toxicity is increased among obese patients receiving full weight–based doses. Most data indicate that myelosuppression is the same or less pronounced among the obese than the non-obese who are administered full weight-based doses. Clinicians should respond to all treatment-related toxicities in obese patients in the same ways they do for non-obese patients. The use of fixed-dose chemotherapy is rarely justified, but the Panel does recommend fixed dosing for a few select agents. The Panel recommends further research into the role of pharmacokinetics and pharmacogenetics to guide appropriate dosing of obese patients with cancer.

▶ This article reports the results of the deliberations of an American Society of Clinical Oncology expert panel on the questions surrounding appropriate dosing for the obese patients. Traditionally, these patients have had doses of chemotherapeutic agents capped usually at a body surface area of either 2 or 2.2 m^2. The panel concluded that obese patients should be treated with full doses based on either weight or body surface area as calculated by standard formulae. These recommendations seem relatively straightforward but deserve a cautionary note. As noted in the panel's report, the conclusions are based on a very limited number of randomized clinical trials, and it seems unlikely that there will be more data forthcoming addressing these questions. Most oncologists recognize the importance of maintaining relative dose intensity at least up to a point, but if the recommendations are to be followed, the patient should be informed of the potential risk of being overdosed. Furthermore, the oncologist must be prepared to deal with anticipated toxicity and to adjust doses as needed based on observed toxicity.

J. T. Thigpen, MD

17 Gastrointestinal

Long-term risk of colorectal cancer after negative colonoscopy
Brenner H, Chang-Claude J, Seiler CM, et al (German Cancer Res Ctr, Heidelberg, Germany)
J Clin Oncol 29:3761-3767, 2011

Purpose.—Colonoscopy is thought to be a powerful and cost-effective tool to reduce colorectal cancer (CRC) incidence and mortality. Empirical evidence for overall and risk group-specific definition of screening intervals is sparse. We aimed to assess the risk of CRC according to time since negative colonoscopy, overall, and by sex, smoking, and family history of CRC, in a large population-based case-control study.

Patients and Methods.—In all, 1,945 patients with CRC and 2,399 population controls were recruited in 22 hospitals and through population registers in the Rhine-Neckar region of Germany from 2003 to 2007. Data on history of colonoscopy and important covariates were obtained by personal interviews and from medical records.

Results.—Compared with people who had never undergone colonoscopy, people with a previous negative colonoscopy had a strongly reduced risk of CRC. Adjusted odds ratios for time windows of 1 to 2, 3 to 4, 5 to 9, 10 to 19, and 20+ years after negative colonoscopy were 0.14 (95% CI, 0.10 to 0.20), 0.12 (95% CI, 0.08 to 0.19), 0.26 (95% CI, 0.18 to 0.39), 0.28 (95% CI, 0.17 to 0.45), and 0.40 (95% CI, 0.24 to 0.66), respectively. Low risks even beyond 10 years after negative colonoscopy were observed for both left- and right-sided CRC and in all risk groups assessed except current smokers, who had a risk similar to that of never smokers with no previous colonoscopy 10 or more years after a negative colonoscopy.

Conclusion.—These results support suggestions that screening intervals for CRC screening by colonoscopy could be longer than the commonly recommended 10 years in most cases, perhaps even among men and people with a family history of CRC, but probably not among current smokers.

▶ The use of screening colonoscopy has become a very important tool to decrease the incidence and mortality associated with colorectal cancer. Few patients, physicians, and even insurers question the need for this screening examination. Yet once a patient has a colonoscopy and the results are negative, what is the next appropriate interval for subsequent ones? The answer to this question is not known with certainty and is very important from a cost, patient convenience, and colorectal cancer risk perspective.

We know as physicians that the current answer to the question of timing of subsequent screening colonoscopies after an initial negative one has been 10 years. The data to verify that 10 years is the correct timeframe are lacking. These authors have attempted to answer the question through the use of population-based registries in Germany. Based on their data, especially in nonsmokers, the interval could be every 20 years. These results need to be evaluated in a larger cohort of patients, but they do provide tantalizing data to encourage us to pursue this important question.

C. Lawton, MD

18 Genitourinary

Cost-Effectiveness of Prostate Specific Antigen Screening in the United States: Extrapolating From the European Study of Screening for Prostate Cancer
Shteynshlyuger A, Andriole GL (Washington Univ School of Medicine, St Louis, MO)
J Urol 185:828-832, 2011

Purpose.—Preliminary results of the European Randomized Study of Screening for Prostate Cancer showed a decrease in prostate cancer specific mortality associated with prostate specific antigen screening. We evaluated the cost-effectiveness of prostate specific antigen screening using data from the European Randomized Study of Screening for Prostate Cancer protocol when extrapolated to the United States.

Materials and Methods.—We used previously reported Surveillance, Epidemiology and End Results-Medicare data and a nationwide sample of employer provided estimates of costs of care for patients with prostate cancer. The European data were used in accordance with the study protocol to determine the costs and cost-effectiveness of prostate specific antigen screening.

Results.—The lifetime cost of screening with prostate specific antigen, evaluating abnormal prostate specific antigen and treating identified prostate cancer to prevent 1 death from prostate cancer was $5,227,306 based on the European findings and extrapolated to the United States. If screening achieved a similar decrease in overall mortality as the decrease in prostate cancer specific mortality in the European study, such intervention would cost $262,758 per life-year saved. Prostate specific antigen screening reported in the European study would become cost effective when the lifelong treatment costs were below $1,868 per life-year, or when the number needed to treat was lowered to 21 or fewer men.

Conclusions.—The lifelong costs of screening protocols are determined by the cost of treatment with an insignificant contribution from screening costs. We established a model that predicts the minimal requirements that would make screening a cost-effective measure for population based implementation.

▶ Prostate cancer claims the lives of over 32 000 US males annually, and unfortunately, it is too often thought of as an indolent disease that requires little concern much less treatment or screening. Breast cancer in women, on the other hand, claims the lives of approximately 40 000 US women annually and is considered an epidemic that must be stopped at all cost, with mammography screening and breast examinations remaining imperative. Given this disproportional concern, the role of prostate-specific antigen (PSA) screening for prostate cancer is constantly evaluated and often debunked as too expensive, given that virtually no one dies of this disease!

Since thousands of men do die of this disease, it is important that we continue to evaluate the role of digital rectal examination and PSA screening for prostate cancer. The goal is to define a population of men for which digital rectal examinations and PSA help diagnose those prostate cancers that do impact survival. These authors suggest such a model, which takes into account the age of the patient, life expectancy, and costs of evaluating men in the age range of 50 to 80 years. We simply must work with models like this to establish the role of digital rectal examinations and PSA screening so as to decrease the risk of prostate cancer deaths in the United States, which are second only to lung cancer deaths.

C. Lawton, MD

Fifteen-year biochemical relapse-free survival, cause-specific survival, and overall survival following I^{125} prostate brachytherapy in clinically localized prostate cancers: Seattle experience

Sylvester JE, Grimm PD, Wong J, et al (Lakewood Ranch Oncology, FL; Prostate Cancer Treatment Ctr, Seattle, WA; Univ California, Irvine, et al)
Int J Radiat Oncol Biol Phys 81:376-381, 2011

Purpose.—To report 15-year biochemical relapse–free survival (BRFS), cause-specific survival (CSS), and overall survival (OS) outcomes of patients treated with I^{125} brachytherapy monotherapy for clinically localized prostate cancer early in the Seattle experience.

Methods and Materials.—Two hundred fifteen patients with clinically localized prostate cancer were consecutively treated from 1988 to 1992 with I^{125} monotherapy. They were prospectively followed as a tight cohort. They were evaluated for BRFS, CSS, and OS. Multivariate analysis was used to evaluate outcomes by pretreatment clinical prognostic factors. BRFS was analyzed by the Phoenix (nadir + 2 ng/mL) definition. CSS and OS were evaluated by chart review, death certificates, and referring physician follow-up notes. Gleason scoring was performed by general pathologists at a community hospital in Seattle. Time to biochemical failure (BF) was calculated and compared by Kaplan-Meier plots.

Results.—Fifteen-year BRFS for the entire cohort was 80.4%. BRFS by D'Amico risk group classification cohort analysis was 85.9%, 79.9%, and 62.2% for low, intermediate, and high-risk patients, respectively. Follow-up ranged from 3.6 to 18.4 years; median follow-up was 15.4 years for biochemically free of disease patients. Overall median follow-up was 11.7 years. The median time to BF in those who failed was 5.1 years. CSS was 84%. OS was 37.1%. Average age at time of treatment was 70 years. There was no significant difference in BRFS between low and intermediate risk groups.

Conclusion.—I^{125} monotherapy results in excellent 15-year BRFS and CSS, especially when taking into account the era of treatment effect.

▶ Treatment options for organ-confined prostate cancer, especially those patients with low or intermediate risk disease, are numerous. Surgery is available robotically or as an open procedure. Watchful waiting or active surveillance is appropriate for many low-risk patients (eg, < clinical T2a, < Gleason Score 6, and < prostate-specific antigen 10). Radiation is available as external beam or brachytherapy, both low-dose rate (LDR) and high-dose rate.

The team of physicians from Seattle who pioneered the resurgence of I-125 LDR brachytherapy for these patients has reported their results with 15-year follow-up. This report is important for a number of reasons: First, it confirms that the long-term outcome in terms of disease control for these patients is very good. Second, it confirms that many patients with intermediate-risk disease are also very appropriate candidates for LDR brachytherapy. Third, it shows that patients who fail generally do so within 8 to 10 years. Finally, although a thorough review of toxicity is not available in this article, there were no treatment-related deaths or other serious complications, such as deep venous thrombosis or strokes. The take-home message here is that this option for patients with low- or intermediate-risk prostate cancer should be offered, as it appears to be effective and certainly is cost effective.

C. Lawton, MD

19 Gynecology

Management of recurrent cervical cancer: A review of the literature
Peiretti M, Zapardiel I, Zanagnolo V, et al (European Inst of Oncology, Milan, Italy; La Paz Univ Hosp, Madrid, Spain; et al)
Surg Oncol 21:e59-e66, 2012

Objective.—The aim of this narrative review is to update the current knowledge on the treatment of recurrent cervical cancer based on a literature review.

Material and Methods.—A web based search in Medline and CancerLit databases has been carried out on recurrent cervical cancer management and treatment. All relevant information has been collected and analyzed, prioritizing randomized clinical trials.

Results.—Cervical cancer still represents a significant problem for public health with an annual incidence of about half a million new cases worldwide. Percentages of pelvic recurrences fluctuate from 10% to 74% depending on different risk factors. Accordingly to the literature, it is suggested that chemoradiation treatment (containing cisplatin and/or taxanes) could represent the treatment of choice for locoregional recurrences of cervical cancer after radical surgery. Pelvic exenteration is usually indicated for selected cases of central recurrence of cervical cancer after primary or adjuvant radiation and chemotherapy with bladder and/or rectum infiltration neither extended to the pelvic side walls nor showing any signs of extrapelvic spread of disease. Laterally extended endopelvic resection (LEER) for the treatment of those patients with a locally advanced disease or with a recurrence affecting the pelvic wall has been described.

Conclusions.—The treatment of recurrences of cervical carcinoma consists of surgery, and of radiation and chemotherapy, or the combination of different modalities taking into consideration the type of primary therapy, the site of recurrence, the disease-free interval, the patient symptoms, performance status, and the degree to which any given treatment might be beneficial.

▶ Carcinoma of the cervix is the third most common gynecologic malignancy in the United States. In developed countries with widespread Pap smear screening programs, the frequency of deaths has declined remarkably since the 1950s. In less developed countries, however, this disease remains a major killer. This article reviews in detail the management of recurrent carcinoma of the cervix. In particular, the article reviews studies of systemic therapy for disseminated recurrence and points out that a taxane/platinum regimen appears to be the optimal regimen currently available for the treatment of the disease. More recent information suggests that paclitaxel/carboplatin is an acceptable regimen in those patients who have previously received cisplatin in the setting of concurrent chemoradiation for locally advanced disease, but in those patients who have not been previously exposed to cisplatin, it remains the platinum agent of choice to combine with a taxane. The article is worth reading in detail for the discussion of the role of surgery and radiation in patients with recurrent carcinoma of the cervix.

J. T. Thigpen, MD

A systematic review evaluating the relationship between progression free survival and post progression survival in advanced ovarian cancer
Sundar S, Wu J, Hillaby K, et al (City Hosp, UK; Univ of Birmingham, UK)
Gynecol Oncol 125:493-499, 2012

Objective.—Although overall survival is the ultimate goal of cancer therapy, many clinical and health economic decisions are taken when only progression free survival (PFS) data are available. This study evaluates the relationship between PFS and post progression survival (i.e. the time between disease progression and death) to estimate how many months a new drug for ovarian cancer might add to overall survival if the number of months the drug added to PFS (relative to a standard drug) was already known.

Methods.—A literature search was conducted over Medline for randomised controlled trials published between January 1990 and July 2010 that evaluated the effect of a drug treatment in comparison to alternative drug treatment in patients with either advanced stage primary or recurrent ovarian cancer. A systematic review of progression free and post progression survival (PPS) was performed. The relationship between PFS and PPS was evaluated by a graphical method and standard statistical tests.

Results.—Thirty-seven trials involving 15,850 patients met the inclusion criteria. The review found that increases in median PFS generally lead to little change in post-progression survival. Percentage gains in PFS are generally associated with no percentage gains or with very slight percentage gains or losses in post-progression survival.

Conclusion.—If the effect of a new drug treatment for ovarian cancer is to extend median PFS by *x* months, then it is reasonable to estimate that the treatment will also extend median overall survival by *x* months. This information will be useful for individual and collective decision making.

▶ The issue of endpoints in ovarian cancer has become an important and controversial issue over the past several years. The Food and Drug Administration (FDA) has generally taken the position that only overall survival (OS) will suffice as a regulatory endpoint in ovarian cancer for at least 2 stated reasons. First, they feel that progression-free survival (PFS) cannot be measured accurately because of the perceived difficulty in determining the point of progression. Second, they contend that PFS does not reflect patient benefit. This puts the FDA at odds with a number of other regulatory agencies worldwide that accept PFS as a valid regulatory endpoint. For ovarian cancers, this is a major problem. The patient with ovarian cancer has many options for further treatment upon progression, with the literature showing at least 22 agents with documented activity at least in phase II trials. In the United States, most patients receive multiple lines of additional therapy, including in many instances crossover to the experimental agent. This postprogression therapy blurs the survival endpoint and for practical purposes renders it uninterpretable. This study illustrates this with the observation that the changes in median PFS led to little change in postprogression survival. Prior to 1990, 13 of 15 phase III trials showed a clear correlation between PFS and OS with similar hazard ratios for both PFS and OS (see FDA website, 2006 endpoints in ovarian cancer conference). Given that very few options were available for the patient with progression of disease in that era, it seems clear that, in the absence of effective postprogression therapy, PFS and OS correlate. Furthermore, in 4 recent trials of bevacizumab added to chemotherapy (total patients over 4000), a very consistent PFS benefit is observed and suggests that PFS can be consistently and accurately measured. These facts argue for PFS as a valid regulatory endpoint and as an indicator of patient benefit.

J. T. Thigpen, MD

CA-125 can be part of the tumour evaluation criteria in ovarian cancer trials: experience of the GCIG CALYPSO trial
Alexandre J, Brown C, Coeffic D, et al (Université Paris Descartes, France; NHMRC Clinical Trials Centre, Sydney, Australia; Hôpital des Diaconesses, Paris, France; et al)
Br J Cancer 106:633-637, 2012

Background.—CA-125 as a tumour progression criterion in relapsing ovarian cancer (ROC) trials remains controversial. CALYPSO is a large randomised trial incorporating CA-125 (GCIG criteria) and symptomatic deterioration in addition to Response Evaluation Criteria in Solid Tumours (RECIST) criteria (radiological) to determine progression.

Methods.—In all, 976 patients with platinum-sensitive ROC were randomised to carboplatin—paclitaxel (C-P) or carboplatin-pegylated liposomal doxorubicin (C-PLD). CT-scan and CA-125 were performed every 3 months until progression.

Results.—In all, 832 patients (85%) progressed, with 60% experiencing a first radiological progression, 10% symptomatic progression, and 28% CA-125 progression without evidence of radiological or symptomatic progression. The benefit of C-PLD *vs* C-P in progression-free survival was not influenced by type of first progression (hazard ratio 0.85 (95% confidence interval (CI): 0.66—1.10) and 0.84 (95% CI: 0.72—0.98) for

CA-125 and RECIST, respectively). In patients with CA-125 first progression who subsequently progressed radiologically, a delay of 2.3 months was observed between the two progression types. After CA-125 first progression, median time to new treatment was 2.0 months. In all, 81% of the patients with CA-125 or radiological first progression and 60% with symptomatic first progression received subsequent treatment.

Conclusion.—CA-125 and radiological tests performed similarly in determining progression with C-PLD or C-P. Additional follow-up with CA-125 measurements was not associated with overtreatment.

▶ The CALYPSO trial was a Gynecologic Cancer Intergroup study that randomized patients with platinum-sensitive recurrent ovarian carcinoma to treatment with carboplatin plus either paclitaxel or pegylated liposomal doxorubicin (PLD). The final results of the study showed a small advantage for the PLD-containing regimen in terms of progression-free survival and no difference in overall survival. Because of the controversy over whether progression-free survival can be measured accurately in ovarian carcinoma, the investigators in this article look at determination of progression by scan as opposed to cancer antigen-125 (CA-125). The data suggest that both methods can accurately determine the onset of progression and that use of CA-125 as a criterion does not lead to overtreatment of the patients. As has been reported before, they also observed that CA-125 can determine the onset of progression a median of 2.3 months earlier in about 30% of the patients. This study is part of a growing body of evidence suggesting that progression-free survival can be an accurate endpoint for ovarian carcinoma trials and that CA-125 is a reliable marker of progression and thus can be a part of the approach to determining onset of progression.

J. T. Thigpen, MD

Final overall survival results of phase III GCIG CALYPSO trial of pegylated liposomal doxorubicin and carboplatin *vs* paclitaxel and carboplatin in platinum-sensitive ovarian cancer patients
Wagner U, Marth C, Largillier R, et al (Univ Hosp of Gießen and Marburg, Germany; Med Univ Innsbruck, Austria; Centre Azuréen de Cancérologie, Mougins, France; et al)
Br J Cancer 1-4, 2012

Background.—The CALYPSO phase III trial compared CD (carboplatin-pegylated liposomal doxorubicin (PLD)) with CP (carboplatin-paclitaxel) in patients with platinum-sensitive recurrent ovarian cancer (ROC). Overall survival (OS) data are now mature.

Methods.—Women with ROC relapsing > 6 months after first- or second-line therapy were randomised to CD or CP for six cycles in this international, open-label, non-inferiority trial. The primary endpoint was progression-free survival. The OS analysis is presented here.

Results.—A total of 976 patients were randomised (467 to CD and 509 to CP). With a median follow-up of 49 months, no statistically significant difference was observed between arms in OS (hazard ratio = 0.99 (95% confidence interval 0.85, 1.16); log-rank $P = 0.94$). Median survival times were 30.7 months (CD) and 33.0 months (CP). No statistically significant difference in OS was observed between arms in predetermined subgroups according to age, body mass index, treatment-free interval, measurable disease, number of lines of prior chemotherapy, or performance status. Post-study cross-over was imbalanced between arms, with a greater proportion of patients randomised to CP receiving post-study PLD (68%) than patients randomised to CD receiving post-study paclitaxel (43%; $P < 0.001$).

Conclusion.—Carboplatin-PLD led to delayed progression and similar OS compared with carboplatin-paclitaxel in platinum-sensitive ROC.

▶ Two previously reported phase III trials have established the value of carboplatin-based doublets over single-agent carboplatin for platinum-sensitive recurrent ovarian carcinoma: ICON4 (carboplatin paclitaxel) and AGO-OVAR 2.5 (carboplatin gemcitabine). This study randomized patients with platinum-sensitive recurrent ovarian carcinoma to either paclitaxel/carboplatin or pegylated liposomal doxorubicin (PLD)/carboplatin. The study was conducted by the Gynecologic Cancer Intergroup and involved over 900 patients. The PLD-containing regimen demonstrated a superior progression-free survival in an earlier report. This article presents the overall survival data, which show no difference between the 2 regimens. The bottom line of this study is that oncologists can now choose any of the 3 carboplatin-based doublets as systemic therapy for the patient with platinum-sensitive recurrent ovarian carcinoma and be well within the standard of care. Given the small advantage of PLD/carboplatin in terms of progression-free survival, one could even argue that PLD/carboplatin would be preferred over paclitaxel/carboplatin; thus the choice becomes either PLD/carboplatin or gemcitabine/carboplatin based on available evidence.

J. T. Thigpen, MD

Evolution of surgical treatment paradigms for advanced-stage ovarian cancer: Redefining 'optimal' residual disease
Chang S-J, Bristow RE (Ajou Univ School of Medicine, Suwon, Republic of Korea; Univ of California, Orange)
Gynecol Oncol 125:483-492, 2012

Over the past 40 years, the survival of patients with advanced ovarian cancer has greatly improved due to the introduction of combination chemotherapy with platinum and paclitaxel as standard front-line treatment and the progressive incorporation of increasing degrees of maximal cytoreductive surgery. The designation of "optimal" surgical cytoreduction has evolved from residual disease ≤1 cm to no gross residual disease.

There is a growing body of evidence that patients with no gross residual disease have better survival than those with optimal but visible residual disease. In order to achieve this, more radical cytoreductive procedures such as radical pelvic resection and extensive upper abdominal procedures are increasingly performed. However, some investigators still suggest that tumor biology is a major determinant in survival and that optimal surgery cannot fully compensate for tumor biology. The aim of this review is to outline the theoretical rationale and historical evolution of primary cytoreductive surgery, to re-evaluate the preferred surgical objective and procedures commonly required to achieve optimal cytoreduction in the platinum/taxane era based on contemporary evidence, and to redefine the concept of "optimal" residual disease within the context of future surgical developments and analysis of treatment outcomes.

▶ This is an excellent review of surgical studies that have led to the conclusion that surgical bulk reduction improves outcome in ovarian cancer. The review provides a solid rationale for evolving our understanding of what constitutes appropriate goals for bulk reduction. The authors present evidence that those patients who do best with surgical bulk reduction are those in whom all gross disease can be resected. Based on this, they suggest replacing the old terminology of optimal cytoreduction (defined in the literature initially as no residual disease greater than 2 cm diameter, then later as 1 cm) and suboptimal cytoreduction (> 2 cm disease remaining) with a newer classification with 3 categories (no gross residual, gross residual [GR] less than 1 cm or GR-1, and bulky gross residual or GR-B). These considerations were also discussed at the Fourth Ovarian Cancer Consensus Conference in Vancouver, Canada, by the Gynecologic Cancer InterGroup member groups with strong support for such a new classification. If accepted generally by the practicing community, this new understanding would mean the performance of more aggressive surgery to achieve no gross residual disease status. Such aggressive surgery is already done routinely in the United States by well-trained gynecologic oncologists, but such an understanding would represent for much of the rest of the world a relatively substantial departure from current practice. The article is well worth reading for a complete understanding of the problem.

J. T. Thigpen, MD

Incorporation of Bevacizumab in the Primary Treatment of Ovarian Cancer
Burger RA, for the Gynecologic Oncology Group (Fox Chase Cancer Ctr, Philadelphia, PA; et al)
N Engl J Med 365:2473-2483, 2011

Background.—Vascular endothelial growth factor is a key promoter of angiogenesis and disease progression in epithelial ovarian cancer. Bevacizumab, a humanized anti–vascular endothelial growth factor monoclonal antibody, has shown single-agent activity in women with recurrent tumors. Thus, we aimed to evaluate the addition of bevacizumab to standard front-line therapy.

Methods.—In our double-blind, placebo-controlled, phase 3 trial, we randomly assigned eligible patients with newly diagnosed stage III (incompletely resectable) or stage IV epithelial ovarian cancer who had undergone debulking surgery to receive one of three treatments. All three included chemotherapy consisting of intravenous paclitaxel at a dose of 175 mg per square meter of body-surface area, plus carboplatin at an area under the curve of 6, for cycles 1 through 6, plus a study treatment for cycles 2 through 22, each cycle of 3 weeks' duration. The control treatment was chemotherapy with placebo added in cycles 2 through 22; bevacizumab-initiation treatment was chemotherapy with bevacizumab (15 mg per kilogram of body weight) added in cycles 2 through 6 and placebo added in cycles 7 through 22. Bevacizumab-throughout treatment was chemotherapy with bevacizumab added in cycles 2 through 22. The primary end point was progression-free survival.

Results.—Overall, 1873 women were enrolled. The median progression-free survival was 10.3 months in the control group, 11.2 in the bevacizumab-initiation group, and 14.1 in the bevacizumab-throughout group. Relative to control treatment, the hazard ratio for progression or death was 0.908 (95% confidence interval [CI], 0.795 to 1.040; $P = 0.16$) with bevacizumab initiation and 0.717 (95% CI, 0.625 to 0.824; $P < 0.001$) with bevacizumab throughout. At the time of analysis, 76.3% of patients were alive, with no significant differences in overall survival among the three groups. The rate of hypertension requiring medical therapy was higher in the bevacizumab-initiation group (16.5%) and the bevacizumab-throughout group (22.9%) than in the control group (7.2%). Gastrointestinal-wall disruption requiring medical intervention occurred in 1.2%, 2.8%, and 2.6% of patients in the control group, the bevacizumab-initiation group, and the bevacizumab-throughout group, respectively.

Conclusions.—The use of bevacizumab during and up to 10 months after carboplatin and paclitaxel chemotherapy prolongs the median progression-free survival by about 4 months in patients with advanced epithelial ovarian cancer. (Funded by the National Cancer Institute and Genentech; ClinicalTrials.gov number, NCT00262847.)

▶ This article presents the results of the first phase III trial of the addition of bevacizumab to paclitaxel/carboplatin in the treatment of patients with newly diagnosed advanced ovarian carcinoma (GOG 218). The study was designed as a blinded placebo-controlled trial with 3 arms: paclitaxel/carboplatin/placebo followed by placebo maintenance out to 15 months, paclitaxel/carboplatin/bevacizumab followed by placebo maintenance out to 15 months, or paclitaxel/carboplatin/bevacizumab followed by bevacizumab maintenance out to 15 months. The trial involved more than 1800 patients and showed a statistically significant superior progression-free survival (PFS) with the paclitaxel/carboplatin/bevacizumab followed by bevacizumab maintenance with a hazard ratio of 0.71. No difference in overall survival was observed, but this is not surprising when one considers that patients, upon progression, are treated with up to 8 additional lines of therapy chosen from among the more than 20 additional active agents in ovarian carcinoma. The only significantly increased adverse effects were hypertension and proteinuria. This trial is 1 of 2 large phase III studies evaluating bevacizumab added to chemotherapy in newly diagnosed advanced ovarian carcinoma. The major differences between the 2 studies were inclusion of patients with stages I—II disease in the other trial (ICON 7) and no blinding or placebo control in ICON 7, and a lower dose of bevacizumab in ICON 7 (7.5 mg/kg every 3 weeks in ICON 7 vs 15 mg/kg every 3 weeks in GOG 218). The results across these 2 trials are in addition to a third trial in platinum-sensitive recurrent disease (OCEANS) and a fourth trial in platinum-resistant recurrent disease (AURELIA). More than 4000 patients thus show the consistent improvement in PFS with the addition of bevacizumab to standard chemotherapy for ovarian carcinoma.

J. T. Thigpen, MD

A Phase 3 Trial of Bevacizumab in Ovarian Cancer

Perren TJ, for the ICON7 Investigators (St James's Univ Hosp, Leeds, UK; et al)
N Engl J Med 365:2484-2496, 2011

Background.—Angiogenesis plays a role in the biology of ovarian cancer. We examined the effect of bevacizumab, the vascular endothelial growth factor inhibitor, on survival in women with this disease.

Methods.—We randomly assigned women with ovarian cancer to carbo-platin (area under the curve, 5 or 6) and paclitaxel (175 mg per square meter of body-surface area), given every 3 weeks for 6 cycles, or to this regimen plus bevacizumab (7.5 mg per kilogram of body weight), given concurrently every 3 weeks for 5 or 6 cycles and continued for 12 additional cycles or until progression of disease. Outcome measures included progression-free survival, first analyzed per protocol and then updated, and interim overall survival.

Results.—A total of 1528 women from 11 countries were randomly assigned to one of the two treatment regimens. Their median age was 57 years; 90% had epithelial ovarian cancer, 69% had a serous histologic type, 9% had high-risk early-stage disease, 30% were at high risk for progression, and 70% had stage IIIC or IV ovarian cancer. Progression-free survival (restricted mean) at 36 months was 20.3 months with standard therapy, as compared with 21.8 months with standard therapy plus bevaci-zumab (hazard ratio for progression or death with bevacizumab added, 0.81; 95% confidence interval, 0.70 to 0.94; $P = 0.004$ by the log-rank test). Nonproportional hazards were detected (i.e., the treatment effect was not consistent over time on the hazard function scale) ($P < 0.001$), with a maximum effect at 12 months, coinciding with the end of planned bevacizumab treatment and diminishing by 24 months. Bevacizumab was associated with more toxic effects (most often hypertension of grade 2 or higher) (18%, vs. 2% with chemotherapy alone). In the updated analyses, progression-free survival (restricted mean) at 42 months was 22.4 months without bevacizumab versus 24.1 months with bevacizumab ($P = 0.04$ by log-rank test); in patients at high risk for progression, the benefit was greater with bevacizumab than without it, with progression-free survival (restricted mean) at 42 months of 14.5 months with standard therapy alone and 18.1 months with bevacizumab added, with respective median overall survival of 28.8 and 36.6 months.

Conclusions.—Bevacizumab improved progression-free survival in women with ovarian cancer. The benefits with respect to both progression-free and overall survival were greater among those at high risk for disease progression. (Funded by Roche and others; ICON7 Controlled-Trials.com number, ISRCTN91273375.)

▶ This article presents the results of the second phase III trial of the addition of bevacizumab to paclitaxel/carboplatin in the treatment of patients with newly diagnosed advanced ovarian carcinoma (ICON 7). The study was designed as a 2-arm randomized phase III study: paclitaxel/carboplatin followed by no maintenance versus paclitaxel/carboplatin/bevacizumab followed by bevacizumab maintenance out to12 months. The trial involved more than 1500 patients and found a statistically significant superior progression-free survival (PFS) with the paclitaxel/carboplatin/bevacizumab followed by bevacizumab maintenance with a hazard ratio of 0.87. No difference in overall survival was observed, but this is not surprising when one considers that patients, upon progression, are treated with up to 8 additional lines of therapy chosen from among the more than 20 additional active agents in ovarian carcinoma. The only significantly increased adverse effects were hypertension and proteinuria. This trial is 1 of 2 large phase III studies evaluating bevacizumab added to chemotherapy in newly diagnosed advanced ovarian carcinoma. The major differences between the 2 studies were: inclusion of patients with stages I—II disease in this trial (ICON 7) and no blinding or placebo control in this study, and a lower dose of bevacizumab in this trial (7.5 mg/kg every 3 weeks in ICON 7 vs 15 mg/kg every 3 weeks in GOG 218). The results across these 2 trials are in addition to a third trial in platinum-sensitive recurrent disease (OCEANS) and a fourth trial in platinum-resistant recurrent disease (AURELIA). More than 4000 patients thus demonstrate the consistent improvement in PFS with the addition of bevacizumab to standard chemotherapy for ovarian carcinoma.

J. T. Thigpen, MD

OCEANS: A Randomized, Double-Blind, Placebo-Controlled Phase III Trial of Chemotherapy With or Without Bevacizumab in Patients With Platinum-Sensitive Recurrent Epithelial Ovarian, Primary Peritoneal, or Fallopian Tube Cancer

Aghajanian C, Blank SV, Goff BA, et al (Memorial Sloan-Kettering Cancer Ctr and Weill Cornell Med College, NY; New York Univ School of Medicine; Univ of Washington School of Medicine, Seattle; et al)
J Clin Oncol 30:2039-2045, 2012

Purpose.—This randomized, multicenter, blinded, placebo-controlled phase III trial tested the efficacy and safety of bevacizumab (BV) with gemcitabine and carboplatin (GC) compared with GC in platinum-sensitive recurrent ovarian, primary peritoneal, or fallopian tube cancer (ROC).

Patients and Methods.—Patients with platinum-sensitive ROC (recurrence ≥ 6 months after front-line platinum-based therapy) and measurable disease were randomly assigned to GC plus either BV or placebo (PL) for six to 10 cycles. BV or PL, respectively, was then continued until disease progression. The primary end point was progression-free survival (PFS) by RECIST; secondary end points were objective response rate, duration of response (DOR), overall survival, and safety.

Results.—Overall, 484 patients were randomly assigned. PFS for the BV arm was superior to that for the PL arm (hazard ratio [HR], 0.484; 95% CI, 0.388 to 0.605; log-rank $P < .0001$); median PFS was 12.4 v 8.4 months, respectively. The objective response rate (78.5% v 57.4%; $P < .0001$) and DOR (10.4 v 7.4 months; HR, 0.534; 95% CI, 0.408 to 0.698) were significantly improved with the addition of BV. No new safety concerns were noted. Grade 3 or higher hypertension (17.4% v <1%) and proteinuria (8.5% v <1%) occurred more frequently in the BV arm. The rates of neutropenia and febrile neutropenia were similar in both arms. Two patients in the BV arm experienced GI perforation after study treatment discontinuation.

Conclusion.—GC plus BV followed by BV until progression resulted in a statistically significant improvement in PFS compared with GC plus PL in platinum-sensitive ROC.

▶ This article reports the results of a third phase III randomized trial evaluating bevacizumab in combination with chemotherapy in ovarian carcinoma. This study randomized patients with platinum-sensitive recurrent ovarian carcinoma to gemcitabine/carboplatin bevacizumab for 6 cycles followed by bevacizumab maintenance in the regimen containing bevacizumab. The primary endpoint of the trial was progression-free survival. Just as in the 2 frontline trials (Gynecologic Oncology Group study GOG218 and Gynecologic Cancer InterGroup study ICON7), the results show that the addition of bevacizumab followed by bevacizumab maintenance achieved a statistically significantly improved progression-free survival (hazard ratio = 0.484). This result is absolutely consistent with the results of the 2 frontline trials, which each showed an improved progression-free survival. None of the 3 trials show, as of yet, any improvement in overall survival. This is not surprising when one considers the large number of additional lines of therapy these patients receive when they relapse. In 2012 the American Society of Clinical Oncology initiated a fourth trial (Aurelia), this one in the platinum-resistant setting, also showing exactly the same thing: an improved progression-free survival with the addition of bevacizumab in the absence of an improved overall survival. We thus have 4 studies involving a total of over 4200 patients with ovarian carcinoma showing a consistent clinical benefit in the form of an improved progression-free survival with chemo/bevacizumab followed by maintenance bevacizumab. These data should be consistent to prompt the inclusion of bevacizumab in the treatment of these patients.

J. T. Thigpen, MD

Ovarian low-grade serous carcinoma: A comprehensive update
Diaz-Padilla I, Malpica AL, Minig L, et al (Univ of Toronto, Ontario, Canada; The Univ of Texas M.D. Anderson Cancer Ctr, Houston; Hosp Universitario Madrid, Spain; et al)
Gynecol Oncol 126:279-285, 2012

Ovarian low-grade serous ovarian carcinoma (OvLGSCa) comprises a minority within the heterogeneous group of ovarian carcinomas. Despite biological differences with their high-grade serous counterparts, current treatment guidelines do not distinguish between these two entities. OvLGSCas are characterized by an indolent clinical course. They usually develop from serous tumors of low malignant potential, although they can also arise *de novo*. When compared with patients with ovarian high grade serous carcinoma (OvHGSCa) patients with OvLGSCa are younger and have better survival outcomes. Current clinical and treatment data available for OvLGSCa come from retrospective studies, suggesting that optimal cytoreductive surgery remains the cornerstone in treatment, whereas chemotherapy has a limited role. Molecular studies have revealed the preponderance of the RAS—RAF—MAPK signaling pathway in the pathogenesis of OvLGSCa, thereby representing an attractive therapeutic target for patients affected by this disease. Improved clinical trial designs and international collaboration are required to optimally address the unmet medical treatment needs of patients affected by this disease.

▶ This article is a further discussion of the now-in-place 2-tiered system for grading serous carcinomas of the ovary. The authors discuss the molecular difference between the 2 categories of serous carcinomas as a basis for future trials with targeted agents, particularly in the low-grade group of cancers for which there are few systemic therapeutic options that appear to be effective. Some of these trials are already under way within the Gynecologic Oncology Group and in intergroup settings in the Gynecologic Cancer Intergroup. Because the majority (> 80%) of ovarian cancers entered into Gynecologic Oncology Group trials are high-grade serous carcinomas, there should be sufficient numbers of patients available for study to permit continued phase III trials evaluating the standard of care for these more common lesions. The studies of low-grade serous carcinomas will of necessity be primarily phase II studies because this population of patients is too small to permit phase III trials, but will serve as a basis for a more rational approach to the management of these cancers than simply lumping them in with the high-grade serous cancers.

J. T. Thigpen, MD

Reclassification of Serous Ovarian Carcinoma by a 2-Tier System: A Gynecologic Oncology Group Study
Bodurka DC, Deavers MT, Tian C, et al (The Univ of Texas MD Anderson Cancer Ctr, Houston; Roswell Park Cancer Inst, Buffalo, NY; et al)
Cancer 118:3087-3094, 2012

Background.—A study was undertaken to use the 2-tier system to reclassify the grade of serous ovarian tumors previously classified using the International Federation of Gynecology and Obstetrics (FIGO) 3-tier system and determine the progression-free survival (PFS) and overall survival (OS) of patients treated on Gynecologic Oncology Group (GOG) Protocol 158.

Methods.—The authors retrospectively reviewed demographic, pathologic, and survival data of 290 patients with stage III serous ovarian carcinoma treated with surgery and chemotherapy on GOG Protocol 158, a cooperative multicenter group trial. A blinded pathology review was performed by a panel of 6 gynecologic pathologists to verify histology and regrade tumors using the 2-tier system. The association of tumor grade with PFS and OS was assessed.

Results.—Of 241 cases, both systems demonstrated substantial agreement when combining FIGO grades 2 and 3 (overall agreement, 95%; kappa statistic, 0.68). By using the 2-tier system, patients with low-grade versus high-grade tumors had significantly longer PFS (45.0 vs 19.8 months, respectively; $P = .01$). By using FIGO criteria, median PFS for patients with grade 1, 2, and 3 tumors was 37.5, 19.8, and 20.1 months, respectively ($P = .07$). There was no difference in clinical outcome in patients with grade 2 or 3 tumors in multivariate analysis. Woman with high-grade versus low-grade tumors demonstrated significantly higher risk of death (hazard ratio, 2.43; 95% confidence interval, 1.17-5.04; $P = .02$).

Conclusions.—Women with high-grade versus low-grade serous carcinoma of the ovary are 2 distinct patient populations. Adoption of the 2-tier grading system provides a simple yet precise framework for predicting clinical outcomes.

▶ Serous ovarian carcinoma is by far the most common histology of epithelial ovarian carcinomas. These lesions account for more than 80% of patients entered into Gynecologic Oncology Group studies. The vast majority of these serous cancers are, under the current grading system, grade 2 or grade 3, with a small minority being classified as grade 1 lesions. The current report evaluates 241 cases of advanced stage serous carcinoma. Pertinent findings include the fact that only 6% were classified as grade 1, that these cases demonstrated a markedly superior progression-free survival, and that grade 2 and grade 3 cancers showed no difference in outcome. The investigators recommend that, based on these observations, patients with serous ovarian carcinomas be classified into a 2-tiered system of low-grade and high-grade cancers. Because the prognosis and the response to therapy differ substantially for the low-grade cancers, these should be studied in separate trials from the high-grade lesions. The Gynecologic Oncology Group has already acted on these recommendations and now pursues separate trials for the 2 groups.

J. T. Thigpen, MD

J. T. Thigpen, MD

20 Supportive Care

Impact of Awareness of Terminal Illness and Use of Palliative Care or Intensive Care Unit on the Survival of Terminally Ill Patients With Cancer: Prospective Cohort Study

Yun YH, Lee MK, Kim SY, et al (Natl Cancer Ctr, Gyeonggi-do, Korea)
J Clin Oncol 29:2474-2480, 2011

Purpose.—We conducted this study to evaluate the validity of the perception that awareness of their terminal prognosis and use of palliative care or nonuse of an intensive care unit (ICU) causes patients to die sooner than they would otherwise.

Patients and Methods.—In this prospective cohort study at 11 university hospitals and the National Cancer Center in Korea, we administered questionnaires to 619 consecutive patients immediately after they were determined by physicians to be terminally ill. We followed patients during 6 months after enrollment and assessed how their survival was affected by the disclosure of terminal illness and administration of palliative care or nonuse of the ICU.

Results.—In a follow-up of 481 patients and 163.8 person-years, we identified 466 deceased patients. Nineteen percent of the patients died within 1 month, while 41.3% lived for 3 months, and 17.7% lived for 6 months. Once the cancer was judged terminal, the median survival time was 69 days. On multivariate analysis, neither patient awareness of terminal status at baseline (adjusted hazard ratio [aHR], 1.20; 95% CI, 0.96 to 1.51), use of a palliative care facility (aHR, 0.96; 95% CI, 0.76 to 1.21), nor general prostration (aHR, 1.23; 95% CI, 0.96 to 1.57) was associated with reduced survival. Use of the ICU (aHR, 1.47; 95% CI, 1.06 to 2.05) and poor Eastern Cooperative Oncology Group performance status (aHR, 1.37; 95% CI, 1.10 to 1.71) were significantly associated with poor survival.

Conclusion.—Patients' being aware that they are dying and entering a palliative care facility or ICU does not seem to influence patients' survival.

▶ Oncologists are routinely presented with patients whose prognosis is poor and there are few if any reasonable treatment options left. Yet we struggle in our ability to verbalize this to patients, thinking that if we say "you are terminal; we have no other treatments to offer," it will hasten their demise. Slowly but surely more data are emerging to support this frank communication with our patients and the use of the palliative care option.

The data presented in this prospective cohort study are another example of the appropriate use of this ever-emerging field of medicine. Patients who are told they are terminal and have access to palliative care personnel do not die sooner, as shown in this study. In fact these and other data looking at the role of palliative care services show that not only do patients not die sooner, their quality of life can improve given appropriate palliative care. We as oncologists need to access this option sooner rather than later for our terminal patients and their families.

C. Lawton, MD

21 Thoracic Cancer

Impact on disease-free survival of adjuvant erlotinib or gefitinib in patients with resected lung adenocarcinomas that harbor EGFR mutations

Janjigian YY, Park BJ, Zakowski MF, et al (Weill Med College of Cornell Univ, NY)

J Thorac Oncol 6:569-575, 2011

Background.—Patients with stage IV lung adenocarcinoma and epidermal growth factor receptor (EGFR) mutation derive clinical benefit from treatment with EGFR tyrosine kinase inhibitors (TKIs). Whether treatment with TKI improves outcomes in patients with resected lung adenocarcinoma and EGFR mutation is unknown.

Methods.—Data were analyzed from a surgical database of patients with resected lung adenocarcinoma harboring EGFR exon 19 or 21 mutations. In a multivariate analysis, we evaluated the impact of treatment with adjuvant TKI.

Results.—The cohort consists of 167 patients with completely resected stages I to III lung adenocarcinoma. Ninety-three patients (56%) had exon 19 del, 74 patients (44%) had exon 21 mutations, and 56 patients (33%) received perioperative TKI. In a multivariate analysis controlling for sex, stage, type of surgery, and adjuvant platinum chemotherapy, the 2-year disease-free survival (DFS) was 89% for patients treated with adjuvant TKI compared with 72% in control group (hazard ratio $= 0.53$; 95% confidence interval: 0.28-1.03; $p = 0.06$). The 2-year overall survival was 96% with adjuvant EGFR TKI and 90% in the group that did not receive TKI (hazard ratio: 0.62; 95% confidence interval: 0.26-1.51; $p = 0.296$).

Conclusions.—Compared with patients who did not receive adjuvant TKI, we observed a trend toward improvement in DFS among individuals with resected stages I to III lung adenocarcinomas harboring mutations in EGFR exon 19 or 21 who received these agents as adjuvant therapy. Based on these data, 320 patients are needed for a randomized trial to prospectively validate this DFS benefit.

▶ This retrospective study conducted by the Memorial Sloan-Kettering Cancer Center evaluated stages I to III non–small-cell lung cancer (NSCLC) patients who had epidermal growth factor receptor (EGFR) mutations and analyzed the survival outcomes of these patients after adjuvant erlotinib for 2 years. In this analysis, patients with EGFR mutations were more likely to have a higher stage

(stage III) and they had a trend toward an improved progression-free survival (hazard ratio [HR] 0.53; $P = .06$). This stands in contrast to the prospective Canadian BR.19 trial, which reported a detrimental effect for disease-free survival (DFS) and overall survival (OS) for adjuvant gefitinib for 2 years. The Canadian BR.19 enrolled stage IB through stage IIIA NSCLC patients and randomized them after surgery to gefitinib versus placebo for 2 years (presented by American Society of Clinical Oncology 2010). Unfortunately, for the EGFR mutations patients, there was no benefit to receiving adjuvant gefitinib (HR 1.58) and a detrimental effect for DFS and OS was seen. This is consistent with the detrimental effect of adjuvant gefitinib after chemo-external radiation therapy on the Southwest Oncology Group's study SWOG-0023. There are 2 trials that are ongoing or pending analysis (SELECT and RADIANT), which are prospective studies with adjuvant erlotinib, and will hopefully clarify the role of adjuvant erlotinib in EGFR mutation patients. The Massachusetts General Hospital is conducting a phase II trial (SELECT) of 100 patients with EGFR mutation and determining the role of adjuvant erlotinib therapy. The RADIANT trial is for unselected NSCLC stages I through IIIA patients and gives them up to 2 years of erlotinib adjuvant therapy after resection with or without radiation therapy. This trial has completed accrual but has not released survival outcomes yet. For now, until further data are known, the clinical recommendation is to not give any adjuvant EGFR tyrosine kinase inhibitor in resected NSCLC patients who have EGFR mutations.

A. S. Tsao, MD

Prospective Molecular Marker Analyses of *EGFR* and *KRAS* From a Randomized, Placebo-Controlled Study of Erlotinib Maintenance Therapy in Advanced Non—Small-Cell Lung Cancer
Brugger W, Triller N, Blasinska-Morawiec M, et al (Univ of Freiburg, Germany; Clinic for Respiratory and Allergic Diseases, Golnik, Slovenia, Europe; Copernicus Memorial Hosp, Lodz, Poland, Europe; et al)
J Clin Oncol 29:4113-4120, 2011

Purpose.—The phase III, randomized, placebo-controlled Sequential Tarceva in Unresectable NSCLC (SATURN; BO18192) study found that erlotinib maintenance therapy extended progression-free survival (PFS) and overall survival in patients with advanced non—small-cell lung cancer (NSCLC) who had nonprogressive disease following first-line platinum-doublet chemotherapy. This study included prospective analysis of the prognostic and predictive value of several biomarkers.

Patients and Methods.—Mandatory diagnostic tumor specimens were collected before initiating first-line chemotherapy and were tested for epidermal growth factor receptor (EGFR) protein expression by using immunohistochemistry (IHC), *EGFR* gene copy number by using fluorescent in situ hybridization (FISH), and *EGFR* and *KRAS* mutations by using DNA sequencing. An *EGFR* CA simple sequence repeat in intron 1 (CA-SSR1) polymorphism was evaluated in blood.

Results.—All 889 randomly assigned patients provided tumor samples. EGFR IHC, *EGFR* FISH, *KRAS* mutation, and *EGFR* CA-SSR1 repeat length status were not predictive for erlotinib efficacy. A profound predictive effect on PFS of erlotinib relative to placebo was observed in the EGFR mutation—positive subgroup (hazard ratio [HR], 0.10; $P < .001$). Significant PFS benefits were also observed with erlotinib in the wild-type EGFR subgroup (HR, 0.78; $P = .0185$). *KRAS* mutation status was a significant negative prognostic factor for PFS.

Conclusion.—This large prospective biomarker study found that patients with activating *EGFR* mutations derive the greatest PFS benefit from erlotinib maintenance therapy. No other biomarkers were predictive for outcomes with erlotinib, although the study was not powered for clinical outcomes in biomarker subgroups. EGFR IHC—positive *KRAS* mutations were prognostic for reduced PFS. The study demonstrated the feasibility of prospective tissue collection for biomarker analyses in NSCLC.

▶ The Sequential Tarceva in Unresectable Non—Small Cell-Lung Cancer (NSCLC) (SATURN) trial was a phase III study comparing maintenance erlotinib to placebo after chemo-naive NSCLC patients were treated with a platinum doublet. Patients went on to receive maintenance erlotinib or placebo only if they did not progress after front-line doublet therapy. All patients were required to have tumor tissue biopsies, and the following biomarkers were assessed: epidermal growth factor receptor (EGFR) immunohistochemistry, EGFR fluorescent in situ hybridization, *EGFR* mutation, *KRAS* mutation, and EGFR CA simple sequence repeat in intron 1. The only biomarker with predictive benefit to maintenance erlotinib was the *EGFR* mutation (hazard ratio [HR] 0.10; $P < .001$). *KRAS* mutation was not predictive in any way for erlotinib, but was a prognostic factor for a worse progression-free survival for the entire group (HR 1.5; $P = .02$). The important aspects of this analysis are first, that patients with *EGFR*-sensitive mutations derive significant benefits from early treatment with EGFR tyrosine kinase inhibitors (TKIs). It is highly recommended to give these patients EGFR TKIs either frontline or as maintenance therapy. For quality-of-life purposes, I recommend treating these patients in the frontline setting if their *EGFR* mutation status is known. Second, patients who have wild-type EGFR still gain benefit from maintenance erlotinib (HR 0.81; $P = .0088$). Although the benefit is not as dramatic as that seen in the *EGFR* mutant population, the survival benefit is still significant for EGFR wild-type patients. Lastly, patients with *KRAS* mutations did not have a detrimental effect with the use of erlotinib. Although it did not reach statistical significance, patients with *KRAS* mutations had an HR of 0.77 with the addition of erlotinib maintenance. Taken together, patients who are reasonable candidates for maintenance therapy (regardless of biomarker status or histology) can be considered for switch maintenance. If a patient has a known sensitive *EGFR* mutation, they should receive EGFR TKIs as early as possible in therapy.

A. S. Tsao, MD

Longitudinal Perceptions of Prognosis and Goals of Therapy in Patients With Metastatic Non–Small-Cell Lung Cancer: Results of a Randomized Study of Early Palliative Care

Temel JS, Greer JA, Admane S, et al (Massachusetts General Hosp Cancer Ctr, Boston, MA; State Univ of New York, Buffalo; Yale Cancer Ctr, New Haven, CT)
J Clin Oncol 29:2319-2326, 2011

Purpose.—Understanding of prognosis among terminally ill patients impacts medical decision making. The aims of this study were to explore perceptions of prognosis and goals of therapy in patients with metastatic non–small-cell lung cancer (NSCLC) and to examine the effect of early palliative care on these views over time.

Patients and Methods.—Patients with newly diagnosed metastatic NSCLC were randomly assigned to receive either early palliative care integrated with standard oncology care or standard oncology care alone. Participants completed baseline and longitudinal assessments of their perceptions of prognosis and the goals of cancer therapy over a 6-month period.

Results.—We enrolled 151 participants on the study. Despite having terminal cancer, one third of patients (46 of 145 patients) reported that their cancer was curable at baseline, and a majority (86 of 124 patients) endorsed getting rid of all of the cancer as a goal of therapy. Baseline perceptions of prognosis (ie, curability) and goals of therapy did not differ significantly between study arms. A greater percentage of patients assigned to early palliative care retained or developed an accurate assessment of their prognosis over time (82.5% v 59.6%; $P = .02$) compared with those receiving standard care. Patients receiving early palliative care who reported an accurate perception of their prognosis were less likely to receive intravenous chemotherapy near the end of life (9.4% v 50%; $P = .02$).

Conclusion.—Many patients with newly diagnosed metastatic NSCLC hold inaccurate perceptions of their prognoses. Early palliative care significantly improves patient understanding of prognosis over time, which may impact decision making about care near the end of life.

► This study provides important confirmation of what we all know in the clinic: patients are less likely to choose aggressive end-of-life chemotherapy and additional treatment if they are well educated and accepting of their situation. However, busy clinicians rarely have the time to provide extended counseling and education during a clinic visit. The integration of palliative care specialists to work with patients on this specific issue is a luxury and arguably a financially sound investment in clinical oncology. End-of-life treatment decisions for more aggressive yet futile therapy are often the most significant financial burden for the patient, the patient's family, and health care institutions alike. For terminal oncology patients, this trial clearly shows the benefit of the early integration of palliative care. This trial is important as it is the first to document specific outcome measures and scientifically demonstrate that early palliative care can positively affect treatment decisions later.

A. S. Tsao, MD

Phase III Comparison of Prophylactic Cranial Irradiation Versus Observation in Patients With Locally Advanced Non–Small-Cell Lung Cancer: Primary Analysis of Radiation Therapy Oncology Group Study RTOG 0214

Gore EM, Bae K, Wong SJ, et al (Med College of Wisconsin, Milwaukee; Radiation Therapy Oncology Group, Philadelphia, PA; Thomas Jefferson Univ Hosp, Philadelphia, PA; et al)

J Clin Oncol 29:272-278, 2011

Purpose.—This study was conducted to determine if prophylactic cranial irradiation (PCI) improves survival in locally advanced non–small-cell lung cancer (LA-NSCLC).

Patients and Methods.—Patients with stage III NSCLC without disease progression after treatment with surgery and/or radiation therapy (RT) with or without chemotherapy were eligible. Participants were stratified by stage (IIIA *v* IIIB), histology (nonsquamous *v* squamous), and therapy (surgery *v* none) and were randomly assigned to PCI or observation. PCI was delivered to 30 Gy in 15 fractions. The primary end point of the study was overall survival (OS). Secondary end points were disease-free survival (DFS), neurocognitive function (NCF), and quality of life (QoL). Kaplan-Meier and log-rank analyses were used for OS and DFS. The incidence of brain metastasis (BM) was evaluated with the logistic regression model.

Results.—Overall, 356 patients were accrued of the targeted 1,058. The study was closed early because of slow accrual; 340 of the 356 patients were eligible. The 1-year OS ($P = .86$; 75.6% *v* 76.9% for PCI *v* observation) and 1-year DFS ($P = .11$; 56.4% *v* 51.2% for PCI *v* observation) were not significantly different. The hazard ratio for observation versus PCI was 1.03 (95% CI, 0.77 to 1.36). The 1-year rates of BM were significantly different ($P = .004$; 7.7% *v* 18.0% for PCI *v* observation). Patients in the observation arm were 2.52 times more likely to develop BM than those in the PCI arm (unadjusted odds ratio, 2.52; 95% CI, 1.32 to 4.80).

Conclusion.—In patients with stage III disease without progression of disease after therapy, PCI decreased the rate of BM but did not improve OS or DFS.

▶ Historically, locally advanced non–small-cell lung cancer was a devastating disease with dismal outcomes in terms of survival. Although we clearly need to advance the field of treatment for this disease, there have been improvements in surgery, radiation therapy, and chemotherapy that now result in median survivals of 3 years or more.

Surviving longer increases the risk of these patients for developing intracranial metastatic disease, which can be devastating to the patient's quality of life. Decreasing the risk of brain metastases, therefore, is an important endeavor for oncologists. To that end, the Radiation Therapy Oncology Group launched this trial in 2002 hoping to accrue over 1000 patients with stage III lung cancer without disease progression after surgery and/or radiation therapy chemotherapy.

Patients were randomized to prophylactic radiation therapy to the whole brain versus observation.

Unfortunately, the study did not accrue well, but 356 patients did enter the trial, of which the 340 eligible patients showed that the addition of prophylactic cranial irradiation (PCI) decreased the incidence of brain metastases statistically. Yet this change did not affect overall survival or disease-free survival. Patients who did not receive PCI had a 2.52-fold increase in the development of brain metastases. It is hard to believe that with longer follow-up, this trial will not reveal a survival benefit given the differences in development of brain metastases. Until that time though, these data do not support PCI in these patients. We look forward to a future analysis with longer follow-up to see whether improvement in survival endpoint is achieved.

C. Lawton, MD

Randomized Phase III Study of Thoracic Radiation in Combination With Paclitaxel and Carboplatin With or Without Thalidomide in Patients With Stage III Non–Small-Cell Lung Cancer: The ECOG 3598 Study

Hoang T, Dahlberg SE, Schiller JH, et al (Wisconsin Inst for Med Res, Madison)

J Clin Oncol 30:616-622, 2012

Purpose.—The primary objective of this study was to compare the survival of patients with unresectable stage III non–small-cell lung cancer (NSCLC) treated with combined chemoradiotherapy with or without thalidomide.

Patients and Methods.—Patients were randomly assigned to the control arm (PC) involving two cycles of induction paclitaxel 225 mg/m^2 and carboplatin area under the curve (AUC) 6 followed by 60 Gy thoracic radiation administered concurrently with weekly paclitaxel 45 mg/m^2 and carboplatin AUC 2, or to the experimental arm (TPC), receiving the same treatment in combination with thalidomide at a starting dose of 200 mg daily. The protocol allowed an increase in thalidomide dose up to 1,000 mg daily based on patient tolerability.

Results.—A total of 546 patients were eligible, including 275 in the PC arm and 271 in the TPC arm. Median overall survival, progression-free survival, and overall response rate were 15.3 months, 7.4 months, and 35.0%, respectively, for patients in the PC arm, in comparison with 16.0 months ($P = .99$), 7.8 months ($P = .96$), and 38.2% ($P = .47$), respectively, for patients in the TPC arm. Overall, there was higher incidence of grade 3 toxicities in patients treated with thalidomide. Several grade 3 or higher events were observed more often in the TPC arm, including thromboembolism, fatigue, depressed consciousness, dizziness, sensory neuropathy, tremor, constipation, dyspnea, hypoxia, hypokalemia, rash, and edema. Low-dose aspirin did not reduce the thromboembolic rate.

Conclusion.—The addition of thalidomide to chemoradiotherapy increased toxicities but did not improve survival in patients with locally advanced NSCLC.

▶ Thalidomide is an oral agent with antiangiogenic properties. E3598 was a randomized phase III trial comparing stage III non—small-cell lung cancer (NSCLC) patients receiving neoadjuvant chemotherapy then chemoradiation ± thalidomide. Patients received neoadjuvant carboplatin (area under the curve [AUC] 6) and paclitaxel (225 mg/m^2) for 2 cycles followed by weekly carboplatin (AUC 2) + paclitaxel (45 mg/m^2) with radiation. Half the patients received thalidomide (200 mg daily that was titrated up to 1000 mg daily) added to the chemoradiation and as maintenance therapy for 2 years. This trial showed no difference in response rate, progression-free survival, or overall survival and was stopped at the third interim analysis for futility. Patients who were on the thalidomide arm had more toxicities, especially thromboembolic events; 3 deaths occurred from thromboembolism before an amendment for prophylactic aspirin was put into place. Although no further deaths occurred, there was still an increase in thromboembolic events in the thalidomide arm (11% vs 3%, $P < .001$). This study clearly demonstrated that thalidomide does not have a role in combined modality therapy for stage III NSCLC.

A. S. Tsao, MD

Carboplatin- or Cisplatin-Based Chemotherapy in First-Line Treatment of Small-Cell Lung Cancer: The COCIS Meta-Analysis of Individual Patient Data

Rossi A, Di Maio M, Chiodini P, et al (S.G. Moscati Hosp, Avellino, Italy; Natl Cancer Inst, Naples, Italy; Second Univ, Naples, Italy; et al)
J Clin Oncol 30:1692-1698, 2012

Purpose.—Since treatment efficacy of cisplatin- or carboplatin-based chemotherapy in the first-line treatment of small-cell lung cancer (SCLC) remains contentious, a meta-analysis of individual patient data was performed to compare the two treatments.

Patients and Methods.—A systematic review identified randomized trials comparing cisplatin with carboplatin in the first-line treatment of SCLC. Individual patient data were obtained from coordinating centers of all eligible trials. The primary end point was overall survival (OS). All statistical analyses were stratified by trial. Secondary end points were progression-free survival (PFS), objective response rate (ORR), and treatment toxicity. OS and PFS curves were compared by using the log-rank test. ORR was compared by using the Mantel-Haenszel test.

Results.—Four eligible trials with 663 patients (328 assigned to cisplatin and 335 to carboplatin) were included in the analysis. Median OS was 9.6 months for cisplatin and 9.4 months for carboplatin (hazard ratio [HR], 1.08; 95% CI, 0.92 to 1.27; $P = .37$). There was no evidence of treatment difference between the cisplatin and carboplatin arms according to sex, stage, performance status, or age. Median PFS was 5.5 and 5.3 months for cisplatin and carboplatin, respectively (HR, 1.10; 95% CI, 0.94 to 1.29; $P = .25$). ORR was 67.1% and 66.0%, respectively (relative risk, 0.98; 95% CI, 0.84 to 1.16; $P = .83$). Toxicity profile was significantly different for each of the arms: hematologic toxicity was higher with carboplatin, and nonhematologic toxicity was higher with cisplatin.

Conclusion.—Our meta-analysis of individual patient data suggests no differences in efficacy between cisplatin and carboplatin in the first-line treatment of SCLC, but there are differences in the toxicity profile.

▶ This study was designed to duplicate the CISCA (cisplatin vs carboplatin) meta-analysis in non—small cell lung cancer (NSCLC), which demonstrated that cisplatin had an improved response rate and trend toward improved survival over carboplatin. The CISCA meta-analysis led to the recommendation in early stage NSCLC to use cisplatin-based regimens for any curative intent adjuvant or neoadjuvant or combined modality therapy if tolerated. This meta-analysis in SCLC (n = 663) showed no difference in clinical outcome between carboplatin and cisplatin in all SCLC patients. The subgroup analysis interestingly showed that while the limited-stage SCLC (who all received concurrent thoracic radiotherapy) had no difference in overall survival (OS), the extensive-stage SCLC patients had a nonstatistically significant trend toward improved OS with cisplatin ($P = .17$). Younger patients (younger than age 70) had an improved progression-free survival with cisplatin ($P = .005$). However, while this meta-analysis was well conducted, it has several limitations: (1) different dosages of platinum agents; (2) different schedules of agents given; (3) mixed limited- and extensive-stage SCLC patients with the confounding factor of radiotherapy in the limited-stage patients; and (4) the time frame (1987—2004) when these trials were conducted was not during the era of improved antiemetics. Also the numbers of limited-stage SCLC patients were small. So I would not change my clinical practice based on the results of this study; in limited-stage SCLC patients, I still prefer cisplatin-etoposide when proceeding with curative intent, and in extensive-stage SCLC, I choose the platinum agent based on comorbidities, performance status, and age but will still prefer cisplatin if it can be well tolerated.

A. S. Tsao, MD

PART FOUR

KIDNEY, WATER, AND ELECTROLYTES

RENEE GARRICK, MD

Introduction

The nephrology literature continues to focus our attention on the risks, incidence, progression, and mitigation of chronic kidney disease (CKD), on access to care, and on the need to clearly communicate the complex clinical issues of renal disease to our patients, other providers, and to payer groups.

Topical Summaries

CHRONIC KIDNEY DISEASE AND CLINICAL NEPHROLOGY

The selections regarding CKD and clinical nephrology begin with a focus on the methodology used to estimate glomerular filtration rate and the significance of those estimates as predictors of morbidity and mortality. Current data suggest that across a broad range of populations, the CKD-EPI equation, as compared with the MDRD equation, may more accurately categorize the risks for mortality and end-stage renal disease (ESRD). The ability to categorize mortality risk is emphasized by the observation of Perkins and colleagues who demonstrated that among patients with CKD, the change in eGFR over time adds important prognostic information to traditional mortality risk predictors. The next articles are drawn from The National Kidney Foundation's Kidney Early Evaluation Program (KEEP) and the African-American study of Kidney Disease and Hypertension (AASK) studies. The observations from the KEEP program demonstrate that despite the widespread attention now being focused on the incidence and significance of CKD, there are many barriers that prevent access to care among patients with CKD. The importance of this is reinforced by the findings of the Agrawal and colleagues, using additional data from KEEP. These investigators noted that despite the high prevalence of CKD and associated cardiovascular risk factors (hypertension, diabetes, and hypercholesterolemia) among KEEP participants, the control of cardiovascular risk factors was poor and only a small percentage of the patients had been seen by a nephrologist or other subspecialist. The findings of the KEEP program are made even more compelling when evaluated against the backdrop of the most recent findings of the AASK trial, which demonstrated that kidney function can improve in patients with hypertensive CKD. These findings teach us that a nihilistic approach to CKD and disease progression is not warranted and steps need to be taken to improve access to care for all individuals with CKD. The study by Wright Nunes is particularly interesting. It clearly demonstrates that among patients with CKD, there is a lack of concordance between patients' perceived knowledge and objective knowledge and their understanding and satisfaction with physician communication. This finding is particularly important. It is clear that the care of patients with CKD and associated comorbidities is complex. Patient education endeavors should be objectively assessed, and the link between these activities and patient compliance and outcomes should be scientifically measured.

The foregoing selections are especially interesting in light of the data by Baek and a separate article by O'Hare and colleagues, which demonstrate that the rate of progression of CKD is patient specific. Baek demonstrated approximately half of the patients with CKD stage III progressed to stage 4 to 5 over 10 years, and O'Hare demonstrated substantial heterogeneity of kidney loss and discovered at least 4 distinct trajectories of declining GFR. For resources to be most appropriately marshaled, it will be necessary to determine which patients are truly at risk for progression and to identify the factors that can be manipulated to modify the rate of disease progression. This theme is concluded with selections by Tangri and colleagues, who used routine laboratory tests to develop a predictive model for the progression of CKD to ESRD, and O'Seaghdha and colleagues, who used readily available clinical data to develop a risk score identifying those individuals in the general population at high risk for developing CKD.

This section is completed with articles which focused on 3 very common clinical scenarios in patients with kidney disease: renal cysts, hyperkalemia, and the risk of stroke in patients with atrial fibrillation and CKD.

MEDIATORS AND MODIFIERS OF RENAL DISEASE

Research this year continued to focus on potential mediators and modifiers of the progression of CKD. Interesting observations included the finding that dietary acid reduction with fruits and vegetables appears to attenuate kidney injury in patients with a moderate reduction in eGFR. Other investigators demonstrated that markers of inflammation can predict the long-term risk of developing CKD, and a separate group of investigators demonstrated that a high dietary fiber intake is associated with a reduction in inflammation and all-cause mortality in patients with CKD. Finally, elegant studies by Jelakovic and colleagues extended our understanding of endemic (Balkan) nephropathy and so-called Chinese-herbal nephropathy. Their impressive body of evidence clearly demonstrates that in genetically susceptible individuals, these seemingly disparate conditions and the associated upper tract urinary carcinomas are clearly related to dietary exposure to aristolochic acid, and are best referred to as aristolochic acid nephropathies.

DIABETIC NEPHROPATHY

The initial series of selections focus on the results of the Diabetes Complications and Control Trial regarding the effects of intensive diabetic therapy on the rate of decline of renal function in type I diabetics, on the failure of once-promising sulodexide in slowing the progression of type II diabetic nephropathy, and on predicting the progression of diabetic nephropathy. Niewczas and colleagues[1] demonstrated that in patients with type II diabetics with and without proteinuria, baseline circulating levels of TNF Receptors 1 and 2 can predict the progression to ESRD over a follow-up period of 12 years. In a similar investigation in patients with type I diabetes without proteinuria, the investigators demonstrated that the circulating levels of TNF receptor 1 and 2 measured at study entry were predictive of an early decline in renal function. The long-range predictive nature of these findings is particularly intriguing and raises the possibility that these markers of inflammation may factor in the decline in renal function. The study by Berhane and colleagues was performed in the Pima Indian population, where type II diabetes is almost endemic. The results demonstrated that the incorporating albuminuria data (defined as albumin to creatinine ratio), together with the eGFR, markedly strengthened the prognostic ability to predict the risk of advanced diabetic renal disease and death.

It is commonly believed that patients with underlying diabetic nephropathy and cardiovascular disease will die from their illness before they reach ESRD and dialysis. The study by Packham and colleagues was drawn from 2 prospective controlled trials that included over 3000 patients with type II diabetic nephropathy who were randomized to treatment with or without angiotensin receptor blockade. The results are quite important as they demonstrated that during a mean follow-up period of 3 years, type II diabetics with over 1 gram of protein spillage/day were actually more likely to reach ESRD than to die. Given the incidence and prevalence of type II diabetes, these findings certainly indicate that the clinical resources required for the care of these patients will need careful assessment.

ACUTE KIDNEY INJURY

An episode of acute kidney injury (AKI) has been shown to increase mortality risk (especially in the elderly) and the risk of developing CKD. Against this backdrop the public health impact of an episode of acute renal failure becomes readily apparent. The selections begin with a review of the current definitions and suggested classification systems for AKI, followed by a novel risk model to predict the 60-day mortality in critically ill patients with AKI. If this model proves to be widely applicable, it may help practitioners align clinical resources to those with greatest need. The next several selections focus on the role of urinary biomarkers in the diagnosis and treatment of AKI. A very interesting article by Heller and colleagues demonstrates that urinary calprotectin, in the absence of a urinary obstruction and infection, can accurately discriminate prerenal azotemia from acute intrinsic renal injury. If this noninvasive test stands the test of time, it will be extremely useful, as the predictive power of the currently available tests (such as the FeNa, Fe Urea, urine osmolality, etc) is not robust enough to provide a fail-safe approach to therapy.

Final selections focus on the importance of appropriate long-term follow-up of patients who have had an episode of AKI. This is especially true for patients with acute and chronic kidney injury, where an episode of AKI significantly increases the long-term risks of both dialysis and mortality as compared with patients without preexisting CKD. The data of Meier and colleagues from the tertiary care center in Lausanne, Switzerland, suggest that among noncritically ill patients with AKI, in-hospital mortality and renal outcomes may be improved by early referral to a nephrologist. In view of the personal and public health ramifications of kidney injury, these findings warrant additional study.

TRANSPLANTATION

This year's selections conclude with 2 articles on renal transplantation. Cantarovich and colleagues demonstrated that early changes in kidney function in patients who have received a liver transplant predict both long-term kidney disease and mortality. These findings are of obvious importance to both patients and practitioners. Hall and colleagues analyzed first-time renal transplant data drawn from the Scientific Registry of Transplant Recipients from 1995 to 2007. Their findings suggest that racial disparity in obtaining a living donor kidney transplant exists at every transplant center in the country. Although the explanations for this finding remain incomplete, the data make clear the need to fully examine the distinct patient-, donor-, and center-specific reasons for this disturbing finding.

R. Garrick, MD

Reference

1. Niewczas MA, Gohda T, Skupien J, et al. Circulating TNF receptors 1 and 2 predict ESRD in type 2 diabetes. *J Am Soc Nephrol.* 2012;23:507-515.

22 Chronic Kidney Disease and Clinical Nephrology

Comparison of Risk Prediction Using the CKD-EPI Equation and the MDRD Study Equation for Estimated Glomerular Filtration Rate

Matsushita K, for the Chronic Kidney Disease Prognosis Consortium (Johns Hopkins Univ, Baltimore, MD; et al)

JAMA 307:1941-1951, 2012

Context.—The Chronic Kidney Disease Epidemiology Collaboration (CKD-EPI) equation more accurately estimates glomerular filtration rate (GFR) than the Modification of Diet in Renal Disease (MDRD) Study equation using the same variables, especially at higher GFR, but definitive evidence of its risk implications in diverse settings is lacking.

Objective.—To evaluate risk implications of estimated GFR using the CKD-EPI equation compared with the MDRD Study equation in populations with a broad range of demographic and clinical characteristics.

Design, Setting, and Participants.—A meta-analysis of data from 1.1 million adults (aged ≥ 18 years) from 25 general population cohorts, 7 high-risk cohorts (of vascular disease), and 13 CKD cohorts. Data transfer and analyses were conducted between March 2011 and March 2012.

Main Outcome Measures.—All-cause mortality (84 482 deaths from 40 cohorts), cardiovascular mortality (22 176 events from 28 cohorts), and end-stage renal disease (ESRD) (7644 events from 21 cohorts) during 9.4 million person-years of follow-up; the median of mean follow-up time across cohorts was 7.4 years (interquartile range, 4.2-10.5 years).

Results.—Estimated GFR was classified into 6 categories (≥ 90, 60-89, 45-59, 30-44, 15-29, and < 15 mL/min/1.73 m^2) by both equations. Compared with the MDRD Study equation, 24.4% and 0.6% of participants from general population cohorts were reclassified to a higher and lower estimated GFR category, respectively, by the CKD-EPI equation, and the prevalence of CKD stages 3 to 5 (estimated GFR < 60 mL/min/1.73 m^2) was reduced from 8.7% to 6.3%. In estimated GFR of 45 to 59 mL/min/1.73 m^2 by the MDRD Study equation, 34.7% of participants were reclassified to estimated GFR of 60 to 89 mL/min/1.73 m^2 by the CKD-EPI equation and had lower incidence rates (per 1000 person-years) for the outcomes of interest (9.9 vs 34.5 for all-cause mortality, 2.7 vs 13.0 for cardiovascular mortality, and 0.5 vs 0.8 for ESRD) compared with those not reclassified. The corresponding adjusted hazard ratios were 0.80 (95% CI, 0.74-0.86) for all-cause mortality, 0.73 (95% CI, 0.65-0.82) for cardiovascular mortality, and 0.49 (95% CI, 0.27-0.88) for ESRD. Similar findings were observed in other estimated GFR categories by the MDRD Study equation. Net reclassification improvement based on estimated GFR categories was significantly positive for all outcomes (range, 0.06-0.13; all $P < .001$). Net reclassification improvement was similarly positive in most subgroups defined by age (< 65 years and ≥ 65 years), sex, race/ethnicity (white, Asian, and black), and presence or absence of diabetes and hypertension. The results in the high-risk and CKD cohorts were largely consistent with the general population cohorts.

Conclusion.—The CKD-EPI equation classified fewer individuals as having CKD and more accurately categorized the risk for mortality and ESRD than did the MDRD Study equation across a broad range of populations.

▶ Nephrologists and epidemiologists have been searching for ways to identify patients at risk for progression and death from chronic kidney disease (CKD). The Chronic Kidney Disease Epidemiology Collaboration (CKD-EPI) generated the CKD-EPI equation for estimating glomerular filtration rate (GFR). The meta-analysis presented here is drawn from data from 1.1 million patients from 25 population cohorts. Overall, the CKD-EPI equation classified fewer individuals as having CKD and more accurately categorized the risk for mortality and progression to dialysis than did the Modification of Diet in Renal Disease (MDRD)[1] equation.

For clinicians to better care for individual patients at risk for CKD and end-stage renal disease, and for health care planners to most appropriately marshal the resources needed for that care, it is necessary to first accurately identify those at greatest risk. During the past several years, a variety of biomarkers and comorbid conditions, both alone and in combination, have been evaluated to determine how to best identify individuals at risk for CKD progression. Estimated GFR is generally derived from the widely used MDRD equation, and eGFR-based, CKD stage-specific patient care management guidelines have been implemented. Accurate estimates, widely applicable over the wide range of GFR levels are important for patient and physician compliance with the guidelines and because these GFR determinations are used for other critical applications such as eligibility for life and health insurance. Accurate estimate equations are also useful in guiding clinicians as to when to obtain more detailed data, including more advanced biomarkers. The data from this extremely large meta-analysis suggest that the CKD-EPI equation is more robust than the widely used MDRD equation. Practitioners should become familiar with the use and application of the CKD-EPI equation because it is likely to become more generally applied in both research and clinical medicine.

R. Garrick, MD

Reference

1. Levey AS, Coresh J, Greene T, et al. Using standardized serum creatinine values in the modification of diet in renal disease study equation for estimating glomerular filtration rate. *Ann Intern Med.* 2006;145:247-254.

GFR Decline and Mortality Risk among Patients with Chronic Kidney Disease

Perkins RM, Bucaloiu ID, Kirchner HL, et al (Geisinger Med Ctr, Danville, PA)
Clin J Am Soc Nephrol 6:1879-1886, 2011

Background and Objectives.—Estimates of the effect of estimated GFR (eGFR) decline on mortality have focused on populations with normal kidney function, or have included limited information on factors previously shown to influence the risk of death among patients with CKD.

Design, Setting, Participants, & Measurements.—We retrospectively assessed the effect of rate of eGFR decline on survival of patients with CKD receiving primary care through a large integrated health care system in central Pennsylvania between January 1, 2004, and December 31, 2009.

Results.—A total of 15,465 patients were followed for a median of 3.4 years. Median rates of eGFR change by those in the lower, middle, and upper tertiles of eGFR slope were −4.8, −0.6, and 3.5 ml/min per 1.73 m^2/yr, respectively. In Cox proportional hazard modeling for time to death, adjusted for baseline proteinuria, changes in nutritional parameters, and episodes of acute kidney injury during follow-up (among other covariates), the hazard ratio for those in the lower (declining) and upper (increasing) eGFR tertiles (relative to the middle, or stable, tertile) was 1.84 and 1.42, respectively. Longitudinal changes in nutritional status as well as episodes of acute kidney injury attenuated the risk only modestly. These findings were consistent across subgroups.

Conclusions.—eGFR change over time adds prognostic information to traditional mortality risk predictors among patients with CKD. The utility of incorporating eGFR trends into patient-risk assessment should be further investigated.

▶ Impaired renal function has been clearly associated with adverse cardiovascular outcomes over time, especially in people with preexisting vascular disease.[1] However, the rate of decline in glomerular filtration rate (GFR) over time as an independent risk for adverse outcomes has only been demonstrated in a few retrospective studies.[2] For the most part, these studies were not structured to incorporate well-known prognostic parameters such as malnutrition, proteinuria, or acute kidney injury into their models. As a result, the true independent significance of declining renal function may not have been accurately demonstrated.

This study by Perkins et al retrospectively evaluated 15 000 subjects with complete medical records over a 5-year period for the rate of GFR decline as correlated with outcomes. They looked at 3 major tertiles of changing GFR. Specifically, they examined those with declining, stable, and improving renal function as determined by estimated GFR. The average rate of change in eGFR in millimeters per minute were −4.8, −0.6, and +3.5, respectively. They demonstrated an association between all-cause mortality and the tertiles of functional decline. Specifically, 34.7, 17.5, and 24 deaths per 1000 were noted in the respective groups. This association was demonstrated to be independent of other seemingly important parameters such as nutritional status, proteinuria, and diabetes. As can be seen, the third cohort with improving GFR surprisingly showed a higher hazard ratio for mortality than the stable group. Whether this was due to unrecognized acute kidney injury or decreasing creatinine from volume overload and/or loss of body mass was not evaluated. This trend was noted in the Matsushita data as well.[2]

This article nicely adds to our understanding about the effect of renal dysfunction on outcomes. An impaired estimated GFR portends a poor prognosis, but a rapidly declining estimated GFR worsens that prognosis, apparently independent of malnutrition, diabetes, or proteinuria. That an improving estimated GFR suggested a poorer prognosis is an interesting observation that requires further study.

M. Klein, MD

References

1. Weiner DE, Tighiouart H, Stark PC, et al. Kidney disease as a risk factor for recurrent cardiovascular disease and mortality. *Am J Kidney Dis.* 2004;44:198-206.
2. Matsushita K, Selvin E, Bash LD, Franceschini N, Astor BC, Coresh J. Change in estimated GFR associates with coronary heart disease and mortality. *J Am Soc Nephrol.* 2009;20:2617-2624.

Access to Health Care Among Adults Evaluated for CKD: Findings From the Kidney Early Evaluation Program (KEEP)
Agrawal V, on behalf of the KEEP Investigators (Fletcher Allen Health Care, Burlington, VT; et al)
Am J Kidney Dis 59:S5-S15, 2012

Background.—Data are scant regarding access to health care in patients with chronic kidney disease (CKD). We performed descriptive analyses using data from the National Kidney Foundation's Kidney Early Evaluation Program (KEEP), a nationwide health screening program for adults at high risk of CKD.

Methods.—From 2000-2010, a total of 122,502 adults without end-stage renal disease completed KEEP screenings; 27,927 (22.8%) met criteria for CKD (10,082, stages 1-2; 16,684, stage 3; and 1,161, stages 4-5). CKD awareness, self-rated health status, frequency of physician visits, difficulty obtaining medical care, types of caregivers, insurance status, and medication coverage and estimated costs were assessed.

Results.—Participants with CKD were more likely to report fair/poor health status than those without CKD. Health care utilization increased at later CKD stages; ∼95% of participants at stages 3-5 had visited a physician during the preceding year compared with 83.7% of participants without CKD. More Hispanic and African American than white participants at all CKD stages reported not having a physician. Approximately 40% of participants younger than 65 years reported fair/poor health status at stages 4-5 compared with ~30% who were 65 years and older. Younger participants at all stages were more likely to report extreme or somewhat/moderate difficulty obtaining medical care. Comorbid conditions (diabetes, hypertension, and prior cardiovascular events) were associated with increased utilization of care. Utilization of nephrology care was poor at all CKD stages; <6% of participants at stage 3 and <30% at stages 4-5 reported ever seeing a nephrologist.

Conclusions.—Lack of health insurance and perceived difficulty obtaining medical care with lower health care utilization, both of which are consistent with inadequate access to health care, are more likely for KEEP participants who are younger than 65 years, nonwhite, and without previously diagnosed comorbid conditions. Nephrology care is infrequent in elderly participants with advanced CKD who are nonwhite, have comorbid disease, and have high-risk states for cardiovascular disease (Table 3).

▶ Prior studies have demonstrated that reduced access to care is linked to a higher rate of end-stage renal disease in African American patients as compared to whites.[1,2] Additionally, a lack of health insurance has been reported as a risk factor for chronic kidney disease (CKD) progression.[3] It has been suggested that, in general, access to health care represents a significant obstacle. However, scant data are available regarding access to care in patients with CKD. This article is interesting because it evaluates over 122 000 adults of whom approximately 28 000 met the criteria for CKD stages. These data demonstrate that utilization of nephrology specialty care is poor at all levels of CKD. In fact, as shown in Table 3, only 34% of patients with albuminuria over 300 mg/g creatinine and an estimated glomerular filtration rate of less than 29 mL/min/1.73 m^2 were seen by a nephrologist. Comorbid conditions were associated with increased utilization of care, but even among patients with underlying diabetes, hypertension, or cardiovascular disease in conjunction with CKD, approximately 12% of patients reported it was extremely or moderately difficult to obtain access to care.

TABLE 3.—Nephrologist Care by eGFR and Albuminuria

| | ACR = 0-29 mg/g | | ACR = 30-299 mg/g | | ACR ≥300 mg/g | |
	No.	Nephrologist Care	No.	Nephrologist Care	No.	Nephrologist Care
eGFR						
≥90 mL/min/1.73 m^2	46,319	461 (1.0)	4,338	93 (2.1)	269	13 (4.8)
60-89 mL/min/1.73 m^2	48,256	720 (1.5)	5,043	133 (2.6)	432	26 (6.0)
45-59 mL/min/1.73 m^2	10,024	361 (3.6)	1,825	108 (5.9)	250	28 (11.2)
30-44 mL/min/1.73 m^2	3,213	298 (9.3)	1,108	144 (13.0)	264	41 (15.5)
<29 mL/min/1.73 m^2	438	82 (18.7)	431	135 (31.3)	292	100 (34.2)
Total	108,250	1,922 (1.8)	12,745	613 (4.8)	1,507	208 (13.8)

Note: Number of missing values in source of care, 14,474.
Abbreviations: ACR, albumin-creatinine ratio; eGFR, estimated glomerular filtration rate.

Participants with comorbid conditions were more likely to have seen a nephrologist than were those without concomitant comorbidities; but even among this group, less than 10% were under the routine care of nephrologists. Reduced access to care was most marked among the young, nonwhites, and those who lacked health insurance. Screening activities and earlier intervention related to blood pressure control, cardiovascular therapy, and diabetes may help slow the progression of CKD. This study clearly demonstrates that greater attention needs to be focused on access to health care among patients with CKD.

R. Garrick, MD

References

1. Perneger TV, Whelton PK, Klag MJ. Race and end-stage renal disease. Socioeconomic status and access to health care as mediating factors. *Arch Intern Med.* 1995;155:1201-1208.
2. Ward MM. Access to care and the incidence of end-stage renal disease due to diabetes. *Diabetes Care.* 2009;32:1032-1036.
3. Hall YN, Rodriguez RA, Boyko EJ, Chertow GM, O'Hare AM. Characteristics of uninsured Americans with chronic kidney disease. *J Gen Intern Med.* 2009;24: 917-922.

Physician Utilization, Risk-Factor Control, and CKD Progression Among Participants in the Kidney Early Evaluation Program (KEEP)

Jurkovitz CT, on behalf of the KEEP Investigators (Ctr for Outcomes Res, Newark, DE; et al)
Am J Kidney Dis 59:S24-S33, 2012

Background.—Chronic kidney disease (CKD) is a well-known risk factor for cardiovascular mortality, but little is known about the association between physician utilization and cardiovascular disease risk-factor control in patients with CKD. We used 2005-2010 data from the National Kidney Foundation's Kidney Early Evaluation Program (KEEP) to examine this association at first and subsequent screenings.

Methods.—Control of risk factors was defined as control of blood pressure, glycemia, and cholesterol levels. We used multinomial logistic regression to examine the association between participant characteristics and seeing a nephrologist after adjusting for kidney function and paired *t* tests or McNemar tests to compare characteristics at first and second screenings.

Results.—Of 90,009 participants, 61.3% had a primary care physician only, 2.9% had seen a nephrologist, and 15.3% had seen another specialist. The presence of 3 risk factors (hypertension, diabetes, and hypercholesterolemia) increased from 26.8% in participants with CKD stages 1-2 to 31.9% in those with stages 4-5. Target levels of all risk factors were achieved in 7.2% of participants without a physician, 8.3% of those with a primary care physician only, 9.9% of those with a nephrologist, and 10.3% of those with another specialist. Of up to 7,025 participants who met at least one criterion for nephrology consultation at first screening, only 12.3% reported seeing a nephrologist. Insurance coverage was associated strongly with seeing a nephrologist. Of participants who met criteria for nephrology consultation, 406 (5.8%) returned for a second screening, of whom 19.7% saw a nephrologist. The percentage of participants with all risk factors controlled was higher at the second screening (20.9% vs 13.3%).

Conclusion.—Control of cardiovascular risk factors is poor in the KEEP population. The percentage of participants seeing a nephrologist is low, although better after the first screening. Identifying communication barriers between nephrologists and primary care physicians may be a new focus for KEEP.

▶ The investigators of KEEP sought to evaluate the association between physician usage and the control of cardiovascular risk factors (hypertension, diabetes, and hypercholesterolemia) in patients with underlying chronic kidney disease (estimated glomerular filtration rate lower than 60 mL/min). This study is important because the incidence of chronic kidney disease (CKD) is clearly rising.[1] In addition, as demonstrated by other studies,[2] the education required to increase patient awareness and understanding of kidney disease and the associated comorbid risk factors, can be somewhat daunting. Moreover, despite the fact many,[3,4] but not all studies,[5] have suggested that timely referral to a nephrologist is associated with improved outcomes and delayed disease progression, the frequency and predictors of nephrology consultation remain incompletely characterized.

Approximately 90 000 patients eligible for this evaluation were enrolled in the KEEP database between 2005 and 2010. Of the 7025 participants meeting at least 1 criterion for nephrology referral, only 12.3% actually reported seeing a nephrologist. A potential contributing factor to this observation was the patient's health insurance. Of the patients who saw a nephrologist and returned for at least 1-second screening, the percentage of participants with all risk factors controlled was higher at the second screening follow-up visit.

The study limitations are common to any population-based registry. However, the KEEP data certainly suggest that, at least in this cohort of patients, control of cardiovascular risk factors in patients with underlying CKD is suboptimal. A better understanding of the issues that surround the care and referral of patients with CKD and related comorbid conditions is required. This will become even more important as new structures and payment systems (such as accountable care organizations) evolve for both primary care and specialty referrals.

R. Garrick, MD

References

1. United States Renal Data System: USRDS 2011 Atlas of CKD and ESRD: incidence, prevalence, patient characteristics and modalities. http://www.USDS.orb/Atlas.aspx. Accessed January 5, 2012.
2. Wright Nunes JA, Wallston KA, Eden SK, Shintani AK, Ikizler TA, Cavanaugh KL. Associations among perceived and objective disease knowledge and satisfaction with physician communication in patients with chronic kidney disease. *Kidney Int.* 2011;80:1344-1351.
3. Black C, Sharma P, Scotland G, et al. Early referral strategies for management of people with markers of renal disease: a systematic review of the evidence of clinical

effectiveness, cost-effectiveness and economic analysis. *Health Technol Assess.* 2010;14:1-184.
4. Chan MR, Dall AT, Fletcher KE, Lu N, Trivedi H. Outcomes in patients with chronic kidney disease referred late to nephrologists: a meta-analysis. *Am J Med.* 2007;120:1063-1070.
5. Winkelmayer WC, Liu J, Chertow GM, Tamura MK. Predialysis nephrology care of older patients approaching end-stage renal disease. *Arch Intern Med.* 2011;171: 1371-1378.

Kidney Function Can Improve in Patients with Hypertensive CKD

Hu B, for the African-American Study of Kidney Disease and Hypertension Group (Cleveland Clinic, OH; et al)
J Am Soc Nephrol 23:706-713, 2012

The typical assumption is that patients with CKD will have progressive nephropathy. Methodological issues, such as measurement error and regression to the mean, have made it difficult to document whether kidney function might improve in some patients. Here, we used data from 12 years of follow-up in the African American Study of Kidney Disease and Hypertension to determine whether some patients with CKD can experience a sustained improvement in GFR. We calculated estimated GFR (eGFR) based on serum creatinine measurements during both the trial and cohort phases. We defined clearly improved patients as those with positive eGFR slopes that we could not explain by random measurement variation under Bayesian mixed-effects models. Of 949 patients with at least three follow-up eGFR measurements, 31 (3.3%) demonstrated clearly positive eGFR slopes. The mean slope among these patients was +1.06 (0.12) ml/min per 1.73 m^2 per yr, compared with −2.45 (0.07) ml/min per 1.73 m^2 per yr among the remaining patients. During the trial phase, 24 (77%) of these 31 patients also had clearly positive slopes of ^{125}I-iothalamate−measured GFR during the trial phase. Low levels of proteinuria at baseline and randomization to the lower BP goal (mean arterial pressure ≤ 92 mmHg) associated with improved eGFR. In conclusion, the extended follow-up from this study provides strong evidence that kidney function can improve in some patients with hypertensive CKD.

▶ The African-American Study of Kidney Disease and Hypertension (AASK) trial[1] was a multicenter randomized clinical trial among African Americans aged 18 to 70 with a glomerular filtration rate (GFR) between 20 and 65 mL/min/1.73 m^2. The trial involved a 3-by-2 factorial design to 1 of 3 drug regimens (ramipril, amlodipine, metoprolol) and to 1 of 2 levels of blood pressure control: mean arterial pressure less than 92 mm Hg or 102 to 107 mm Hg. The study terminated in September 2001, and 691 enrolled in the cohort study for an additional 5 years. This study represents the 12-year follow-up data drawn from both the trial and the cohort phase (941 patients had at least 3 follow-up estimated GFR determinations) and is aimed at determining whether renal function can improve in some patients or if renal disease progression is universal, as is typically believed. As shown in Fig 2 in the original article, a positive slope represents an improved estimated GFR and using a Bayesian probability model: 31 patients (3.3%) had a 95% probability of having a positive slope and 94 patients (10%) had a probability of at least 50% of having a positive slope.

A weakness of the study is that serum creatinine rather than histological parameters or direct measurements of GFR was used to estimate the improvement in renal function. The authors did control for changes in body weight over time, which could have affected serum creatinine levels independently of a change in renal function.

Baseline urinary protein excretion (measured by spot time collections and by urinary protein-to-creatinine ratio) was lower in those who improved, and more patients with improved renal function were assigned to the low blood pressure group. It must be noted that this is a *post hoc* analysis, and these findings should not be overinterpreted as meaning that lower blood pressures should be targeted as a way of improving renal function in hypertensive patients with low levels of proteinuria. That will require additional study in an appropriately selected cohort. Overall, however, the results are encouraging as they do suggest that, at least in some patients with hypertensive chronic kidney disease, renal function can not only stabilize but even improve.

R. Garrick, MD

Reference

1. Agodoa LY, Appel L, Bakris GL, et al; African American Study of Kidney Disease and Hypertension (AASK) Study Group. Effect of ramipril vs amlodipine on renal outcomes in hypertensive nephrosclerosis: a randomized controlled trial. *JAMA.* 2001;285:2719-2728.

Associations among perceived and objective disease knowledge and satisfaction with physician communication in patients with chronic kidney disease
Wright Nunes JA, Wallston KA, Eden SK, et al (Vanderbilt Univ Med Ctr, Nashville, TN)
Kidney Int 80:1344-1351, 2011

It is likely that patients with chronic kidney disease (CKD) have a limited understanding of their illness. Here we studied the relationships between objective and perceived knowledge in CKD using the Kidney Disease Knowledge Survey and the Perceived Kidney Disease Knowledge Survey. We quantified perceived and objective knowledge in 399 patients at all stages of non-dialysis-dependent CKD. Demographically, the patient median age was 58 years, 47% were women, 77% had stages 3—5 CKD, and 83% were Caucasians. The overall median score of the perceived knowledge survey was 2.56 (range: 1—4), and this new measure exhibited excellent reliability and construct validity. In unadjusted analysis, perceived knowledge was associated with patient characteristics defined a *priori*, including objective knowledge and patient satisfaction with physician communication. In adjusted analysis, older age, male gender, and limited health literacy were associated with lower perceived knowledge. Additional analysis revealed that perceived knowledge was associated with significantly higher odds (2.13), and objective knowledge with lower odds (0.91), of patient satisfaction with physician communication. Thus, our results present a mechanism to evaluate distinct forms of patient kidney knowledge and identify specific opportunities for education tailored to patients with CKD (Table 2).

▶ These are very interesting data. Kidney disease is common and complex.

The authors designed this cross-sectional study to measure patients' perceptions of their knowledge (perceived knowledge), their objective disease knowledge, and their satisfaction with provider communication. The study was conducted at a single academic medical center and included patients 18 years of age and older with chronic kidney disease (CKD)[1-5] (pre−end-stage renal disease population) as defined by the National Kidney Foundation Disease Outcome Quality Initiative (NKF-KDOQI) guidelines.[1] Objective knowledge was assessed using a kidney disease knowledge survey that was previously validated.[2] Perceived knowledge was assessed with a 9-question tool (Table 2), which was validated for internal consistency and reliability.

Interestingly, the data showed a correlation of 0.32 between perceived and objective knowledge among the patients being followed up for their renal disease. Surprisingly, higher objective knowledge scores were associated with lower odds of satisfaction with provider communication. What do these data tell us? Patients who have a mismatch between their perceived knowledge and objective (actual) knowledge are both educationally and clinically challenging. For example, patients who perceive their knowledge base as robust may portray this to the physician when in fact, their objective knowledge is actually insufficient. In this case, the nephrologist could fail to adequately educate the patient, who then in turn may make incorrect self-management decisions. The data also demonstrate that in some clinically crucial areas (especially those related to diet, medications, and disease symptoms), even perceived knowledge is distressingly low.

Previous studies have found that renal disease education is often challenging for both physicians and patients.[3-5] Taken together, these findings suggest that

TABLE 2.—Perceived Kidney Knowledge Survey Item Responses

Perceived Kidney Knowledge Survey Item	N	n (%) of Patients Reporting Little or No Knowledge
Knowledge of medications that help the kidney	396	285 (72%)
Knowledge of medications that can hurt the kidney	396	248 (63%)
Knowledge of foods to avoid if kidney function is low	396	240 (61%)
Knowledge of blood pressure goal	393	89 (23%)
Knowledge of treatment options if kidney function gets worse	393	193 (49%)
Knowledge of symptoms of chronic kidney disease	395	240 (61%)
Knowledge of how kidney function is checked	396	144 (36%)
Knowledge of the functions of the kidney	398	201 (51%)
Knowledge of why patient was sent to a kidney doctor	398	96 (25%)

N indicates the number of nonmissing values.

for this paradigm to shift, physicians should be assessing patients' perceived and objective knowledge both before and after educational interventions occur. Such data would allow physicians to more fully appreciate each patient's actual baseline and then appropriately individualize educational interventions. This study was performed in a single clinic with a fairly homogeneous population of patients and it should be replicated in other populations. Additionally, as the authors note, the next step will be to assess whether improvements in patients' perceived and objective knowledge base are linked to improved clinical outcomes.

R. Garrick, MD

References

1. KDOQI. KDOQI clinical practice guidelines and clinical practice recommendations for diabetes and chronic kidney disease. *Am J Kidney Dis*. 2007;49:S12-S154.
2. Wright JA, Wallston K, Elasy TA, Ikizler TA, Cavanaugh KL. Development and results of a kidney disease knowledge survey given to patients with CKD. *Am J Kidney Dis*. 2011;57:387-395.
3. Plantinga LC, Tuot DS, Powe NR. Awareness of chronic kidney disease among patients and providers. *Adv Chronic Kidney Dis*. 2010;17:225-236.
4. Schatell D, Ellstrom-Calder A, Alt PS, Garland JS. Survey of CKD patients reveals significant GAPS in knowledge about kidney disease. Part 1. *Nephrol News Issues*. 2003;17:23-26.
5. Schatell D, Ellstrom-Calder A, Alt PS, Garland JS. Survey of CKD patients reveals significant gaps in knowledge about kidney disease. Part 2. *Nephrol News Issues*. 2003;17:17-19.

Does stage III chronic kidney disease always progress to end-stage renal disease? A ten-year follow-up study
Baek SD, Baek CH, Kim JS, et al (Univ of Ulsan, Seoul, South Korea)
Scand J Urol Nephrol 46:232-238, 2012

Objective.—Clinically, it may be appropriate to subdivide patients with stage 3 chronic kidney disease (CKD) into two subgroups, as they show different risks for kidney outcomes. This study evaluated the proportion of patients with stage 3 CKD who progressed to stage 4 or 5 CKD over 10 years and independent predictors of progression of renal dysfunction. It sought to validate whether stage 3 CKD patients should be subdivided.

Material and Methods.—This retrospective cohort study enrolled 347 stage 3 CKD patients between January 1997 and December 1999, who were followed up through June 2010. The baseline clinical characteristics and outcomes were compared in patients with stage 3A [45 <estimated glomerular filtration rate (eGFR) <60 ml/min/1.73 m^2] and stage 3B (30 < eGFR < 45 ml/min/1.73 m^2) CKD.

Results.—Of the 347 patients, 196 (58.2%) were in stage 3A. The only difference in baseline characteristics between stages 3A and 3B patients was the degree of albuminuria. During follow-up, 167 patients (48.1%) did not progress, 60 (17.3%) progressed to stage 4 and 120 (34.6%) progressed to stage 5, with 91 (26.2%) starting dialysis. Multivariate Cox regression analysis showed that macroalbuminuria [(hazard ratio (HR) 3.06, 95% confidence interval (CI) 1.48−2.89, $p < 0.001$], microalbuminuria (HR 1.99 95% CI 1.04−3.85, $p = 0.038$), microscopic haematuria (HR 2.07 95% CI 1.48−2.89, $p < 0.001$) and stage 3B CKD (HR 2.99 95% CI 2.19−4.10, $p < 0.001$) were independent predictors of progression of renal dysfunction. Stage 3B patients had higher risks of adverse renal and cardiovascular outcomes than stage 3A patients.

Conclusions.—About half of the patients with stage 3 CKD progressed to stage 4 or 5, as assessed by eGFR, over 10 years. Degree of albuminuria, stage 3 subgroup and microscopic haematuria were important risk factors for progression of stage 3 CKD. It would be appropriate to divide the present stage 3 CKD into two subgroups (Fig 1).

▶ As previously suggested,[1] chronic kidney disease (CKD) comprises a very heterogeneous population of patients. In addition, estimated glomerular filtration rate (eGFR), as calculated by the Modification of Diet in Renal Disease[2] equation, may overestimate the population of patients with progressive renal disease. These authors performed a retrospective cohort study on 347 patients classified with stage 3 (as defined by the staging criteria of the National Kidney Foundation[3]) for a mean of 11.8 years. Patients with evidence of acute flares of chronic disease or interceding episodes of acute renal failure were excluded from analysis. The primary outcome endpoint was progression of renal dysfunction to stage 4 or 5 CKD, and secondary outcomes included deaths, cardiovascular events, and initiation of dialysis. CKD stage 3A patients had an eGFR between 45 and 59, whereas stage 3B patients had an eGFR between 30 and 45 mL/min/1.73 m^2.

At the end of 10 years, approximately 48% of the patients had maintained or improved renal function and close to 52% of the patients with stage 3 CKD had progressed to stage 4 or 5, with 26% beginning dialysis. Multivariate analysis demonstrated that the presence of albuminuria, microscopic hematuria, and

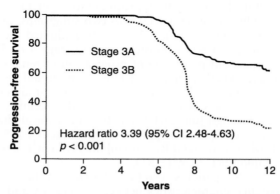

FIGURE 1.—Progression-free survival in groups of patients with stage 3A and 3B chronic kidney disease at baseline. (Reprinted from Baek SD, Baek CH, Kim JS, et al. Does stage III chronic kidney disease always progress to end-stage renal disease? A ten-year follow-up study. *Scand J Urol Nephrol.* 2012;46:232-238, reprinted by permission of the publisher (Taylor & Francis Ltd, http://www.tandf.co. uk/journals).)

CKD stage 3B at initiation were independent predictors of progression of renal dysfunction. Univariant analysis demonstrated that a low hemoglobin and hyperphosphatemia were also suggestive of risk progression. Fig 1 demonstrates 2 fairly distinct populations and rates of progression in patients with stage 3 CKD.

One weakness of the study is its size and another is that the treatment effects of various medications could not be assessed. However, these findings are reminiscent of those of O'Hare et al,[1] which demonstrated diverse cohorts of CKD patients, and Packham et al,[4] who demonstrated that patients with diabetes and proteinuria were more likely to progress to dialysis than to succumb to cardiovascular disease.

The results are important from the perspective of clinical research since the diverse population of patients with CKD should be taken into account when studies are planned and outcomes evaluated. From the clinical care perspective, the results reinforce the concept that clinicians need to be particularly cautious about making global predictions regarding the likelihood of progression for their patients with stage 3 CKD. The findings regarding specific risk factors for progression (eg, proteinuria, hematuria, hyperphosphatemia, etc) may help clinicians focus their attention and resources more specifically on those patients with stage 3 CKD who are more likely to progress.

R. Garrick, MD

References

1. O'Hare AM, Batten A, Burrows NR, et al. Trajectories of kidney function decline in the 2 years before initiation of long-term dialysis. *Am J Kidney Dis*. 2012;59: 513-522.
2. Levey AS, Bosch JP, Lewis JB, Greene T, Rogers N, Roth D. A more accurate method to estimate glomerular filtration rate from serum creatinine: a new prediction equation. Modification of Diet in Renal Disease Study Group. *Ann Intern Med*. 1999;130:461-470.
3. National Kidney Foundation. K/DOQI clinical practice guidelines for chronic kidney disease: evaluation, classification, and stratification. *Am J Kidney Dis*. 2002;39:S1-S266.
4. Packham DK, Alves TP, Dwyer JP, et al. Relative incidence of ESRD versus cardiovascular mortality in proteinuric type 2 diabetes and nephropathy: results from the DIAMETRIC (Diabetes Mellitus Treatment for Renal Insufficiency Consortium) database. *Am J Kidney Dis*. 2012;59:75-83.

Trajectories of Kidney Function Decline in the 2 Years Before Initiation of Long-term Dialysis
O'Hare AM, Batten A, Burrows NR, et al (VA Puget Sound Healthcare System and Univ of Washington, Seattle; VA Puget Sound Healthcare System, Seattle, WA; Ctrs for Disease Control and Prevention, Atlanta, GA; et al)
Am J Kidney Dis 59:513-522, 2012

Background.—Little is known about patterns of kidney function decline leading up to the initiation of long-term dialysis.
Study Design.—Retrospective cohort study.

Setting & Participants.—5,606 Veterans Affairs patients who initiated long-term dialysis in 2001-2003.

Predictor.—Trajectory of estimated glomerular filtration rate (eGFR) during the 2-year period before initiation of long-term dialysis.

Outcomes & Measurements.—Patient characteristics and care practices before and at the time of dialysis initiation and survival after initiation.

Results.—We identified 4 distinct trajectories of eGFR during the 2-year period before dialysis initiation: 62.8% of patients had persistently low level of eGFR < 30 mL/min/1.73 m^2 (mean eGFR slope, 7.7 ± 4.7 [SD] mL/min/1.73 m^2 per year), 24.6% had progressive loss of eGFR from levels of approximately 30-59 ml/min/1.73 m^2 (mean eGFR slope, 16.3 ± 7.6 mL/min/1.73 m^2 per year), 9.5% had accelerated loss of eGFR from levels > 60 mL/min/1.73 m^2 (mean eGFR slope, 32.3 ± 13.4 mL/min/1.73 m^2 per year), and 3.1% experienced catastrophic loss of eGFR from levels > 60 mL/min/1.73 m^2 within 6 months or less. Patients with steeper eGFR trajectories were more likely to have been hospitalized and have an inpatient diagnosis of acute kidney injury. They were less likely to have received recommended predialysis care and had a higher risk of death in the first year after dialysis initiation.

Conclusions.—There is substantial heterogeneity in patterns of kidney function loss leading up to the initiation of long-term dialysis perhaps

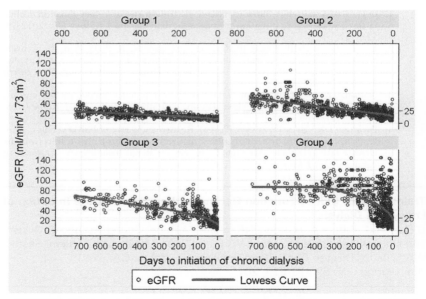

FIGURE 2.—Scatterplots of all estimated glomerular filtration rate (eGFR) measurements during the 2-year period before dialysis initiation for 25 randomly selected members of each trajectory group. (Reprinted from American Journal of Kidney Diseases, O'Hare AM, Batten A, Burrows NR, et al. Trajectories of kidney function decline in the 2 years before initiation of long-term dialysis. *Am J Kidney Dis.* 2012;59:513-522. Copyright 2012 with permission from the National Kidney Foundation.)

TABLE 1.—Information for Kidney Function During the 2-Year Period Before Initiation of Long-term Dialysis

Parameter	All Patients (n = 5,606)	Trajectory Group			
		Persistently Low eGFR (Group 1, n = 3,520)	Progressive eGFR Loss (Group 2, n = 1,379)	Accelerated eGFR Loss (Group 3, n = 535)	Catastrophic eGFR Loss (Group 4, n = 172)
eGFR slope[a]	10.0 (5.8, 16.6)	7.2 (4.5, 10.5)	16.0 (11.6, 20.9)	31.7 (23.8, 40.2)	47.7 (29.1, 64.6)
eGFR slope[a]	13.5 ± 13.1	7.8 ± 4.7	16.3 ± 7.6	32.3 ± 13.4	50.7 ± 30.4
SCr measures, median[b]					
All	20 (12, 34)	18 (12, 30)	24 (11, 46)	24 (12, 44)	25 (8, 42)
Outpatient	12 (7, 18)	13 (7, 19)	8 (5, 14)	6 (3, 10)	6 (3, 10)
Inpatient	6 (0, 17)	4 (0, 12)	9 (1, 23)	14 (3, 32)	15 (2, 33)
Quarters with ≥1SCr measure[b]	5.4 ± 2	5.6 ± 2.1	5.5 ± 1.8	4.8 ± 1.8	4.1 ± 1.9

Note: Values shown are median (25th, 75th percentile) or mean ± standard deviation.
Abbreviations: SCr, serum creatinine; eGFR estimated glomerular filtration rate.
[a]Based on all inpatient and outpatient SCr measurements during the 2-year period before dialysis initiation.
[b]During the 2-year period (8 quarters) before dialysis initiation.

calling for a more flexible approach toward preparing for end-stage renal disease (Fig 2, Table 1).

▶ Using a robust Veterans Affairs data system, O'Hare and colleagues report the trajectory to end-stage renal disease on more than 5000 individuals who started dialysis between 2001 and 2003 and had at least 2 years of data available. This is the first time such comprehensive data tracking the entry to end-stage renal disease have been studied. As shown in Table 1 and Fig 2, patients could be divided into 4 groups with distinct trajectories. Groups 1 and 2 are of particular interest. In patients in group 1 (persistently low estimated glomerular filtration rate [eGFR]), the time between an eGFR of less than 20 mL/min/1.73 m^2 (the point at which patients can accrue time on the transplant list and fistula should be placed), and the initiation of dialysis was approximately 18 months. For patients in group 2 (progressive loss of eGFR), the time between an eGFR of less than 20 mL/min/1.73 m^2 and the initiation dialysis was 6 months.

The Veterans database obviously has some limitations. The data cannot be easily generalized to all patients (woman are very underrepresented), the comorbidities affecting the renal trajectory may be incomplete, and the data, of course, have survivor bias. This effect is important, as many patients die from comorbid events before reaching dialysis. This fact makes the timing of interventions (such as fistula placement) even more difficult, especially in patients with a slow eGFR trajectory (group 1).

These trajectory data are the first of their kind and are extremely important, as they demonstrate that there is a great deal of variability and clinical heterogeneity among these patients. Of concern is the finding that 32% of patients in group 2 (progressive loss of GFR) were not seen by a nephrologist in the 2-year period before dialysis initiation. This is of special concern in view of their trajectory to renal replacement therapy and the need to plan appropriate therapeutic interventions, such as fistula placement, for example, where all available data suggest that initiation of dialysis with a fistula rather than a temporary catheter significantly improves mortality, especially within the first 90 days of dialysis therapy.[1] The ability to predict which patients are in which cohort requires careful assessment and critical interpretation of serial clinical findings and laboratory data. Substantial clinical skill, flexibility, and experience are clearly required to appropriately guide patients though these uncharted waters.

R. Garrick, MD

Reference

1. Al-Aly Z, Zeringue A, Fu J, et al. Rate of kidney function decline associates with mortality. *J Am Soc Nephrol.* 2010;21:1961-1969.

A Predictive Model for Progression of Chronic Kidney Disease to Kidney Failure

Tangri N, Stevens LA, Griffith J, et al (Tufts Med Ctr, Boston, MA; et al)
JAMA 305:1553-1559, 2011

Context.—Chronic kidney disease (CKD) is common. Kidney disease severity can be classified by estimated glomerular filtration rate (GFR) and albuminuria, but more accurate information regarding risk for progression to kidney failure is required for clinical decisions about testing, treatment, and referral.

Objective.—To develop and validate predictive models for progression of CKD.

Design, Setting, and Participants.—Development and validation of prediction models using demographic, clinical, and laboratory data from 2 independent Canadian cohorts of patients with CKD stages 3 to 5 (estimated GFR, 10-59 mL/min/1.73 m^2) who were referred to nephrologists between April 1, 2001, and December 31, 2008. Models were developed using Cox proportional hazards regression methods and evaluated using C statistics and integrated discrimination improvement for discrimination, calibration plots and Akaike Information Criterion for goodness of fit, and net reclassification improvement (NRI) at 1, 3, and 5 years.

Main Outcome Measure.—Kidney failure, defined as need for dialysis or preemptive kidney transplantation.

Results.—The development and validation cohorts included 3449 patients (386 with kidney failure [11%]) and 4942 patients (1177 with kidney failure [24%]), respectively. The most accurate model included age, sex, estimated GFR, albuminuria, serum calcium, serum phosphate, serum bicarbonate, and serum albumin (C statistic, 0.917; 95% confidence interval [CI], 0.901-0.933 in the development cohort and 0.841; 95% CI, 0.825-0.857 in the validation cohort). In the validation cohort, this model was more accurate than a simpler model that included age, sex, estimated GFR, and albuminuria (integrated discrimination improvement, 3.2%; 95% CI, 2.4%-4.2%; calibration [Nam and D'Agostino χ^2 statistic, 19 vs 32]; and reclassification for CKD stage 3 [NRI, 8.0%; 95% CI, 2.1%-13.9%] and for CKD stage 4 [NRI, 4.1%; 95% CI, −0.5% to 8.8%]).

Conclusion.—A model using routinely obtained laboratory tests can accurately predict progression to kidney failure in patients with CKD stages 3 to 5.

► O'Seaghdha and colleagues[1] have developed a risk score to estimate an individual's absolute incident risk of developing chronic kidney disease (CKD). Packham and colleagues[2] and O'Hare and colleagues[3] have data to suggest that patients with CKD are a very heterogeneous population, and that rate of progression is quite different among various cohorts of patients with CKD.[3] The findings of Packham et al[2] suggest that many patients with combined diabetes and cardiac disease will in fact advance to dialysis rather than succumbing to a comorbid condition. Within this context, the analysis of Tangri and colleagues is particularly appealing. These investigators have developed a predictive model for the progression of CKD to kidney failure. The utility of such a model is obvious, and it is especially attractive in its simplicity, as it uses laboratory tests (phosphorous, bicarbonate, calcium, albumin), obtained as part of routine care to predict progression to dialysis in patients with CKD 3 and beyond.

The need for clinicians to be able to reliably predict which patients will progress and therefore require additional procedures and preparation (eg, vascular access placement) versus those patients less likely to progress is readily apparent. The current study presents a statistically validated risk-prediction model for progression to kidney failure among patients with moderate to severe CKD.

The model was developed using cohorts from British Columbia and Toronto and, of course, will need to be confirmed in other more heterogeneous populations of CKD patients. In addition, the model may be strengthened by including modeling for mortality, along with the modeling for progression to renal replacement therapy. The details computerized application are available online.[4]

R. Garrick, MD

References

1. O'Seaghdha CM, Lyass A, Massaro JM, et al. A risk score for chronic kidney disease in the general population. *Am J Med*. 2012;125:270-277.
2. Packham DK, Alves TP, Dwyer JP. Relative incidence of ESRD versus cardiovascular mortality in proteinuric type 2 diabetes and nephropathy: results from the diametric (diabetes mellitus treatment for renal insufficiency consortium) database. *Am J Kidney Dis*. 2012;59:75-83.
3. O'Hare AM, Batten A, Burrows NR. Trajectories of kidney function decline in the 2 years before initiation of long-term dialysis. *Am J Kidney Dis*. 2012;59:513-522.
4. QxMD. Kidney failure risk equation. *American Medical Association*. http://www.qxmd.com/calculate-online/nephrology/kidney-failure-risk-equation. Accessed September 27, 2012.

A Risk Score for Chronic Kidney Disease in the General Population

O'Seaghdha CM, Lyass A, Massaro JM, et al (Natl Heart, Lung and Blood Inst's Framingham Heart Study, MA; Boston Univ, MA; Boston Univ School of Public Health, MA; et al)
Am J Med 125:270-277, 2012

Background.—Stratification of individuals at risk for chronic kidney disease may allow optimization of preventive measures to reduce disease incidence and complications. We sought to develop a risk score that estimates an individual's absolute risk of incident chronic kidney disease.

Methods.—Framingham Heart Study participants free of baseline chronic kidney disease, who attended a baseline examination in 1995-1998 and follow-up in 2005-2008, were included in the analysis (n = 2490). Chronic kidney disease was defined as an estimated glomerular filtration rate < 60 mL/min/1.73 m^2 using the Modification of Diet in Renal Disease equation. Participants were assessed for the development of chronic kidney disease at 10 years follow-up. Stepwise logistic regression was used to identify chronic kidney disease risk factors, and these were used to construct a risk score predicting 10-year chronic kidney disease risk. Performance characteristics were assessed using calibration and discrimination measures. The final model was externally validated in the bi-ethnic Atherosclerosis Risk in Communities Study (n = 1777).

Results.—There were 1171 men and 1319 women at baseline, and the mean age was 57.1 years. At follow-up, 9.2% (n = 229) had developed chronic kidney disease. Age, diabetes, hypertension, baseline estimated glomerular filtration rate, and albuminuria were independently associated with incident chronic kidney disease (*P* <.05), and these covariates were incorporated into a risk function (c-statistic 0.813). In external validation in the ARIC study, the c-statistic was 0.74 in whites (n = 1353) and 0.75 in blacks (n = 424).

Conclusion.—Risk stratification for chronic kidney disease is achievable using a risk score derived from clinical factors that are readily accessible in primary care. The utility of this score in identifying individuals in the community at high risk of chronic kidney disease warrants further investigation (Tables 1 and 4).

▶ In 2009, we reported on a study by Kshirsagar et al[1] that used the Atherosclerosis Risk in Communities (ARIC) and the Cardiovascular Health Study (CHS)

TABLE 1.—Baseline Characteristics of Participants in the FHS and ARIC Studies*

	FHS	ARIC
Number of participants	2490	1777
Age, years	57.1 (8.9)	62.4 (5.4)
Female sex, %	53.0 (1319)	50.6 (900)
Ethnicity		
White, %	100 (2490)	76.1 (1353)
Black, %	NA	23.9 (424)
Diabetes, %	7.4 (184)	13.4 (239)
Systolic blood pressure, mm Hg	126 (18)	128 (18)
Hypertension, %	35.3 (878)	46.1 (819)
High density lipoprotein cholesterol, mg/dL	52 (16)	50 (17)
Triglycerides, mg/dL	137 (98)	139 (82)
Obesity (body mass index ≥30 kg/m²), %	27.1 (673)	31.0 (552)
Current smoking, %	14.3 (355)	14.2 (252)
Cardiovascular disease, %[†]	8.3 (206)	7.3 (130)
Estimated glomerular filtration rate, mL/min/1.73m²	92 (23)	85 (16)
Categorical eGFR, mL/min/1.73m²		
60-74 mL/min/1.73m², %	20.0 (499)	30.9 (549)
75-89 mL/min/1.73m², %	35.4 (882)	32.2 (572)
90-119 mL/min/1.73m², %	35.0 (238)	34.1 (605)
≥120 mL/min/1.73m², %	9.6 (871)	2.9 (51)
Dipstick proteinuria,[‡] %	17.1 (422)	NA
Albuminuria[§], %	9.2 (197)	5.7 (101)

ARIC = Atherosclerosis Risk in Communities; eGFR = estimated glomerular filtration rate; FHS = Framingham Heart Study.

SI conversion factors: to convert cholesterol level to millimoles per liter, multiply by 0.0259 and triglyceride level to millimoles per liter, multiply by 0.0113. Data were ≥ 99.7% complete for all variables except albumin-to-creatinine ratio, which was 86% complete.

*Data presented as mean with SD in parentheses for continuous variables or percentage with number in parentheses for categorical variables.

[†]Includes coronary heart disease and congestive heart failure.

[‡]Defined as trace or above.

[§]Defined as spot urine albumin to creatinine ratio of ≥30 mg/g.

TABLE 4.—Risk of Chronic Kidney Disease at 10 Years in the Development (FHS) Cohort According to Risk Category

Risk Factor	Points Awarded	Risk Score*	10-Year Risk of Chronic Kidney Disease
Age (years)		0	0%
30-34	0	1	0%
35-39	1	2	1%
40-44	2	3	1%
45-49	3	4	2%
50-54	4	5	3%
55-59	4	6	5%
60-64	5	7	9%
65-69	6	8	14%
70-74	7	9	20%
75-79	8	10	30%
80-85	9	11	41%
		12	54%
Diabetes (yes)	1	13	66%
		14	76%
Hypertension (yes)	1	15	84%
Dipstick proteinuria (trace or above)[†]	1		
Estimated glomerular filtration rate			
60-74 mL/min/1.73m^2	3		
75-89 mL/min/1.73m^2	1		
90-119 mL/min/1.73m^2	0		
Above 120 mL/min/1.73m^2	0		

FHS = Framingham Heart Study.
C-statistic for overall score is 0.813.
*The risk score is calculated by adding the points for each risk factor from column 2 (points awarded).
†Dipstick proteinuria may be substituted with quantitative albuminuria, defined as urine albumin to creatinine ratio ≥30 mg/g.

cohorts to predict the likelihood that over the ensuing 9 years an individual patient with identified risk factors would develop clinically significant kidney disease (defined as a glomerular filtration rate [GFR] of less than 60 mL/min/1.73 m^2). This study uses the Framingham Heart Study participants who underwent a baseline evaluation between 1995 and 1998 and a follow-up evaluation between 2005 and 2008 (N = 2490) to develop a risk score to estimate an individual's absolute risk over a 10-year period of incident chronic kidney disease. The model was externally validated in the biethnic Atherosclerosis Risk in Communities (ARIC) studies[2] (Table 1). Based on logistic regression analysis, age, albuminuria, diabetes, hypertension, and baseline estimated GFR were independently associated with incident chronic kidney disease. The risk of chronic kidney disease derived from the Framingham cohort at 10 years is shown in Table 4.

The strengths of this study include the long follow-up, the community-based sample, the detailed assessment of risk factors and baseline, and follow-up data regarding creatinine and proteinuria. The major limitations are that data regarding family history (which can be a risk factor for renal disease) were not available; baseline and follow-up creatinine were based on a single value; and estimated GRF was used, which can underestimate GFR in both healthy individuals and in those with advanced disease. However, the population size and length of follow-up population help mitigate these limitations. The bedside risk tool is appealing as it is based on readily available clinical information and can clearly help the clinician prioritize attention and arrange for timely specialty-care referral, as required. The long-term use of the tool to identify specific individuals at high risk of chronic kidney disease certainly deserves further study.

R. Garrick, MD

References

1. Kshirsagar AV, Bang H, Bomback AS, et al. A simple algorithm to predict incident kidney disease. *Arch Intern Med.* 2008;168:2466-2473.
2. The Atherosclerosis Risk in Communities (ARIC) study: design and objectives. The ARIC investigators. *Am J Epidemiol.* 1989;129:687-702.

Predictors of Hyperkalemia and Death in Patients With Cardiac and Renal Disease
Jain N, Kotla S, Little BB, et al (Veterans Affairs North Texas Health Care System, Dallas; Univ of Texas Southwestern Med School at Dallas; Tarleton State Univ, Stephenville, TX)
Am J Cardiol 109:1510-1513, 2012

Predictors of hyperkalemia in patients with cardiovascular disease (CVD; defined as patients with hypertension and heart failure) and associated chronic kidney disease (CKD) are not well established. The aim of this study was to ascertain risk factors of hyperkalemia (defined as serum potassium concentration >5.0 mEq/L) and associated all-cause mortality in patients with CVD treated with antihypertensive drugs that impair potassium homeostasis. In a retrospective analysis using a logistic regression model, risk factors for hyperkalemia and all-cause mortality were analyzed in 15,803 patients with CVD treated with antihypertensive drugs. The mean estimated glomerular filtration rate and mean serum potassium concentration were 55.55 ml/min/1.73 m^2 and 4.06 mEq/L, respectively. Hyperkalemia was observed in 24.5% of study patients and 1.7% of total hospital admissions. Compared to patients with normokalemia, those with hyperkalemia had a higher percentage of death (6.25% *vs* 2.92%, $p = 0.0001$) and admissions (7.80% *vs* 5.04%, $p = 0.0001$). Predictors of hyperkalemia were CKD stage (odds ratio [OR] 2.14, 95% confidence interval [CI] 2.02 to 2.28), diabetes mellitus (OR 1.59, 95% CI 1.47 to 1.72), coronary artery disease (OR 1.32, 95% CI 1.21 to 1.43), and peripheral vascular disease (OR 1.55, 95% CI 1.36 to 1.77). Predictors of all-cause mortality were CKD stage (OR 1.26, 95% CI 1.12 to 1.43), hyperkalemic event (OR 1.56, 95% CI 1.30 to 1.88), age (OR 1.04, 95% CI 1.03 to 1.05), and hospitalization (OR 1.04, 95% CI 1.04 to 1.05). In conclusion, hyperkalemia is encountered frequently in patients with established CVD who are taking antihypertensive drugs and is associated with increases in all-cause mortality and hospitalizations. Advanced CKD, diabetes mellitus, coronary artery disease, and peripheral vascular disease are independent predictors of hyperkalemia.

▶ These authors evaluated the predictors of hyperkalemia (over 5.0 mEq/L) and mortality in patients with chronic kidney disease (estimated glomerular filtration rate less than 60 m/min/1.73m^2) and underlying hypertension and heart failure. The study is of interest because prior large population studies such as the Left Ventricular Dysfunction (SOLVD)[1] and the Candesartan Heart Failure-Assessment of Reduction in Mortality and Morbidity (CHARM)[2] excluded patients with a creatinine level greater than 2 mg/dL and 3 mg/dL, respectively. Diabetics and patients on beta-blockers, potassium-sparing diuretics, and angiotensin-converting enzyme inhibitors and receptor blockers were all included in this retrospective review, which encompassed 15 803 patients drawn from Veterans Affairs North Texas Health Care System.

In addition to diabetes (which was an anticipated finding), coronary artery disease and peripheral vascular disease were both found to be independent predictors of hyperkalemia, within the range of kidney function study. Chronic kidney disease stage, a hyperkalemia event, age, and hospitalization were all predictors of all-cause mortality.

The results are important because they highlight the fact that even a moderate degree of chronic kidney disease poses a risk for a hyperkalemia event. The data demonstrate that this is especially true in patients with underlying coronary artery disease, peripheral vascular disease, or diabetes, a constellation of disorders frequently encountered in clinical medicine.

Potential limitations of the study are that it was a retrospective analysis and therefore dependent on the quality of the database, and potential confounders could not be evaluated. However, the patients included are representative of those encountered in real-world medicine, and as such, it is important for practitioners to be aware of the risk factors that have been linked to a hyperkalemia event and the associated increased risk in all-cause mortality.

R. Garrick, MD

References

1. de Denus S, Tardif JC, White M, et al. Quantification of the risk and predictors of hyperkalemia in patients with left ventricular dysfunction: a retrospective analysis of the Studies of Left Ventricular Dysfunction (SOLVD) trials. *Am Heart J.* 2006; 152:705-712.
2. Desai AS, Swedberg K, McMurray JJ, et al. Incidence and predictors of hyperkalemia in patients with heart failure: an analysis of the CHARM Program. *J Am Coll Cardiol.* 2007;50:1959-1966.

Warfarin in Atrial Fibrillation Patients with Moderate Chronic Kidney Disease

Hart RG, Pearce LA, Asinger RW, et al (Univ of Texas Health Sciences Ctr, San Antonio; Minot, ND; Hennepin County Med Ctr, Minneapolis, MN)
Clin J Am Soc Nephrol 6:2599-2604, 2011

Background and Objectives.—The efficacy of adjusted-dose warfarin for prevention of stroke in atrial fibrillation patients with stage 3 chronic kidney disease (CKD) is unknown.

Design, Setting, Participants, & Measurements.—Patients with stage 3 CKD participating in the Stroke Prevention in Atrial Fibrillation 3 trials were assessed to determine the effect of warfarin anticoagulation on stroke and major hemorrhage, and whether CKD status independently contributed to stroke risk. High-risk participants ($n = 1044$) in the randomized trial were assigned to adjusted-dose warfarin (target international normalized ratio 2 to 3) *versus* aspirin (325 mg) plus fixed, low-dose warfarin (subsequently shown to be equivalent to aspirin alone). Low-risk participants ($n = 892$) all received 325 mg aspirin daily. The primary outcome was ischemic stroke (96%) or systemic embolism (4%).

Results.—Among the 1936 participants in the two trials, 42% ($n = 805$) had stage 3 CKD at entry. Considering the 1314 patients not assigned to adjusted-dose warfarin, the primary event rate was double among those with stage 3 CKD (hazard ratio 2.0, 95% CI 1.2, 3.3) *versus* those with a higher estimated GFR (eGFR). Among the 516 participants with stage 3 CKD included in the randomized trial, ischemic stroke/systemic embolism was reduced 76% (95% CI 42, 90; $P < 0.001$) by adjusted-dose warfarin compared with aspirin/ low-dose warfarin; there was no difference in major hemorrhage (5 patients versus 6 patients, respectively).

Conclusions.—Among atrial fibrillation patients participating in the Stroke Prevention in Atrial Fibrillation III trials, stage 3 CKD was associated with higher rates of ischemic stroke/systemic embolism. Adjusted-dose warfarin markedly reduced ischemic stroke/systemic embolism in high-risk atrial fibrillation patients with stage 3 CKD.

▶ The purpose of this trial was to evaluate the safety and efficacy of warfarin therapy in patients with chronic kidney disease (CKD).[1] Atrial fibrillation is particularly common in patients with CKD. A large population study found that approximately one-third of patients with atrial fibrillation had stage 3 or 4 CKD, and the presence of kidney disease was an independent risk factor for stroke.[2] The risks and benefits of anticoagulation in patients with more advanced kidney disease, however, is less clear.[1,3] The stroke prevention in atrial fibrillation trial (SPAF3) includes a stratification stroke risk, and those deemed to be high risk were eligible for the treatment with warfarin, whereas those deemed to be low risk received 325 mg aspirin a day. Within the high-risk group, patients either received fixed-dose warfarin in combination with 325 mg daily of aspirin (which was subsequently shown to be equivalent to aspirin therapy alone) or adjusted-dose warfarin (target international normalized ratio 2 to 3). The primary outcomes studied were ischemic stroke and systemic emboli, and ischemic stroke comprised 96% of primary events. Of 1936 SPAF3 participants, 805 had stage 3 CKD and 30 had stage 4 CKD. A total of 289 stage 3 CKD patients (average age 67), were categorized as low stroke risk and 516 (average age 72) were categorized as high-risk patients.

The 2-year primary event rates were higher for patients with stage 3 CKD who were not assigned to warfarin. For those assigned to warfarin, the stroke reduction effect was similar to that seen in patients with a glomerular filtration rate (GFR) greater than 60 mL/min/1.73 m^2. Lower estimated GFR (eGFR) was an independent predictor of primary events after adjustment for additional stroke risk factors (CHADS2 congestive heart failure, hypertension, age ≥75, diabetes mellitus with 2 points for prior stroke/transient ischemic attack). The frequency of major hemorrhage in the CKD 3 group on adjusted-dose warfarin was small (5 episodes) and was not increased compared with those with a higher eGFR.

The data are important, as they are the first to show that warfarin therapy is both safe and effective for stroke prevention in patients with stage 3 CKD. This large well-controlled trial should be used to help guide therapy in patients with underlying moderate kidney disease and atrial fibrillation at risk for stroke.

R. Garrick, MD

References

1. Wizemann V, Tong L, Satayathum S, et al. Atrial fibrillation in hemodialysis patients: clinical features and associations with anticoagulant therapy. *Kidney Int.* 2010;77:1098-1106.
2. Go AS, Fang MC, Udaltsova N, et al; ATRIA Study Investigators. Impact of proteinuria and glomerular filtration rate on risk of thromboembolism in atrial fibrillation. the anticoagulation and risk factors in atrial fibrillation (ATRIA) study. *Circulation.* 2009;119:1363-1369.
3. Chan KE, Lazarus JM, Thadhani, et al. Warfarin use associates with increased risk for stroke in hemodialysis patients with atrial fibrillation. *J Am Soc Nephrol.* 2009;20:2223-2233.

Characteristics of Renal Cystic and Solid Lesions Based on Contrast-Enhanced Computed Tomography of Potential Kidney Donors

Rule AD, Sasiwimonphan K, Lieske JC, et al (Mayo Clinic, Rochester, MN)
Am J Kidney Dis 59:611-618, 2012

Background.—The presence of a few renal cysts is considered of little relevance in healthy adults, although acquired renal cystic disease occurs in advanced kidney failure. The objective of this study was to detail renal cystic and solid lesions and identify any association with clinical characteristics.

Study Design.—Clinical-pathologic correlation.

Setting & Participants.—Potential kidney donors undergoing a standardized evaluation at the Mayo Clinic in 2000-2008.

Predictors.—Age, kidney function, and chronic kidney disease risk factors.

Measurements.—Renal cystic and solid lesions by contrast-enhanced computed tomographic images.

TABLE 2.—Cortical and Medullary Cyst and Mass Characteristics in Potential Kidney Donors

Characteristic	Age 18-49 y (n = 1,345)	Ages 50 to 75 y (n = 603)	P[a]
Simple cysts			
Largest cyst 2-4 mm	223 (17)	120 (20)	0.08
Any cyst ≥2 mm	521 (39)	377 (63)	<0.001
Any cyst ≥5 mm	298 (22)	257 (43)	<0.001
Any cyst ≥10 mm	106 (7.9)	134 (22)	<0.001
Any cyst ≥20 mm	21 (1.6)	47 (7.8)	<0.001
No. of cysts ≥5 mm			<0.001[b]
0	1,047 (78)	346 (57)	
1	240 (18)	155 (26)	
2	41 (3.0)	59 (9.8)	
3	13 (0.9)	26 (4.3)	
4	3 (0.2)	7 (1.2)	
≥5	1 (0.1)	10 (1.7)	
Diameter of largest cyst ≥5 mm	10 ± 7.5	15 ± 13	<0.001
Any cortical cysts ≥5 mm	156 (12)	198 (33)	<0.001
Any medullary cyst ≥5 mm	163 (12)	101 (17)	0.007
Unilateral cyst or cysts ≥5 mm	267 (20)	189 (31)	<0.001
Bilateral cysts ≥5 mm	31 (2.3)	68 (11)	<0.001
Any left kidney cyst ≥5 mm	167 (12)	168 (28)	<0.001
Any right kidney cyst ≥5 mm	162 (12)	157 (26)	<0.001
Largest cyst ≥5 mm in upper pole	66 (4.9)	96 (16)	0.001
Largest cyst ≥5 mm in lower pole	78 (5.8)	69 (11)	<0.001
Ravine criteria[c] for ADPKD 1 (≥5 mm cysts)	4 (0.3)	5 (0.8)	0.1
Angiomyolipomas and hyperdense cysts			
Any angiomyolipoma	25 (1.9)	18 (3.0)	0.1
Largest diameter among angiomyolipomas (mm)	5.4 ± 4.4	4.5 ± 2.0	0.8
Any hyperdense cyst without contrast enhancement	12 (0.9)	12 (2.0)	0.04
Largest diameter among hyperdense cysts (mm)	9.6 ± 5.0	9.6 ± 3.2	0.9
Cysts or masses with concerning features for malignancy			
Septa in any of the cysts	149 (11)	129 (21)	<0.001
Any thickened irregular septa	0 (0.0)	1 (0.2)	0.3
Any thickened smooth septa	0 (0.0)	0 (0.0)	0.9
Any enhancement of septa	0 (0.0)	3 (0.5)	0.03
Any irregular cyst walls	0 (0.0)	1 (0.2)	0.3
Any thickened cyst walls (>1 mm)	3 (0.2)	4 (0.7)	0.1
Any fine cyst calcification	2 (0.15)	7 (1.2)	0.005
Any slightly thickened cyst calcification	0 (0.0)	0 (0.0)	0.9
Any thick nodular cyst calcification	0 (0.0)	0 (0.0)	0.9
Any cyst soft-tissue enhancement	0 (0.0)	1 (0.2)	0.3
Any enhancing masses	4 (0.3)	5 (0.8)	0.2
Bosniak classification[d]			<0.001[b]
No cysts	817 (61)	207 (34)	
Category I	372 (28)	257 (43)	
Category II	156 (12)	136 (23)	
Category IIF	0 (0.0)	0 (0.0)	
Category III	0 (0.0)	3 (0.5)	
Category IV	0 (0.0)	0 (0.0)	
Enhancing mass or category III cyst diameter, mm	19.3 ± 8.0	14.0 ± 8.6	0.4

Note: N = 1,948. Categorical variables are given as number (percentage); continuous variables, as mean ± standard deviation.

Abbreviation: ADPKD, autosomal dominant polycystic kidney disease.

Editor's Note: Please refer to original journal article for full references.

[a]Wilcoxon test or Fisher exact test.

[b]Likelihood ratio test.

[c]Ravine criteria for ADPKD are intended for assessing ultrasound cysts in first-degree relatives with ADPKD. Cyst thresholds are age 15-29 years, at least 2 cysts; 30-59 years, at least 2 cysts in each kidney; and 60 years and older, at least 4 cysts in each kidney.[9]

[d]Highest if multiple cysts.

Outcomes.—Cyst number, diameter, and location.

Results.—After excluding 8 with cystic disease, 7 of whom had autosomal dominant polycystic kidney disease, there were 1,948 potential kidney donors (42% men; mean age, 43 years). A cortical, medullary, or parapelvic cyst ≥5 mm was present in 12%, 14%, or 2.8%. For ages 19-49 years, 39%, 22%, 7.9%, and 1.6% had a cortical or medullary cyst ≥2, ≥5, ≥10, and ≥20 mm in diameter. For ages 50-75 years, 63%, 43%, 22%, and 7.8% had a cortical or medullary cyst ≥2, ≥5, ≥10, and ≥20 mm in diameter. The 97.5th percentile for number of cortical and medullary cysts ≥5 mm increased with age (10 for men and 4 for women in the 60- to 69-year group). After age and sex adjustment, cortical and medullary cysts ≥5 mm were associated with higher 24-hour urine albumin excretion, as well as increased body surface area, hypertension, and higher glomerular filtration rate in some analyses. Angiomyolipomas, hyperdense cysts, and enhancing masses or cysts with concerning features for malignancy occurred in 2.2%, 1.2%, and 0.6% and were associated with older age ($P \le 0.05$ for each).

Limitations.—Persons with known chronic kidney disease were excluded.

Conclusions.—Renal cysts are common, particularly in older men, and may be a marker of early kidney injury because they associate with albuminuria, hypertension, and hyperfiltration (Table 2).

▶ Simple renal cysts are an exceedingly common clinical finding, and asymptomatic simple cysts are typically thought to be of little clinical importance. The current population study was conducted over an 8-year timeframe and includes 1957 consecutive potential kidney donors. Typically, renal cysts are not evaluated with CAT scan. However, because these patients were potential renal donors, contrast-enhanced CAT scans were performed. This is the first (and perhaps only) systematic study to use this technology in a healthy population. The scans were characterized for the presence of renal cystic and solid lesions with regard to size, location, internal characteristics, and malignant features, and these features were correlated with clinical data including renal function and blood pressure.

Individuals with probable lithium-induced microcystic disease and autosomal dominant polycystic kidney disease, were excluded from analysis. The features and locations of the other lesions detected, stratified by age, are shown in Table 2. The data confirm that renal cysts are common, and older age and male sex are associated with renal cysts (more commonly in the cortex than the medulla). If associated with albuminuria or hypertension, a renal cyst of greater than 5 mm in either the cortex or the medulla may be a marker of renal injury. However, consistent with their lymphatic origin, parapelvic cysts do not associate with kidney function and do not appear to be a marker for kidney injury. The data also suggest that patients with larger cysts or larger numbers of cysts should be evaluated for the presence of albuminuria and hypertension. Lesions that occur less frequently, such as angiomyolipomas, enhancing cysts, and complex masses, demand additional investigation.

R. Garrick, MD

Fibroblast Growth Factor 23 and Risks of Mortality and End-Stage Renal Disease in Patients With Chronic Kidney Disease

Isakova T, for the Chronic Renal Insufficiency Cohort (CRIC) Study Group (Univ of Miami Miller School of Medicine, FL; et al)
JAMA 305:2432-2439, 2011

Context.—A high level of the phosphate-regulating hormone fibroblast growth factor 23 (FGF-23) is associated with mortality in patients with end-stage renal disease, but little is known about its relationship with adverse outcomes in the much larger population of patients with earlier stages of chronic kidney disease.

Objective.—To evaluate FGF-23 as a risk factor for adverse outcomes in patients with chronic kidney disease.

Design, Setting, and Participants.—A prospective study of 3879 participants with chronic kidney disease stages 2 through 4 who enrolled in the Chronic Renal Insufficiency Cohort between June 2003 and September 2008.

Main Outcome Measures.—All-cause mortality and end-stage renal disease.

Results.—At study enrollment, the mean (SD) estimated glomerular filtration rate (GFR) was 42.8 (13.5) mL/min/1.73 m^2, and the median FGF-23 level was 145.5 RU/mL (interquartile range [IQR], 96-239 reference unit [RU]/mL). During a median follow-up of 3.5 years (IQR, 2.5-4.4 years), 266 participants died (20.3/1000 person-years) and 410 reached end-stage renal disease (33.0/1000 person-years). In adjusted analyses, higher levels of FGF-23 were independently associated with a greater risk of death (hazard ratio [HR], per SD of natural log-transformed FGF-23, 1.5; 95% confidence interval [CI], 1.3-1.7). Mortality risk increased by quartile of FGF-23: the HR was 1.3 (95% CI, 0.8-2.2) for the second quartile, 2.0 (95% CI, 1.2-3.3) for the third quartile, and 3.0 (95% CI, 1.8-5.1) for the fourth quartile. Elevated fibroblast growth factor 23 was independently associated with significantly higher risk of end-stage renal disease among participants with an estimated GFR between 30 and 44 mL/min/1.73 m^2 (HR, 1.3 per SD of FGF-23 natural log-transformed FGF-23; 95% CI, 1.04-1.6) and 45 mL/min/1.73 m^2 or higher (HR, 1.7; 95% CI, 1.1-2.4), but not less than 30 mL/min/1.73 m^2.

Conclusion.—Elevated FGF-23 is an independent risk factor for end-stage renal disease in patients with relatively preserved kidney function and for mortality across the spectrum of chronic kidney disease (Fig 3).

▶ The study of O'Seaghdha and colleagues[1] help define who is at risk for the development of incident chronic kidney disease (CKD); the studies of Packham[2] and O'Hare[3] helped to further clarify the heterogeneity of the population of patients with CKD. The predictive model of Tangri[4] and colleagues did not include an all-cause mortality prediction, but rather defined those patients with mild-moderate to severe CKD who will progress to dialysis. The current study by the Chronic Renal Insufficiency Cohort (CRIC) Study Group is extremely

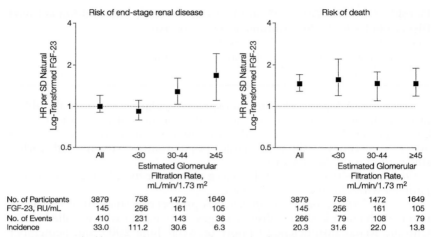

FIGURE 3.—Fibroblast Growth Factor 23 Levels and Risks of End-Stage Renal Disease and Death by Baseline Kidney Function. Multivariable-adjusted risks of end-stage renal disease and death per unit increment in SD of natural logtransformed fibroblast growth factor 23 (FGF-23) in all participants and according to categories of baseline estimated glomerular filtration rate (GFR). See Figure 1 legend for adjusted variables. Error bars indicate 95% confidence intervals. HR indicates hazard ratio. (Reprinted from Isakova T, for the Chronic Renal Insufficiency Cohort (CRIC) Study Group. Fibroblast growth factor 23 and risks of mortality and end-stage renal disease in patients with chronic kidney disease. *JAMA.* 2011;305:2432-2439. Copyright 2011 American Medical Association. All rights reserved.)

interesting because it demonstrates that elevated FGF-23 is an independent risk factor for end-stage renal disease in patients with estimated glomerular filtration rate (eGFR) above 30 mL/min/1.73 m^2. In addition, higher levels of FGF-23 were independently associated with a greater risk of death across the spectrum of CKD (Fig 3).

FGF-23 increases urinary phosphate excretion, and the levels of FGF-23 progressively increase as kidney function declines. This study extends smaller observational studies that suggested that elevated FGF-23 is an independent risk factor for mortality among dialysis patients.[5] Interestingly, despite the previously suggested association between serum phosphorus and mortality,[6] the relationship between FGF-23 and mortality was not confounded or modified by either phosphate or parathyroid hormone. In addition, the relationship between FGF-23 and mortality was not altered after adjustment for eGFR, albuminuria, or cardiovascular risk factors including hypertension, diabetes, dyslipidemia, and heart failure, peripheral vascular disease, or cerebrovascular accident. In contrast to the mortality data, at lower levels of glomerular filtration rate (less than 30 mL/min/1.73 m^2) but not at higher eGFR levels, the relationship between the FGF-23 and progression of CKD was influenced by confounder adjustment. This suggests that the influence of FGF-23 on renal disease progression is modified by the prevailing eGFR.

A strength of this study is the large population or carefully defined patients and the adjustments made for a variety of confounders. Unfortunately, not all suspected urinary biomarkers of progression and mortality (β trace protein, β2 microglobulin, cystatin, among others) were available for analysis. Nonetheless, the data are very interesting. Given the heterogeneity of the kidney disease population as demonstrated by others,[2,3] using FGF-23 as a biomarker for risk stratification for kidney disease progression, especially at high levels of eGFR, may prove clinically useful. Although these FGF-23 data certainly do not prove causality, a biomarker for the prediction of prognosis and mortality in patients with CKD is intriguing, especially when determining the timing and appropriateness of interventions. In addition to testing the clinical applicability of FGF-23, further studies are warranted to determine if clinical maneuvers to reduce FGF-23 levels influence mortality and disease progression.

R. Garrick, MD

References

1. O'Seaghdha CM, Lyass A, Massaro JM. A risk score for chronic kidney disease in the general population. *Am J Med.* 2012;125:270-277.
2. Packham DK, Alves TP, Dwyer JP, et al. Relative incidence of ESRD versus cardiovascular mortality in proteinuric type 2 diabetes and nephropathy: results from the DIAMETRIC (Diabetes Mellitus Treatment for Renal Insufficiency Consortium) database. *Am J Kidney Dis.* 2011;59:75-83.
3. O'Hare AM, Batten A, Burrows NR, et al. Trajectories of kidney function decline in the 2 years before initiation of long-term dialysis. *Am J Kidney Dis.* 2012;59:513-515.
4. Tangri N, Stevens A, Griffith J, et al. A predictive model for progression of chronic kidney disease to kidney failure. *JAMA.* 2011;305:1553-1559.
5. Gutiérrez OM, Mannstadt M, Isakova T, et al. Fibroblast growth factor 23 and mortality among patients undergoing hemodialysis. *N Engl J Med.* 2008;359:584-592.
6. Palmer SC, Hayen A, Macaskill P, et al. Serum levels of phosphorus, parathyroid hormone, and calcium and risks of death and cardiovascular disease in individuals with chronic kidney disease: a systematic review and meta-analysis. *JAMA.* 2011;305:1119-1127.

Novel Markers of Kidney Function as Predictors of ESRD, Cardiovascular Disease, and Mortality in the General Population
Astor BC, Shafi T, Hoogeveen RC, et al (Johns Hopkins Univ, Baltimore, MD; Johns Hopkins School of Medicine, Baltimore, MD; Methodist DeBakey Heart Ctr, Houston, TX; et al)
Am J Kidney Dis 59:653-662, 2012

Background.—Cystatin C level predicts mortality more strongly than serum creatinine level. It is unknown whether this advantage extends to other outcomes, such as kidney failure, or whether other novel renal filtration markers share this advantage in predicting outcomes.

Study Design.—Observational cohort study.

Setting & Participants.—9,988 participants in the Atherosclerosis Risk in Communities (ARIC) Study, a population-based study in 4 US communities, followed for approximately 10 years.

Predictors.—Serum creatinine—based estimated glomerular filtration rate calculated using the Chronic Kidney Disease Epidemiology Collaboration (CKD-EPI) equation (eGFR$_{CKD-EPI}$) and cystatin C, β-trace protein (BTP), and β_2-microglobulin (B2M) levels.

Outcomes.—Mortality, coronary heart disease, heart failure, and kidney failure.

Results.—Higher cystatin C and B2M concentrations were associated more strongly with mortality (n = 1,425) than BTP level and all were associated more strongly than eGFR$_{CKD-EPI}$ (adjusted HR for the upper 6.7 percentile compared with the lowest quintile: 1.6 [95% CI, 1.3-1.9] for eGFR$_{CKD-EPI}$, 2.9 [95% CI, 2.3-3.6] for cystatin C level, 1.9 [95% CI, 1.5-2.4] for BTP level, and 3.0 [95% CI, 2.4-3.8] for B2M level). Similar patterns were observed for coronary heart disease (n = 1,279), heart failure (n = 803), and kidney failure (n = 130). The addition of cystatin C, BTP, and B2M levels to models including eGFR$_{CKD-EPI}$ and all covariates, including urinary albumin-creatinine ratio, significantly improved risk prediction for all outcomes (P < 0.001).

Limitations.—No direct measurement of GFR.

Conclusions.—B2M and, to a lesser extent, BTP levels share cystatin C's advantage over eGFR$_{CKD-EPI}$ in predicting outcomes, including kidney failure. These additional markers may be helpful in improving estimation of risk associated with decreased kidney function beyond current estimates based on eGFR$_{CKD-EPI}$ (Table 4).

▶ Given the prevalence of chronic kidney disease (CKD), it is clear that it is necessary to try to determine ways to predict which individuals will progress to end-stage disease.[1] In addition, defining the outcome, risk, and overall mortality and cardiovascular disease in patients with CKD is of obvious clinical importance.[2-4] It has previously been shown that cystatin C is a better predictor of mortality than is the serum creatinine.[2] These authors evaluated whether the predictive strength of cystatin C extended to other associated outcomes (ie, kidney failure, heart failure, or cardiovascular events) and sought to determine whether the addition of renal biomarkers improved the ability to predict outcomes.

The filtration biomarkers were measured on samples obtained from participants in the Atherosclerosis Risk in Communities (ARIC) study, which included 99 988 participants from 4 US communities followed for approximately 10 years. The glomerular filtration rate (GFR) was estimated using the Chronic Kidney Disease Epidemiology Collaboration equation (CKD-EPI). Cystatin C, β-trace protein (BTP), and β2-microglobulin (B2-M) were also determined.

As shown in Table 4, cystatin C and B2-M levels correlated more strongly with mortality than BTP, and all were associated more strongly than estimated GFR CKD-EPI. Similar patterns were observed for other major clinical outcomes, including coronary heart disease, heart failure, and kidney failure.

One limitation is that the study was drawn from a solitary database and GFR was determined by derivative equations rather than by direct measurement. However, this is a novel approach, and if the data are replicated in other populations, these markers may help better predict those individuals in the general population who are at significant risk for end-stage renal disease, cardiovascular disease, and mortality.

Given the heterogeneity and size of the population of patients at risk for progressive kidney disease, the clinical need for us to better predict individual

TABLE 4.—Adjusted Hazard Ratios for Participants With eGFR$_{CKD-EPI}$ ≥60 mL/min/1.73 m^2 by Quintile of Kidney Function Marker

	1	2	3	4	5a	5b	5c	P Trend
				Quintile				
Mortality (1,201 events/9,320 participants)								
eGFR$_{CKD-EPI}$	Ref	0.88 (0.73-1.07)	0.84 (0.69-1.02)	0.84 (0.69-1.02)	0.87 (0.67-1.13)	1.09 (0.86-1.38)	—	0.8
Cystatin C	Ref	1.20 (0.97-1.49)	1.26[a] (1.02-1.56)	1.44[a] (1.17-1.77)	1.70[b] (1.32-2.20)	1.69[b] (1.31-2.18)	2.56[b] (1.96-3.34)	<0.001
BTP	Ref	1.07 (0.87-1.30)	1.23[a] (1.01-1.50)	1.27[a] (1.04-1.55)	1.21 (0.93-1.58)	1.45[a] (1.13-1.86)	1.49[a] (1.14-1.95)	<0.001
B2M	Ref	1.07 (0.87-1.33)	1.35[a] (1.10-1.67)	1.51[b] (1.23-1.86)	1.45[a] (1.12-1.88)	1.83[b] (1.42-2.37)	2.62[b] (2.00-3.42)	<0.001
CHD (1,115 events/9,320 participants)								
eGFR$_{CKD-EPI}$	Ref	0.95 (0.78-1.16)	0.95 (0.78-1.17)	1.02 (0.84-1.25)	1.13 (0.87-1.46)	1.08 (0.83-1.39)	—	0.2
Cystatin C	Ref	1.07 (0.87-1.33)	0.93 (0.75-1.15)	1.24[a] (1.01-1.52)	1.31[a] (1.01-1.70)	1.14 (0.87-1.49)	1.26 (0.91-1.73)	0.02
BTP	Ref	1.05 (0.85-1.29)	1.02 (0.82-1.26)	1.19 (0.97-1.46)	1.35[a] (1.04-1.76)	1.33[a] (1.04-1.73)	1.22 (0.91-1.62)	0.006
B2M	Ref	1.26[a] (1.02-1.54)	1.10 (0.89-1.37)	1.34 (1.08-1.65)	1.26 (0.96-1.65)	1.30 (0.98-1.71)	1.55[a] (1.13-2.14)	0.01
Heart Failure (672 events/8,840 participants)								
eGFR$_{CKD-EPI}$	Ref	1.24 (0.96-1.62)	0.92 (0.70-1.21)	1.38[a] (1.07-1.79)	1.08 (0.76-1.53)	1.36 (0.99-1.87)	—	0.05
Cystatin C	Ref	0.99 (0.74-1.32)	1.21 (0.91-1.60)	1.38[a] (1.05-1.82)	1.94[b] (1.40-2.69)	1.91[b] (1.38-2.65)	2.94[b] (2.08-4.17)	<0.001
BTP	Ref	0.93 (0.72-1.20)	1.00 (0.77-1.29)	1.08 (0.83-1.39)	1.41[a] (1.02-1.94)	1.26 (0.90-1.76)	1.60[a] (1.14-2.25)	0.001
B2M	Ref	0.94 (0.70-1.26)	1.21 (0.92-1.60)	1.49[a] (1.14-1.95)	1.29 (0.91-1.84)	1.96[b] (1.41-2.74)	2.97[b] (2.10-4.21)	<0.001
ESRD (54 events/9,277 participants)[c]								
eGFR$_{CKD-EPI}$	Ref				3.05 (1.45-6.43)	1.00 (0.30-3.31)	—	0.2
Cystatin C	Ref				0.76 (0.18-3.24)	2.22 (0.96-5.13)	5.73[b] (2.55-12.87)	<0.001
BTP	Ref				0.50 (0.07-3.71)	3.04[a] (1.25-7.36)	4.36[b] (2.04-9.31)	<0.001
B2M	Ref				0.76 (0.18-3.24)	2.22 (0.96-5.13)	5.73[b] (2.55-12.87)	<0.001

Note: Values in parentheses are 95% confidence intervals. Adjusted for age, sex, race, field center, diabetes, prevalent CHD, current smoking, systolic blood pressure, antihypertensive medication use, low- and high-density lipoprotein cholesterol levels, log(triglycerides), log(high-sensitivity C-reactive protein), and log(albumin-creatinine ratio).

Abbreviations: B2M, β_2-microglobulin; BTP, β-trace protein; CHD, coronary heart disease; eGFR$_{CKD-EPI}$, estimated glomerular filtration rate based on serum creatinine level, using Chronic Kidney Disease Epidemiology Collaboration equation; ESRD, end-stage renal disease; ref, reference.

[a]P < 0.05 versus quintile 1.
[b]P < 0.001 versus quintile 1.
[c]For each row, the reference group comprises quintiles 1-4 combined.

outcome has becoming increasingly clear. These data are the first to demonstrate that combining novel biomarkers may improved our predictive acumen.

R. Garrick, MD

References

1. United States Renal Data System: USRDS 2011 Atlas of CKD and ESRD: Incidence, Prevalence, Patient Characteristics and Modalities. http://www.US.DS.orb/Atlas. aspx. Accessed May 1, 2012.
2. Shlipak MG, Sarnak MJ, Katz R, et al. Cystatin C and the risk of death and cardiovascular events among elderly persons. *N Engl J Med.* 2005;352:2049-2060.
3. Astor BC, Levey AS, Stevens LA, Van Lente F, Selvin E, Coresh J. Method of glomerular filtration rate estimation affects prediction of mortality risk. *J Am Soc Nephrol.* 2009;20:2214-2222.
4. Shlipak MG, Sarnak MJ, Katz R, et al. Cystatin C and the risk of death and cardiovascular events among elderly persons. *N Engl J Med.* 2005;352:2049-2060.

Racial and Ethnic Differences in Mortality among Individuals with Chronic Kidney Disease: Results from the Kidney Early Evaluation Program (KEEP)
Jolly SE, Burrows NR, Chen S-C, et al (Cleveland Clinic Medicine Inst, OH; Ctrs for Disease Control and Prevention, Atlanta, GA; Minneapolis Med Res Foundation, MN; et al)
Clin J Am Soc Nephrol 6:1858-1865, 2011

Background and Objectives.—Chronic kidney disease (CKD) is prevalent in minority populations and racial/ethnic differences in survival are incompletely understood.

Design, Setting, Participants, & Measurements.—Secondary analysis of Kidney Early Evaluation Program participants from 2000 through 2008 with CKD, not on dialysis, and without previous kidney transplant was performed. Self-reported race/ethnicity was categorized into five groups: non-Hispanic white, African American, Asian, American Indian/Alaska Native, and Hispanic. CKD was defined as a urinary albumin to creatinine ratio of ≥30 mg/g among participants with an estimated GFR (eGFR) ≥60 ml/min per 1.73 m² or an eGFR of < 60 ml/min per 1.73 m². The outcome was all-cause mortality. Covariates used were age, sex, obesity, diabetes, hypertension, albuminuria, baseline eGFR, heart attack, stroke, smoking, family history, education, health insurance, geographic region, and year screened.

Results.—19,205 participants had prevalent CKD; 55% (n = 10,560) were White, 27% (n = 5237) were African American, 9% (n = 1638) were Hispanic, 5% (n = 951) were Asian, and 4% (n = 813) were American Indian/Alaska Native. There were 1043 deaths (5.4%). African Americans had a similar risk of death compared with Whites (adjusted Hazard Ratio (AHR) 1.07, 95% CI 0.90 to 1.27). Hispanics (AHR 0.66, 95% CI 0.50 to 0.94) and Asians (AHR 0.63, 95% CI 0.41 to 0.97) had a lower mortality risk compared with Whites. In contrast, American Indians/Alaska Natives had a higher risk of death compared with Whites (AHR 1.41, 95% CI 1.08 to 1.84).

TABLE 2.—Adjusted Hazards Ratios of Risk of Death for Participants with Chronic Kidney Disease, by Race/Ethnicity, Kidney Early Evaluation Program, 2000 Through 2009

| | | Adjusted[a] Hazards Ratio (95% CI) | |
| | | Albuminuria and | |
Race/Ethnicity	CKD ($n = 19\ 205$)	eGFR ≥ 60 ($n = 6068$)	eGFR < 60 ($n = 13{,}137$)
White	1.00	1.00	1.00
African American	1.07 (0.90 to 1.27)	1.08 (0.78 to 1.49)	1.03 (0.84 to 1.27)
Hispanic	0.66 (0.50 to 0.94)	0.52 (0.27 to 1.01)	0.70 (0.45 to 1.07)
Asian	0.63 (0.41 to 0.97)	0.44 (0.20 to 0.99)[b]	0.71 (0.41 to 1.20)
American Indian/Alaska Native	1.41 (1.08 to 1.84)[b]	1.22 (0.73 to 2.03)	1.37 (0.99 to 1.89)

Note: KEEP censored on May 31, 2009. CKD, chronic kidney disease; CI, confidence interval; eGFR, estimated glomerular filtration rate (ml/min per 1.73 m²); KEEP, Kidney Early Evaluation Program.
[a]Adjusted for age, sex, obesity, diabetes mellitus, hypertension, albuminuria (macroalbuminuria only for albuminuria and eGFR ≥ 60 group), baseline eGFR, heart attack, stroke, smoking status, family history of diabetes mellitus, family history of hypertension, family history of CKD, education level, presence of health insurance, region where screened, and year screened.
[b]$P < 0.05$.

Conclusions.—Significant differences in mortality among some minority groups were found among persons with CKD detected by community-based screening (Table 2).

▶ The National Kidney Foundation KEEP database is a voluntary screening program designed to detect patients at risk for chronic kidney disease. Risk factors are defined as either a personal diagnosis of diabetes or hypertension or family diagnosis of diabetes, hypertension, or kidney disease. Since its inception in 2000, more than 120 000 individuals have been screened. Using this voluntary database, the authors evaluated individuals (between August 2000 and December 2008; n = 122 716) with an estimated glomerular filtration rate of less than 60 mL/min per 1.73 m² or a urine albumin to creatinine ratio of ≥30 mg/g. Using these definitions, 19 205 participants had prevalent CKD.

Many important observations have been generated from this self-reported community population. The current findings (Table 2) demonstrate interesting differences in the hazard ratios for mortality among minority populations as compared with whites. This pattern persisted in subgroup analyses after adjustment for age (greater than or less than 65 years of age), sex, obesity, diabetes, hypertension education, insurance status, region of the country, and year of screening.

The population of individuals with end-stage renal disease is growing and most noteworthy is that it is growing most rapidly among racial/ethnic minorities. A clear strength of this study is the large population surveyed and that it extends across the entire country. Because it is a self-reported database, there is an inherent possibility for misclassification, including a misclassification of early chronic kidney disease. The outcome was all-cause mortality, rather than cause-specific mortality; therefore, it is not possible to further define all the factors that may have contributed to the differences in survival. However, these limitations aside, it is important that clinicians be aware of these data and patterns of disease to more effectively plan educational and outreach programs in an effort to improve outcomes.

R. Garrick, MD

23 Mediators and Modifiers of Renal Injury

Dietary acid reduction with fruits and vegetables or bicarbonate attenuates kidney injury in patients with a moderately reduced glomerular filtration rate due to hypertensive nephropathy
Goraya N, Simoni J, Jo C, et al (Texas A&M College of Medicine, Temple; Texas Tech Univ Health Sciences Ctr, Lubbock; Scott and White Healthcare, Temple, TX)
Kidney Int 81:86-93, 2012

The neutralization of dietary acid with sodium bicarbonate decreases kidney injury and slows the decline of the glomerular filtration rate (GFR) in animals and patients with chronic kidney disease. The sodium intake, however, could be problematic in patients with reduced GFR. As alkali-induced dietary protein decreased kidney injury in animals, we compared the efficacy of alkali-inducing fruits and vegetables with oral sodium bicarbonate to diminish kidney injury in patients with hypertensive nephropathy at stage 1 or 2 estimated GFR. All patients were evaluated 30 days after no intervention; daily oral sodium bicarbonate; or fruits and vegetables in amounts calculated to reduce dietary acid by half. All patients had 6 months of antihypertensive control by angiotensin-converting enzyme inhibition before and during these studies, and otherwise ate *ad lib*. Indices of kidney injury were not changed in the stage 1 group. By contrast, each treatment of stage 2 patients decreased urinary albumin, N-acetyl β-D-glucosaminidase, and transforming growth factor β from the controls to a similar extent. Thus, a reduction in dietary acid decreased kidney injury in patients with moderately reduced eGFR due to hypertensive nephropathy and that with fruits and vegetables was comparable to sodium bicarbonate. Fruits and vegetables appear to be an effective kidney protective adjunct to blood pressure reduction and angiotensin-converting enzyme inhibition in hypertensive and possibly other nephropathies (Table 2).

▶ Prior studies have suggested that alkali supplementation (or citrate therapy), can slow the progression of renal disease.[1-3] The current interventional study compared the effects of 30 days of added oral daily bicarbonate or added fruits

TABLE 2.—Net Change in Acid-Base Data Pre- and Post-Dietary Intervention (Post–Pre), Expressed as Mean ± S.D

	CKD 1			CKD 2		
	Time Control Mean ± S.D.	HCO₃ Mean ± S.D.	F+V Mean ± S.D.	Time Control Mean ± S.D.	HCO₃ Mean ± S.D.	F+V Mean ± S.D.
Plasma total CO_2 (mmol/l)	0.0 ± 1.2	0.0 ± 0.7	−0.1 ± 1.1	0.0 ± 0.5	0.1 ± 0.6	0.0 ± 0.4
P-value, pre versus post	0.886	0.935	0.687	0.742	0.387	0.604
Potential renal acid load (mmol/day)	0.1 ± 2.5	−0.1 ± 2.7	−20.9 ± 10.9*,**	−0.2 ± 2.6*	0.0 ± 2.5	−21.7 ± 11.9*,**
P-value, pre versus post	0.809	0.865	<0.001	0.688	0.914	<0.001
8-Hour urine net acid excretion (mEq)	0.1 ± 1.1	−6.0 ± 4.8*	−7.9 ± 5.2*,**	0.3 ± 1.7	−7.2 ± 6.0*	−8.1 ± 4.6*
P-value, pre versus post	0.751	<0.001	<0.001	0.333	<0.001	<0.001

Abbreviations: CKD, chronic kidney disease; F+V, 30 days after dietary intervention with fruits + vegetables; HCO₃, 30 days after oral intervention with oral NaHCO₃.
*P < 0.05 versus Time Control in change (Post-Pre).
**P < 0.05, versus HCO₃ in change.

and vegetables (F + V) on markers of renal injury in patients with underlying macroalbuminuria (urine albumin/creatinine ratio > 200 mg/g creatinine) and hypertensive nephropathy with chronic kidney disease (CKD) stage I (estimated glomerular filtration rate (eGFR) > 90 ml/min) or CKD2 (eGFR 60—90 mL/min).

The oral bicarbonate dose was 0.5 mg/kg/d. Increased dietary alkali intake was done by increasing the consumption F + V, which are base inducing, and was assessed by formula based on the consumption reported in a 3-day food diary. As shown in Table 2, the net effect of these simple adjustments was an overall reduction in urinary net acid excretion in patients with CKD2. In addition, patients with CKD2 also had a decrease in urinary albumin, in transforming growth factor-β, and N-acetyl-β-D-glucosaminidase (UNAG a marker of tubular interstitial injury[4]). One weakness was the use of derivative, and, in the case of UNAG, putative, markers of renal injury rather than measurements of creatinine. Additionally, other variables such as systolic blood pressure, which was significantly reduced in both CKD1 and CKD2 by F + V intake, may also have contributed to the improvement noted in the renal parameters. The study was of short duration and the long-term effects of therapy remain to be determined. Certainly, the mechanisms of injury amelioration remain to be more fully elucidated. However, in view of the apparent ability of alkali therapy to stabilize or improve renal injury parameters, acidosis and, in the case of F + V intake, blood pressure, in patients with underlying CKD, the addition of this well-tolerated and readily available therapy to our clinical armamentarium certainly seems reasonable.

R. Garrick, MD

References

1. Mahajan A, Simoni J, Sheather S, Broglio KR, Rajab MH, Wesson DE. Daily oral sodium bicarbonate preserves glomerular filtration rate by slowing its decline in early hypertensive nephropathy. *Kidney Int.* 2010;78:303-309.
2. Phisitkul S, Hacker C, Simoni J, Tran RM, Wesson DE. Dietary protein causes a decline in the glomerular filtration rate of the remnant kidney mediated by metabolic acidosis and endothelin receptors. *Kidney Int.* 2008;73:192-199.
3. Phisitkul S, Khanna A, Simoni J, et al. Amelioration of metabolic acidosis in patients with low GFR reduced kidney endothelin production and kidney injury, and better preserved GFR. *Kidney Int.* 2010;77:617-623.
4. Costigan M, Rustom R, Shenkin A, Bone JM. Origin and significance of urinary N-acetyl-beta-D-glucosaminidase (NAG) in renal patients with proteinuria. *Clin Chim Acta.* 1996;255:133-144.

Markers of inflammation predict the long-term risk of developing chronic kidney disease: a population-based cohort study

Shankar A, Sun L, Klein BEK, et al (West Virginia Univ School of Medicine, Morgantown; Univ of Wisconsin School of Medicine and Public Health, Madison; et al)

Kidney Int 80:1231-1238, 2011

In animal models, inflammatory processes have been shown to have an important role in the development of kidney disease. In humans, however, the independent relation between markers of inflammation and the risk of chronic kidney disease (CKD) is not known. To clarify this, we examined the relationship of several inflammatory biomarker levels (high-sensitivity C-reactive protein, tumor necrosis factor-α receptor 2, white blood cell count, and interleukin-6) with the risk of developing CKD in a population-based cohort of up to 4926 patients with 15 years of follow-up. In cross-sectional analyses, we found that all these inflammation markers were positively associated with the outcome of interest, prevalent CKD. However, in longitudinal analyses examining the risk of developing incident CKD among those who were CKD-free at baseline, only tumor necrosis factor-α receptor 2, white blood cell count, and interleukin-6 levels (hazard ratios comparing highest with the lowest tertile of 2.10, 1.90, and 1.45, respectively), and not C-reactive protein (hazard ratio 1.09), were positively associated with incident CKD. Thus, elevations of most markers of inflammation predict the risk of developing CKD. Each marker should be independently verified (Table 4).

▶ Shankar and colleagues investigated the relationship between several inflammatory markers and the risk of developing chronic kidney disease (CKD) in a cohort of 4926 patients with a 15-year follow-up. The patients were drawn from The Beaver Dam Chronic Kidney Disease Study, which is a prospective cohort study examining risk factors for CKD. That study's hypothesis drawn from experimental animal studies is that inflammation has a role in the pathogenesis and progression of CKD[1-3] In humans, the independent relationship between inflammatory mediators and progression of disease is not so clear-cut, and the specific markers selected were based on those studied in a variety of animal models of inflammatory disease and included high sensitivity C-reactive protein, tumor necrosis factor (TNF)-α receptor 2, interleukin-6, and neutrophilia.

Biomarker determinations were done on stored blood drawn from the various sub-cohorts of the various Beaver Dam trials. The longitudinal association between the biomarkers and the 15-year incidence of CKD are shown in Table 4. Among patients who were CKD-free at baseline TNF-α receptor 2, the white blood cell count, and the interleukin-6 level were associated with risk of developing incident CKD. Of these, the association between TNF-α receptor 2 and incident CKD was the strongest.

There are some weaknesses to the study. Although validated measures of kidney function were available, other important markers of kidney injury such as the urinary albumin excretion rate were not available and so their possible contributory effects are unknown. Similarly, it is possible that intervening events such as an episode of AKI may have confounded the long-term incident data. These weaknesses aside, the data are quite interesting and are similar to the findings by the Joslin group and colleagues, which demonstrated a relationship between plasma levels of TNF-α receptor 2 and progressive kidney disease in patients with type I and type II diabetes (also reviewed here). Taken together, the results suggest that TNF-α receptor 2 levels are an early marker of the inflammatory mechanism. As a group, these results are certainly intriguing and offer

TABLE 4.—Longitudinal Association Between Markers of Inflammation and 15-year Incidence of Chronic Kidney Disease (CKD)

Inflammatory Marker Level	No. at Risk	CKD Cases	Unadjusted Hazard Ratio (95% Confidence Interval)	Age-Sex-Adjusted Hazard Ratio (95% Confidence Interval)	Multivariable-Adjusted Hazard Ratio 1 (95% Confidence Interval)[a]	Multivariable-Adjusted Hazard Ratio 2 (95% Confidence Interval)[a]
Serum C-reactive protein (CRP)[b]						
Tertile 1	960	197	1 (Referent)	1 (Referent)	1 (Referent)	1 (Referent)
Tertile 2	961	234	1.19 (1.00–1.40)	1.13 (0.95–1.33)	1.10 (0.92–1.32)	1.06 (0.89–1.27)
Tertile 3	956	244	1.24 (1.05–1.47)	1.19 (0.97–1.46)	1.14 (0.95–1.37)	1.09 (0.91–1.29)
P-trend			0.001	0.09	0.21	0.42
Serum tumor necrosis factor (TNF)-α receptor 2[c]						
Tertile 1	349	54	1 (Referent)	1 (Referent)	1 (Referent)	1 (Referent)
Tertile 2	350	82	1.51 (1.11–2.06)	1.49 (1.06–2.09)	1.47 (1.01–2.14)	1.40 (0.94–2.09)
Tertile 3	349	132	2.44 (1.85–3.23)	2.68 (1.73–4.15)	2.49 (1.66–3.74)	2.10 (1.55–2.84)
P-trend			<0.0001	<0.0001	<0.0001	<0.0001
Serum white blood cell (WBC) count[d]						
Tertile 1	961	140	1 (Referent)	1 (Referent)	1 (Referent)	1 (Referent)
Tertile 2	960	252	1.80 (1.50–2.17)	1.63 (1.36–1.95)	1.58 (1.29–1.94)	1.41 (1.16–1.70)
Tertile 3	956	293	2.10 (1.76–2.52)	2.04 (1.70–2.45)	1.98 (1.68–2.33)	1.90 (1.59–2.27)
P-trend			<0.0001	<0.0001	0.0011	0.0014
Serum interleukin-6[e]						
Tertile 1	351	51	1 (Referent)	1 (Referent)	1 (Referent)	1 (Referent)
Tertile 2	348	97	1.92 (1.41–2.60)	1.43 (0.98–2.07)	1.39 (0.95–2.03)	1.32 (0.89–1.97)
Tertile 3	349	120	2.37 (1.77–3.17)	1.72 (1.11–2.67)	1.57 (1.04–2.37)	1.45 (0.99–2.14)
P-trend			<0.0001	0.022	0.043	0.073

[a]Multivariable-adjusted hazard ratio 1: adjusted for age (years), sex, education categories (< high school, high school, > high school, smoking (never, former, current), alcohol intake (never, former, current), body mass index (kg/m²), glycosylated hemoglobin (%), mean arterial blood pressure (mm Hg), and serum total cholesterol (mg/dl); Multivariable-adjusted hazard ratio 2: additionally adjusted for diabetes (absent, present) and hypertension (absent, present).

[b]Serum C-reactive protein cutoffs (mg/dl): Tertile 1 (men: <1.13, women: <1.19), Tertile 2 (men: 1.13–2.60, women: 1.19–2.99), and Tertile 3 (men: >2.60, women: >2.99).

[c]Serum TNF-α receptor 2 tertile cutoffs (pg/ml): Tertile 1 (men: <2043.9, women: <2078.5), Tertile 2 (men: 2043.9–2491.5, women: 2078.5–2544.5), and Tertile 3 (men: >2491.5, women: >2544.5).

[d]Serum white blood cell count tertile cutoffs (per 1000 cells/mm³): Tertile 1 (men: <6.2, women: <5.8), Tertile 2 (men: 6.2–7.8, women: 5.8–7.3), and Tertile 3 (men: >7.8, women: >7.3).

[e]Serum interleukin-6 tertile cutoffs (pg/ml): Tertile 1 (men: <1.5, women: <1.6 mg/l), Tertile 2 (men: 1.5–2.6, women: 1.6–2.7), and Tertile 3 (men:> 2.6, women: >2.7).

exciting possibilities for studies into the basic mechanism of inflammation in CKD and for the development of clinical markers to forecast CKD progression.

R. Garrick, MD

References

1. Diamond JR. Analogous pathobiologic mechanisms in glomerulosclerosis and atherosclerosis. *Kidney Int Suppl.* 1991;31:S29-S34.
2. Ross R. Atherosclerosis—an inflammatory disease. *N Engl J Med.* 1999;340: 115-126.
3. Schmidt MI, Duncan BB, Sharrett AR, et al. Markers of inflammation and prediction of diabetes mellitus in adults (Atherosclerosis Risk in Communities study): a cohort study. *Lancet.* 1999;353:1649-1652.

High dietary fiber intake is associated with decreased inflammation and all-cause mortality in patients with chronic kidney disease
Krishnamurthy VM, Wei G, Baird BC, et al (VA Salt Lake City Health Care System, UT; Univ of Utah School of Medicine, Salt Lake City; et al)
Kidney Int 81:300-306, 2012

Chronic kidney disease is considered an inflammatory state and a high fiber intake is associated with decreased inflammation in the general population. Here, we determined whether fiber intake is associated with decreased inflammation and mortality in chronic kidney disease, and whether kidney disease modifies the associations of fiber intake with inflammation and mortality. To do this, we analyzed data from 14,543 participants in the National Health and Nutrition Examination Survey III. The prevalence of chronic kidney disease (estimated glomerular filtration rate less than 60 ml/min per 1.73 m^2) was 5.8%. For each 10-g/day increase in total fiber intake, the odds of elevated serum C-reactive protein levels were decreased by 11% and 38% in those without and with kidney disease, respectively. Dietary total fiber intake was not significantly associated with mortality in those without but was inversely related to mortality in those with kidney disease. The relationship of total fiber with inflammation and mortality differed significantly in those with and without kidney disease. Thus, high dietary total fiber intake is associated with lower risk of inflammation and mortality in kidney disease and these associations are stronger in magnitude in those with kidney disease. Interventional trials are needed to establish the effects of fiber intake on inflammation and mortality in kidney disease (Figs 1, 2, and Table 2).

▶ A number of studies have shown that in patients with prevalent renal disease, C-reactive protein (CRP), a marker of inflammation and a strong predictor of cardiovascular events, is increased.[1-4] A diet high in fiber is believed to reduce inflammation.[5-7] However, because of dietary restrictions, the fiber intake in chronic kidney disease (CKD) patients is often low. The authors used the National Health and Nutrition Examination Survey to evaluate the association between

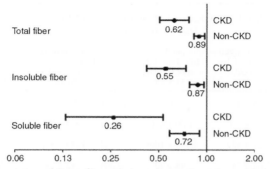

FIGURE 1.—Associations of dietary fiber with elevated serum C-reactive protein (> 3 mg/l) in the non-chronic kidney disease (CKD) and CKD sub-populations. Odds ratio for every 10-g/day increase in each type of fiber intake in CKD and non-CKD sub-populations. Models adjusted for age, gender, race, myocardial infarction, congestive heart failure, stroke, cancer, smoking, alcohol use, leisure-time physical inactivity, systolic blood pressure, diastolic blood pressure, calorie and protein intakes, serum triglycerides, serum high-density lipoprotein cholesterol, and serum low-density lipoprotein cholesterol. (Reprinted with permission from Macmillan Publishers Ltd: Kidney International, Krishnamurthy VM, Wei G, Baird BC, et al. High dietary fiber intake is associated with decreased inflammation and allcause mortality in patients with chronic kidney disease. *Kidney Int.* 2012;81:300-306. Copyright 2012.)

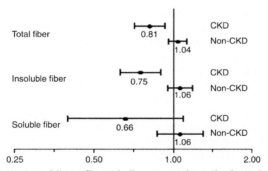

FIGURE 2.—Associations of dietary fiber with all-cause mortality in the chronic kidney disease (CKD) and non-CKD sub-populations. Hazard ratio for every 10-g/day increase in each type of fiber intake in CKD and non-CKD sub-populations. Models adjusted for age, gender, race, smoking, alcohol, leisuretimephysical inactivity, and calorie intake and protein intakes. (Reprinted with permission from MacmillanPublishers Ltd: Kidney International, Krishnamurthy VM, Wei G, Baird BC, et al. High dietary fiberintake is associated with decreased inflammation and all-cause mortality in patients with chronic kidneydisease. *Kidney Int.* 2012;81:300-306. Copyright 2012.)

dietary fiber, CRP (greater than 3 mg/L), and all-cause mortality in both non-CKD and CKD populations. This is the first trial to investigate such an association.

Based on their median total fiber intake (14.6 g/day, Table 2), non-CKD and prevalent CKD patients (5.8% of the study population of 14 533 adult participants) were divided into high and low fiber groups. The results demonstrate that higher dietary fiber intake is associated with lower degrees of inflammation (as measured by CRP and shown in Fig 1), and this association is influenced by the presence of CKD. In addition, the presence of CKD strongly modified the effect of dietary fiber on all cause mortality (Fig 2). Soluble fiber intake had

TABLE 2.—Baseline Dietary Factors[a] of Non-CKD and CKD Participants According to Dietary Total Fiber Intake

| | Non-CKD ($\geq$60 ml/min per 1.73 m^2) | | | CKD (<60 ml/min per 1.73 m^2) | | |
	Low Total Fiber (<14.5 g/day; 48.5%)	High Total Fiber ($\geq$14.6 g/day; 51.5%)	P	Low Total Fiber (<14.5 g/day; 56.4%)	High Total Fiber ($\geq$14.6 g/day; 43.6%)	P
Soluble fiber (g/day)	3.5 ± 1.3	8.2 ± 3.1	<0.001	3.6 ± 1.6	7.7 ± 2.7	<0.001
Insoluble fiber (g/day)	5.9 ± 2.1	16.0 ± 6.4	<0.001	5.9 ± 2.5	14.9 ± 6.1	<0.001
Calorie intake (cal/day)	1721 ± 682	2658 ± 1009	<0.001	1329 ± 558	1987 ± 792	<0.001
Protein intake (g/day)	65 ± 31	98 ± 42	<0.001	52 ± 25	78 ± 37	<0.001

Abbreviations: CKD, chronic kidney disease; cal, calories.
[a]Mean ± s.d. or median (25th to 75th percentiles) for continuous variables and proportion (95% confidence interval) for dichotomous variables are presented.

the most marked effect on both CRP levels and mortality. The authors note that adjustments for serum CRP levels eliminated the association between fiber intake and CKD mortality, suggesting that the influence of dietary fiber is mediated through changes in inflammation.

As reviewed in an elegant accompanying editorial, the mechanisms of this dietary fiber effect may be the result of a change or shift in colonic microbial metabolism from a "proteolytic towards a saccharolytic fermentation pattern."[8] This results in an increase in the production of short chain fatty acids, which, in turn, improves insulin sensitivity and alters the fibrinolytic and cholesterol cascades. A high-fiber intake also results in a reduction in the production of indoles and phenols, which may contribute to cardiovascular disease and renal disease progression. Although the mechanisms of dietary fiber effect remain to be fully elucidated, the effect of fiber on mortality in CKD seems greater than that seen with many other maneuvers studied to date. The data suggest adjustment of dietary fiber intake represents an untapped opportunity to modify outcomes in patients with CKD.

R. Garrick, MD

References

1. Menon V, Wang X, Greene T, et al. Relationship between C-reactive protein, albumin, and cardiovascular disease in patients with chronic kidney disease. *Am J Kidney Dis*. 2003;42:44-52.
2. Kalantar-Zadeh K, Brennan ML, Hazen SL. Serum myeloperoxidase and mortality in maintenance hemodialysis patients. *Am J Kidney Dis*. 2006;48:59-68.
3. Yeun JY, Levine RA, Mantadilok V, Kaysen GA. C-Reactive protein predicts all-cause and cardiovascular mortality in hemodialysis patients. *Am J Kidney Dis*. 2000;35:469-476.
4. Ridker PM, Hennekens CH, Buring JE, Rifai N. C-reactive protein and other markers of inflammation in the prediction of cardiovascular disease in women. *N Engl J Med*. 2000;342:836-843.

5. Ajani UA, Ford ES, Mokdad AH. Dietary fiber and C-reactive protein: findings from national health and nutrition examination survey data. *J Nutr.* 2004;134: 1181-1185.
6. King DE, Egan BM, Geesey ME. Relation of dietary fat and fiber to elevation of C-reactive protein. *Am J Cardio.* 2003;92:1335-1339.
7. Jacobs DR Jr, Meyer KA, Kushi LH, Folsom AR. Is whole grain intake associated with reduced total and cause-specific death rates in older women? The Iowa Women's Health Study. *Am J Public Health.* 1999;89:322-329.
8. Evenepoel P, Meijers BK. Dietary fiber and protein: nutritional therapy in chronic kidney disease and beyond. *Kidney Int.* 2012;81:227-229.

Aristolactam-DNA adducts are a biomarker of environmental exposure to aristolochic acid

Jelaković B, Karanović S, Vuković-Lela I, et al (Univ Hosp Ctr Zagreb, Croatia)
Kidney Int 81:559-567, 2012

Endemic (Balkan) nephropathy is a chronic tubulointerstitial disease frequently accompanied by urothelial cell carcinomas of the upper urinary tract. This disorder has recently been linked to exposure to aristolochic acid, a powerful nephrotoxin and human carcinogen. Following metabolic activation, aristolochic acid reacts with genomic DNA to form aristolactam-DNA adducts that generate a unique TP53 mutational spectrum in the urothelium. The aristolactam-DNA adducts are concentrated in the renal cortex, thus serving as biomarkers of internal exposure to aristolochic acid. Here, we present molecular epidemiologic evidence relating carcinomas of the upper urinary tract to dietary exposure to aristolochic acid. DNA was extracted from the renal cortex and urothelial tumor tissue of 67 patients that underwent nephroureterectomy for carcinomas of the upper urinary tract and resided in regions of known endemic nephropathy. Ten patients from nonendemic regions with carcinomas of the upper urinary tract served as controls. Aristolactam-DNA adducts were quantified by (32)P-postlabeling, the adduct was confirmed by mass spectrometry, and TP53 mutations in tumor tissues were identified by chip sequencing. Adducts were present in 70% of the endemic cohort and in 94% of patients with specific A:T to T:A mutations in TP53. In contrast, neither aristolactam-DNA adducts nor specific mutations were detected in tissues of patients residing in nonendemic regions. Thus, in genetically susceptible individuals, dietary exposure to aristolochic acid is causally related to endemic nephropathy and carcinomas of the upper urinary tract.

▶ Chinese herbal nephropathy (CHN) and Balkan endemic nephropathy (BEN) (a favorite topic of medical school exams) cause chronic tubular interstitial nephropathy and have been associated with uroepithelial carcinoma.

The article by Jelakovic and colleagues is included here because it represents a fascinating modern story of molecular bile epidemiology. The use of *Aristolochia* (birthwort) for medicinal properties dates back more than 2000 years. The modern story began unfolding in the early 1990s when women in Brussels,

Belgium developed kidney failure after ingesting Chinese herbs as part of a weight loss regimen. That potion accidentally contained extract from the *Aristolochia* plant, aristolochic acid (AA).[1] As the story spread, similar cases were noted in other countries, and pathophysiologic similarities were noted between the use of herbal medicines containing AA and the occurrence of end-stage renal disease. Interestingly, as the authors point out, only approximately 5% of the 1800 women exposed in Brussels developed renal disease, suggesting the presence of the genetic susceptibility. Other investigators[2,3] reported that women exposed to AA had developed uroepithelial malignancies and found a link between the overexpression of *p53*, a tumor suppressor gene, and the risk of carcinoma. AA-related DNA adducts were found in the malignancies, and their presence was related to the amount of exposure to the herbal remedy.

Turn the story now to an earlier time, 1969, where Ivić,[4] working in another part of the world, suggested that Balkan nephropathy may be related to exposure to Aristolochia. He postulated that local wheat may have been contaminated with the seeds of the *Aristolochia* plants, which were also present in the local fields. Advanced molecular biology techniques were not available in 1969. However, decades later, Grollman et al[5] demonstrated AA-derived DNA adducts in the uroepithelial tumor tissue of patients with pathophysiologically documented BEN.

We can now fast forward to this article, in which Jelakovic and colleagues used molecular epidemiologic evidence to demonstrate that in genetically susceptible patients, uroepithelial carcinomas are linked to dietary exposure to AA, and this exposure can be demonstrated by the finding of aristalotam-DNA adducts in the renal cortex. The ability to use advanced molecular biological techniques to unravel the causal similarities and demonstrate the link between the seemingly distinct renal disorders of CHN and BEN in geographically and ethnically disparate populations is a modern-day tale of scientific inquiry and application. The combined evidence certainly supports the authors' contention that Balkan endemic nephropathy would be better referred to as Aristolochic acid nephropathy.

R. Garrick, MD

References

1. Vanherweghem JL, Depierreux M, Tielemans C, et al. Rapidly progressive interstitial renal fibrosis in young women: association with slimming regimen including Chinese herbs. *Lancet*. 1993;341:387-391.
2. Cosyns J-P, Dehoux J-P, Guiot Y, et al. Chronic aristolochic acid toxicity in rabbits: a model of Chinese herbs nephropathy? *Kidney Int*. 2001;59:2164-2173.
3. Nortier JL, Martinez MC, Schmeiser HH, et al. Urothelial carcinoma associated with the use of a Chinese herb (Aristolochia fangchi). *N Engl J Med*. 2000;342:1686-1692.
4. Ivić M. [Etiology of endemic nephropathy]. *Lijec Vjesn*. 1969;91:1273-1281.
5. Grollman AP, Shibutani S, Moriya M, et al. Aristolochic acid and the etiology of endemic (Balkan) nephropathy. *Proc Natl Acad Sci USA*. 2007;104:12129-12134.

24 Diabetes

Intensive Diabetes Therapy and Glomerular Filtration Rate in Type 1 Diabetes
The DCCT/EDIC Research Group (Univ of Washington, Seattle; The George Washington Univ, Rockville, MD; et al)
N Engl J Med 365:2366-2376, 2011

Background.—An impaired glomerular filtration rate (GFR) leads to end-stage renal disease and increases the risks of cardiovascular disease and death. Persons with type 1 diabetes are at high risk for kidney disease, but there are no interventions that have been proved to prevent impairment of the GFR in this population.

Methods.—In the Diabetes Control and Complications Trial (DCCT), 1441 persons with type 1 diabetes were randomly assigned to 6.5 years of intensive diabetes therapy aimed at achieving near-normal glucose concentrations or to conventional diabetes therapy aimed at preventing hyperglycemic symptoms. Subsequently, 1375 participants were followed in the observational Epidemiology of Diabetes Interventions and Complications (EDIC) study. Serum creatinine levels were measured annually throughout the course of the two studies. The GFR was estimated with the use of the Chronic Kidney Disease Epidemiology Collaboration formula. We analyzed data from the two studies to determine the long-term effects of intensive diabetes therapy on the risk of impairment of the GFR, which was defined as an incident estimated GFR of less than 60 ml per minute per 1.73 m^2 of body-surface area at two consecutive study visits.

Results.—Over a median follow-up period of 22 years in the combined studies, impairment of the GFR developed in 24 participants assigned to intensive therapy and in 46 assigned to conventional therapy (risk reduction with intensive therapy, 50%; 95% confidence interval, 18 to 69; $P = 0.006$). Among these participants, end-stage renal disease developed in 8 participants in the intensive-therapy group and in 16 in the conventional-therapy group. As compared with conventional therapy, intensive therapy was associated with a reduction in the mean estimated GFR of 1.7 ml per minute per 1.73 m^2 during the DCCT study but during the EDIC study was associated with a slower rate of reduction in the GFR and an increase in the mean estimated GFR of 2.5 ml per minute per 1.73 m^2 ($P < 0.001$ for both comparisons). The beneficial effect of intensive therapy on the risk of an impaired GFR was fully attenuated after adjustment for glycated hemoglobin levels or albumin excretion rates.

TABLE 2.—Incidence of an Impaired Glomerular Filtration Rate (GFR) and Secondary Outcomes*

Outcome	Intensive Diabetes Therapy		Conventional Diabetes Therapy		Risk Reduction with Intensive Therapy[†]	
	No. of Events	Incidence Rate/1000 Person-Yr	No. of Events	Incidence Rate/1000 Person-Yr	% (95% CI)	P Value
Impaired GFR[‡]	24	1.6	46	3.0	50 (18 to 69)	0.006
Onset during DCCT	1		3			
Onset during EDIC	23		43			
Estimated GFR <45 ml/min/1.73 m²	24	1.6	39	2.5	40 (1 to 64)	0.045
Estimated GFR <30 ml/min/1.73 m²[§]	13	0.8	23	1.5	44 (−9 to 72)	0.09
End-stage renal disease[§]	8	0.5	16	1.1	51 (−14 to 79)	0.10
Combined outcome of impaired GFR or death[¶]	53	3.4	80	5.2	37 (10 to 55)	0.01

Editor's Note: Please refer to original journal article for full references.

*Separate models were created to assess the effect of intensive therapy in the DCCT on the risk of each outcome, with the use of Cox proportional-hazards models, with robust estimation of the covariance matrix according to the method of Lin and Wei[16] to compute confidence limits and P values that are valid when proportional-hazards assumptions are violated; models were adjusted for the estimated GFR at baseline in the DCCT.

[†]The reduction in risk associated with intensive diabetes therapy was calculated as (1 − hazard ratio with intensive versus conventional diabetes therapy) × 100.

[‡]An impaired GFR, defined as a sustained estimated GFR of less than 60 ml per minute per 1.73 m² of body-surface area, was the primary study outcome.

[§]All cases of an estimated GFR that was less than 30 ml per minute per 1.73 m² and all cases of end-stage renal disease occurred during the course of the follow-up EDIC study. There were two participants (both assigned to conventional therapy) in whom end-stage renal disease developed without a documented sustained estimated GFR of less than 60 ml per minute per 1.73 m²; it was assumed for the purposes of the analyses that the impaired GFR developed midway between the last available measurement of the estimated GFR and the time of onset of end-stage renal disease.

[¶]This analysis included all 70 instances of renal impairment that were observed (of which 24 occurred among participants in the intensive-therapy group and 46 among participants in the conventional-therapy group), plus an additional 63 deaths that occurred among participants who were still free of renal impairment (of which 29 occurred in the intensive-therapy group and 34 in the conventional-therapy group). There were additional deaths (data not shown) that occurred after renal impairment developed in a participant; these deaths did not constitute a competing risk for renal impairment, and the difference between the groups in the rate of these deaths was insufficient to permit a reliable analysis.

Conclusions.—The long-term risk of an impaired GFR was significantly lower among persons treated early in the course of type 1 diabetes with intensive diabetes therapy than among those treated with conventional diabetes therapy. (Funded by the National Institute of Diabetes and Digestive and Kidney Diseases and others; DCCT/EDIC ClinicalTrials.gov numbers, NCT00360815 and NCT00360893.) (Table 2).

▶ Type I diabetics are at particularly high risk for progressive renal disease. To date, no single intervention has been found to completely stave off the progression of renal disease in those patients at risk for progression. The Diabetes Control and Complications Trial (DCCT) and the observational study that followed it, the Epidemiology of Diabetes Intervention and Complications (EDIC), found that intensive glucose control reduced the risk of micro/macroalbuminuria in patients with type I diabetes. Albuminuria, however, is not universally accepted as a clinical surrogate of renal outcome.[1-4] The current study evaluated the effects of intensive diabetic therapy on the development of impaired renal function as measured by glomerular filtration rate (GFR) with a total follow-up of 22 years. Of note, at the time of 16-year follow-up, the use of angiotensin-converting enzyme inhibitor or angiotensin receptor blocker therapy was not different between the 2 groups. The mean glycated hemoglobin level during the DCCT trial was 7.3% in the intensive therapy group and 9.1% in the conventional therapy group. Table 2 displays the long-term incidence data for GFR and secondary outcomes. For this study, an impaired GFR was defined as an estimated GFR of less than 60 mL/min/1.73 m^2 for 2 consecutive study visits usually a year apart.

An obvious strength of this study is the long-term follow-up of well-defined, randomly assigned treatment groups. A limitation in the trial was a nonrandomized use of medications other than insulin.

Overall, the study found that a risk of an impaired GFR was 50% lower in patients in whom intensive diabetic treatment began early and who received treatment for an average of 6.5 years when compared with those who received conventional glycemic control. As the authors note, these data suggest that treating approximately 29 persons with type I diabetes with intensive therapy for 6.5 years will prevent 1 case of an impaired GFR over a period of 20 years. These results add a direct measure of renal function (creatinine) to the prior surrogate data (albuminuria) and reinforce an HgA1C level of less than 7% as a goal to prevent GFR impairment in patients with type I diabetes.

R. Garrick, MD

References

1. The Diabetes Control and Complications Trial Research Group. The effect of intensive treatment of diabetes on the development and progression of long-term complications in insulin-dependent diabetes mellitus. *N Engl J Med.* 1993;329:977-986.
2. The Diabetes Control and Complications Trial Research Group. Effect of intensive therapy on the development and progression of diabetic nephropathy in the Diabetes Control and Complications Trial. *Kidney Int.* 1995;47:1703-1720.
3. Writing Team for the Diabetes Control and Complications Trial/Epidemiology of Diabetes Interventions and Complications Research Group. Sustained effect of intensive treatment of type 1 diabetes mellitus on development and progression

of diabetic nephropathy: the Epidemiology of Diabetes Interventions and Complications (EDIC) study. *JAMA*. 2003;290:2159-2167.
4. Molitch ME, Steffes M, Sun W, et al. Development and progression of renal insufficiency with and without albuminuria in adults with type 1 diabetes in the diabetes control and complications trial and the Epidemiology of diabetes interventions and complications study. *Diabetes Care*. 2010;33:1536-1543.

Sulodexide fails to demonstrate renoprotection in overt type 2 diabetic nephropathy

Packham DK, Collaborative Study Group (Melbourne Renal Res Group, Victoria, Australia)
J Am Soc Nephrol 23:123-130, 2012

Sulodexide, a mixture of naturally occurring glycosaminoglycan polysaccharide components, has been reported to reduce albuminuria in patients with diabetes, but it is unknown whether it is renoprotective. This study reports the results from the randomized, double-blind, placebo-controlled, sulodexide macroalbuminuria (Sun-MACRO) trial, which evaluated the renoprotective effects of sulodexide in patients with type 2 diabetes, renal impairment, and significant proteinuria (> 900 mg/d) already receiving maximal therapy with angiotensin II receptor blockers. The primary end point was a composite of a doubling of baseline serum creatinine, development of ESRD, or serum creatinine ≥ 6.0 mg/dl. We planned to enroll 2240 patients over approximately 24 months but terminated the study after enrolling 1248 patients. After 1029 person-years of follow-up, we did not detect any significant differences between sulodexide and placebo; the primary composite end point occurred in 26 and 30 patients in the sulodexide and placebo groups, respectively. Side effect profiles were similar for both groups. In conclusion, these data do not suggest a renoprotective benefit of sulodexide in patients with type 2 diabetes, renal impairment, and macroalbuminuria.

▶ The Collaborative Study Group evaluated the renoprotective effect of sulodexide, a noncoagulate heparin naturally occurring glucosaminoglycan, in patients with type II diabetes. Sulodexide has been marketed worldwide for a number of years as treatment for a range of vascular disorders. Initial data suggested that therapy with sulodexide reduced albuminuria in both type I and type II diabetes. The current multinational, randomized, double-blind, placebo-controlled trial studied the effect of sulodexide in patients with type II diabetes and significant proteinuria (> 900 mg/d).

Although the initial plan was to enroll 2409 patients, after enrollment of 1248 patients the study was terminated, unrelated to concerns regarding drug toxicity or adverse clinical outcomes. Evaluation of 1029 person-years of follow-up did not yield any significant differences between sulodexide treatment and placebo with regard to either changes in serum creatinine or the urinary protein creatinine ratio.

The study results are important because early clinical trials, including those by the collaborative study group, yielded promising results regarding its potential antiproteinuric effect in diabetics.[1-3]

Despite its early termination, it is important that clinicians be aware of the results of this trial. Many agents that initially appear promising lose their luster when subjected to more detailed investigation. Unfortunately, this particular drug is especially challenging, as there are no surrogate biomarkers by which to measure its absorption or biopharmacologic effectiveness. Although the early termination precludes definitive analysis, the available data suggest that this agent will not be useful for the treatment of diabetic nephropathy.

R. Garrick, MD

References

1. Heerspink HL, Greene T, Lewis JB, et al; Collaborative Study Group. Effects of sulodexide in patients with type 2 diabetes and persistent albuminuria. *Nephrol Dial Transplant*. 2008;23:1946-1954.
2. Lambers Heerspink HJ, Fowler MJ, Volgi J, et al; Collaborative Study Group. Rationale for and study design of the sulodexide trials in Type 2 diabetic, hypertensive patients with microalbuminuria or overt nephropathy. *Diabet Med*. 2007;24:1290-1295.
3. Lewis E, Lewis J, Greene T, et al; Collaborative Study Group. Sulodexide for kidney protection in type 2 diabetes patients with microalbuminuria: a randomized controlled trial. *Am J Kidney Dis*. 2011;58:729-736.

Circulating TNF Receptors 1 and 2 Predict Stage 3 CKD in Type 1 Diabetes

Gohda T, Niewczas MA, Ficociello LH, et al (Harvard Med School, Boston, MA)

J Am Soc Nephrol 23:516-524, 2012

Elevated plasma concentrations of TNF receptors 1 and 2 (TNFR1 and TNFR2) predict development of ESRD in patients with type 2 diabetes without proteinuria, suggesting these markers may contribute to the pathogenesis of renal decline. We investigated whether circulating markers of the TNF pathway determine GFR loss among patients with type 1 diabetes. We followed two cohorts comprising 628 patients with type 1 diabetes, normal renal function, and no proteinuria. Over 12 years, 69 patients developed estimated GFR less than 60 mL/min per 1.73 m² (16 per 1000 person-years). Concentrations of TNFR1 and TNFR2 were strongly associated with risk for early renal decline. Renal decline was associated only modestly with total TNFα concentration and appeared unrelated to free TNFα. The cumulative incidence of estimated GFR less than 60 mL/min per 1.73 m² for patients in the highest TNFR2 quartile was 60% after 12 years compared with 5%−19% in the remaining quartiles. In Cox proportional hazards analysis, patients with TNFR2 values in the highest quartile were threefold more likely to experience renal decline than patients in the other quartiles (hazard ratio, 3.0; 95% confidence interval, 1.7−5.5). The risk associated with high TNFR1 values was

TABLE 2.—Incidence of CKD ≥ 3 in Patients with T1D During 5- to 12-Year Follow-up According to Quartiles of Distributions of Baseline Circulating TNF Pathway Marker Concentrations

Quartile	Patients (n)	Incidence Per 1000 Person-Years (No. of Events)			
		Free TNFα	Total TNFα	TNFR1	TNFR2
Q1	157	10 (11)	9 (9)	5 (6)	3 (4)
Q2	157	11 (12)	8 (9)	9 (10)	9 (10)
Q3	157	14 (13)	9 (10)	10 (11)	9 (10)
Q4	157	24 (21)	33 (29)	45 (42)	48 (44)
P for trend[a]		0.048	<0.0001	<0.0001	<0.0001

Q1–Q4, quartiles 1–4. Quartile boundaries for 25th, 50th, and 75th percentiles, respectively, are as follows (pg/ml for all values). Free TNFα: 3.3, 4.6, 6.1; total TNFα: 5.5, 8.8, 12.7; TNFR1: 1170, 1371, 1670; TNFR2: 1810, 2197, 2690.
[a]Bonferroni correction was applied.

slightly less than that associated with high TNFR2 values. TNFR levels were unrelated to baseline free TNFα level and remained stable over long periods within an individual. In conclusion, early GFR loss in patients with type 1 diabetes without proteinuria is strongly associated with circulating TNF receptor levels but not TNFα levels (free or total) (Table 2).

▶ Based on their observations that elevated plasma concentrations of tumor necrosis factor (TNF) alpha receptors 1 and 2 can predict the development of end-stage renal disease in type II diabetics with or without proteinuria,[1] the same team of investigators extended their work to type I diabetics. The current trial is based on 2 cohorts from Joslin Clinic studies comprising 628 patients with type I diabetes, no proteinuria, and normal renal function. Over a 12-year period, 69 patients developed stage 3 chronic kidney disease and as shown in Table 2, the plasma concentrations of TNF alpha receptors 1 and 2 were strongly associated with the risk for a decline in renal function. The influence of a variety of other clinical risk markers for diabetic progression such as glycemic control and albuminuria were assessed and the predictive power of TNF alpha receptors 1 and 2 remained intact.

This observation extends the investigators' similar findings regarding the role of TNF alpha receptors in the progression of renal disease in patients with type II diabetes to patients with type I diabetes. Of great interest is that these patients had normal renal function and no proteinuria at the start of the study when the samples for TNF measurements were obtained. The exact mechanism through which circulating TNF alpha receptors may affect kidney function remains to be elucidated, and these exciting human data clearly open a pathway for multiple lines of further investigation.

R. Garrick, MD

Reference

1. Niewczas MA, Gohda T, Skupien J, et al. Circulating TNF receptors 1 and 2 predict ESRD in type 2 diabetes. *J Am Soc Nephrol.* 2012;23:507-515.

Albuminuria and Estimated Glomerular Filtration Rate as Predictors of Diabetic End-Stage Renal Disease and Death

Berhane AM, Weil EJ, Knowler WC, et al (Natl Insts of Health, Phoenix, AZ)
Clin J Am Soc Nephrol 6:2444-2451, 2011

Background and Objectives.—We investigated predictive value of albuminuria and estimated GFR (eGFR) for ESRD in Pima Indians with type 2 diabetes.

Design, Setting, Participants and Measurements.—Beginning in 1982, 2420 diabetic Pima Indians ≥18 years old were followed until they developed ESRD or died or until December 31, 2005. Individuals were classified at baseline by urinary albumin-to-creatinine ratio (ACR) and by eGFR, calculated by the Chronic Kidney Disease Epidemiology Collaboration equation. Predictors of ESRD and mortality were examined by proportional hazards regression.

Results.—During a mean follow-up of 10.2 years, 287 individuals developed ESRD. Incidence of ESRD among individuals with macroalbuminuria (ACR ≥300 mg/g) was 9.3 times that of those with normoalbuminuria (ACR <30 mg/g), controlled for age, gender, and duration of diabetes. Incidence among individuals with eGFR 15 to 29 ml/min per 1.73 m^2 was 81.9 times that of those with eGFR 90 to 119 ml/min per 1.73 m^2. Models that combined albuminuria and eGFR added significant predictive information about risk of ESRD or death compared with models containing eGFR or albuminuria alone. The hazard ratio for ESRD associated with a 10-ml/min per 1.73 m^2 lower eGFR was 1.36, whereas that associated with an increase in albuminuria category was 2.69; corresponding hazard ratios for death were 1.15 and 1.37.

Conclusions.—These results suggest that incorporation of quantitative information about albuminuria into staging systems based on eGFR adds significant prognostic information about risk for diabetic ESRD and death (Table 3).

▶ Significant evidence demonstrates that the presence of albuminuria in addition to an elevated glomerular filtration rate (GFR) confers additional risk for the development of end-stage renal disease (ESRD).[1,2] Most of these data were drawn from heterogeneous population studies, and a relatively small percentage of the total population of each study had diabetes. The Native American Pima is a homogeneous population in which type 2 diabetes is extremely prevalent and represents an opportunity to study the predictive role of albuminuria and elevated GFR, either alone or in combination, on the development of end-stage renal disease. The results are quite impressive: over a 10-year period, slightly more than 12% of the patients studied developed end-stage renal disease. The incidence of end-stage renal disease increased with increasing albuminuria within each GFR category (Table 3). The data demonstrate that in this largely homogeneous population with type 2 diabetes, the combination of albuminuria and estimated GFR is a significantly better predictor of the development of ESRD than either marker is alone. This is the first large database that has focused on the

TABLE 3.—Unadjusted Incidence of ESRD and Mortality per 1000 Person-Years, Along with 95% CI, Stratified Simultaneously by Categories of eGFR and Albuminuria

	Normoalbuminuria			Microalbuminuria			Macroalbuminuria		
	Events	Person-Years	Rate (95% CI)	Events	Person-Years	Rate (95% CI)	Events	Person-Years	Rate (95% CI)
Incidence of ESRD									
eGFR (ml/min per 1.73 m²)									
≥120	34	5561.0	6.1 (4.1, 8.2)	16	2399.7	6.7 (3.8, 10.8)	14	463.9	30.2 (16.5, 50.7)
90 to 119	38	9450.7	4.0 (2.7, 5.3)	47	3503.0	13.4 (9.6, 17.3)	47	1079.6	43.5 (31.1, 56.0)
60 to 89	5	866.6	5.8 (1.9, 13.4)	11	542.3	20.3 (10.1, 36.3)	32	485.8	65.9 (43.0, 88.7)
30 to 59	1	69.9	14.3 (0.4, 79.6)	1	81.6	12.3 (0.3, 68.2)	30	166.3	180.4 (115.8, 245.0)
15 to 29	0	0	—	0	0	—	11	29.3	375.4 (187.3, 672.0)
Mortality rates									
eGFR (ml/min per 1.73 m²)									
≥120	59	5678.4	10.4 (7.7, 13.0)	22	2472.4	8.9 (5.2, 12.6)	15	545.1	27.5 (15.4, 46.2)
90 to 119	146	9583.1	15.2 (12.8, 17.7)	101	3666.7	27.5 (22.2, 32.9)	55	1317.6	41.7 (30.7, 52.8)
60 to 89	36	882.9	40.8 (27.5, 54.1)	29	472.8	50.6 (32.2, 69.1)	45	653.9	68.8 (48.7, 88.9)
30 to 59	4	73.8	54.2 (14.7, 138.7)	8	81.7	97.9 (42.2, 192.9)	37	274.0	135.0 (91.5, 178.5)
15 to 29	0	0	—	0	0	—	13	83.7	155.2 (82.6, 265.5)

Confidence intervals (CIs) are estimated using the exact Poisson multipliers for strata with number of events ≤20 and the normal approximation otherwise (26). eGFR, estimated GFR.

combined effects of eGFR and albuminuria on the risk of progression to ESRD in a homogeneous population of diabetics.

The results of the ADVANCE[3] trial conducted with 10 640 type 2 diabetic patients offer some insight into whether these results will extend to other populations. In ADVANCE, the follow-up was shorter (4.3 years) and the endpoint included doubling the serum creatinine, but as reported in this trial, both a low GFR and albuminuria contributed to the development of adverse renal events. Taken together, in this population, where diabetes and albuminuria are the 2 main contributing confounders, albuminuria and low GFR clearly predict the development of ESRD better than either measure alone. With regard to the general population, the findings suggest that a worsening degree of macroalbuminuria poses a significant risk for progression to ESRD in type 2 diabetics.

R. Garrick, MD

References

1. Hemmelgarn BR, Manns BJ, Lloyd A, et al. Relation between kidney function, proteinuria, and adverse outcomes. *JAMA*. 2010;303:423-429.
2. Hallan SI, Ritz E, Lydersen S, Romundstad S, Kvenild K, Orth SR. Combining GFR and albuminuria to classify CKD improves prediction of ESRD. *J Am Soc Nephrol*. 2009;20:1069-1077.
3. Ninomiya T, Perkovic V, de Galan BE, et al. Albuminuria and kidney function independently predict cardiovascular and renal outcomes in diabetes. *J Am Soc Nephrol*. 2009;20:1813-1821.

Relative Incidence of ESRD Versus Cardiovascular Mortality in Proteinuric Type 2 Diabetes and Nephropathy: Results From the DIAMETRIC (Diabetes Mellitus Treatment for Renal Insufficiency Consortium) Database
Packham DK, Alves TP, Dwyer JP, et al (Royal Melbourne Hosp, Australia; Univ of Texas Health Science Ctr, San Antonio; Vanderbilt Univ Med Ctr, Nashville, TN; et al)
Am J Kidney Dis 59:75-83, 2012

Background.—Previous studies have shown that patients with chronic kidney disease, including those with diabetic nephropathy, are more likely to die of cardiovascular disease than reach end-stage renal disease (ESRD). This analysis was conducted to determine whether ESRD is a more common outcome than cardiovascular death in patients with type 2 diabetic nephropathy, significant proteinuria, and decreased kidney function who were selected for participation in a clinical trial.

Study Design.—Retrospective analysis of the DIAMETRIC (Diabetes Mellitus Treatment for Renal Insufficiency Consortium) database derived from 2 prospective randomized controlled clinical trials (IDNT [Irbesartan Diabetic Nephropathy Trial] and RENAAL [Reduction of Endpoints in Non—Insulin-dependent Diabetes With the Angiotensin II Antagonist Losartan]).

Setting & Participants.—3,228 adult patients with type 2 diabetic nephropathy from IDNT and RENAAL were combined to establish the

DIAMETRIC database. This is the largest global source of clinical information for patients with type 2 diabetic nephropathy who have decreased kidney function and significant proteinuria.

Intervention.—Angiotensin receptor blocker versus non–angiotensin receptor blocker therapy to slow the progression of type 2 diabetic nephropathy (in the prospective trials).

Outcomes & Measurements.—Incidence rates of ESRD, cardiovascular death, and all-cause mortality.

Results.—Mean follow-up was 2.8 years; 19.5% of patients developed ESRD, approximately 2.5 times the incidence of cardiovascular death and 1.5 times the incidence of all-cause mortality. ESRD was more common than cardiovascular death in all subgroups analyzed with the exception of participants with low levels of albuminuria (albumin excretion <1.0 g/g) and well-preserved levels of kidney function (estimated glomerular filtration rate > 45 mL/min/1.73 m^2) at baseline.

Limitations.—All participants were included in a prospective clinical trial.

Conclusions.—Patients with type 2 diabetic nephropathy, characterized by decreased kidney function and significant proteinuria, are more likely to reach ESRD than die during 3 years' mean follow-up. Given the rapidly increasing number of cases of type 2 diabetes worldwide, this has implications for predicting future renal replacement therapy requirements (Fig 2).

▶ Packham and colleagues performed a retrospective analysis of the databases of 2 large randomized, prospective clinical trials involving 3222 adult patients

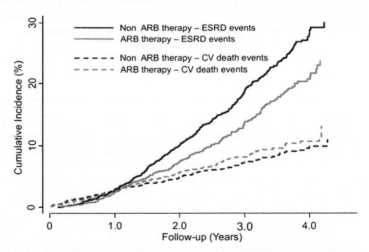

FIGURE 2.—Cumulative incidence plot of end-stage renal disease (ESRD; solid line) and cardiovascular (CV) death (dashed line) events. The black curve represents non–angiotensin receptor blocker (non–ARB)-treated participants and the gray curve represents ARB-treated participants. The plot accounts for the possibility of competing events between ESRD and CV death. (Reprinted from American Journal of Kidney Diseases, Packham DK, Alves TP, Dwyer JP, et al. Relative Incidence of ESRD Versus Cardiovascular Mortality in Proteinuric Type 2 Diabetes and Nephropathy: Results From the DIAMETRIC (Diabetes Mellitus Treatment for Renal Insufficiency Consortium) Database. *Am J Kidney Dis.* 2012;59:75-83. Copyright 2012 with permission from the National Kidney Foundation.)

with type II diabetes. The investigators sought to determine the incident rates of end-stage renal disease (ESRD), cardiovascular death, and all-cause mortality during the 3-year period prior to the onset of dialysis. The question at hand is whether patients with diabetic nephropathy will die before they progress to ESRD and initiate renal replacement therapy. Fig 2 demonstrates that the timing of ESRD and cardiovascular deaths was approximately equal during the first 12 months of follow-up in these large cohorts of type II diabetics. However, the authors report that ESRD becomes progressively more common than cardiovascular death, and after 18 months of follow-up the difference reached statistical significance.

Evaluation of the effective cardiovascular death rate as influenced by baseline albuminuria and estimated glomerular filtration rate (eGFR) found that for patients with an eGFR of less than 30 mL/min/1.73 m^2 and an albumin to creatinine ratio of greater than 2, the ratio of incident ESRD to cardiovascular death was almost 8 to 1.

These data are particularly interesting. Data from the trial UK Prospective Diabetes Study (UKPDS) strongly suggested that for type II diabetics, the likelihood of cardiovascular death was greater than the likelihood of progressing to dialysis.[1] The RENAAL and IDNT cohorts were carefully selected populations; in fact, patients who had a cardiac event in the preceding 3 months were excluded from the trials.[2] When taken in the context of other population studies[3,4] and the data from O'Hare and colleagues[5] regarding the trajectory of the loss of kidney function in the 2 years prior to dialysis (also reviewed here), the data suggest that several different types of patient populations exist. This in turn means that attempts to generalize, rather than individualize, the approach to care can be fraught with hazard. In addition, the data suggest that as the population ages, the number of individuals requiring some form of renal replacement therapy may be much higher than originally believed. This has obvious implications for both physician and national health care resources.

R. Garrick, MD

References

1. Adler AI, Stevens RJ, Manley SE, Bilous RW, Cull CA, Holman RR; UKPDS GROUP. Development and progression of nephropathy in type 2 diabetes: the United Kingdom Prospective Diabetes Study (UKPDS 64). *Kidney Int.* 2003;63:225-232.
2. Foley RN, Parfrey PS, Sarnak MJ. Clinical epidemiology of cardiovascular disease in chronic renal disease. *Am J Kidney Dis.* 1998;32:S112-S119.
3. Keith DS, Nichols GA, Gullion CM, Brown JB, Smith DH. Longitudinal follow-up and outcomes among a population with chronic kidney disease in a large managed care organization. *Arch Intern Med.* 2004;164:659-663.
4. Sarnak MJ, Levey AS, Schoolwerth AC, et al. Kidney disease as a risk factor for development of cardiovascular disease: a statement from the American Heart Association Councils on Kidney in Cardiovascular Disease, High Blood Pressure Research, Clinical Cardiology, and Epidemiology and Prevention. *Hypertension.* 2003;42:1050-1065.
5. O'Hare AM, Batten A, Burrows NR. Trajectories of kidney function decline in the 2 years before initiation of long-term dialysis. *Am J Kidney Dis.* 2012;59:513-522.

25 Selected Issues in Acute Kidney Injury

AKI in the ICU: definition, epidemiology, risk stratification, and outcomes
Singbartl K, Kellum JA (Univ of Pittsburgh, PA)
Kidney Int 81:819-825, 2012

Acute kidney injury (AKI) has emerged as a major public health problem that affects millions of patients worldwide and leads to decreased survival and increased progression of underlying chronic kidney disease (CKD). Recent consensus criteria for definition and classification of AKI have provided more consistent estimates of AKI epidemiology. Patients, in particular those in the ICU, are dying of AKI and not just simply with AKI. Even small changes in serum creatinine concentrations are associated with a substantial increase in the risk of death. AKI is not a single disease but rather a syndrome comprising multiple clinical conditions. Outcomes from AKI depend on the underlying disease, the severity and duration of renal impairment, and the patient's renal baseline condition. The development of AKI is the consequence of complex interactions between the actual insult and subsequent activation of inflammation and coagulation. Contrary to the conventional view, recent experimental and clinical data argue against renal ischemia—reperfusion as a *sine qua non* condition for the development of AKI. Loss of renal function can occur without histological signs of tubular damage or even necrosis. The detrimental effects of AKI are not limited to classical well-known symptoms such as fluid overload and electrolyte abnormalities. AKI can also lead to problems that are not readily appreciated at the bedside and can extend well beyond the ICU stay, including progression of CKD and impaired innate immunity. Experimental and small observational studies provide evidence that AKI impairs (innate) immunity and is associated with higher infection rates (Fig 1).

▶ The frequency and severity of acute kidney injury in the intensive care unit has prompted the need to refine our definitions and classifications standards. The RIFLE system, Fig 1, was initially begun as a research tool. More recently, this tool and other similar tools have been applied to bedside clinical medicine. The use of this approach has become more apparent, and this more clear-cut classification system has allowed us to better define the incidence of significant acute kidney injury (AKI). For example, in Australia between 2000 and 2005, of 120 123 patients admitted to intensive care units, renal injury (RIFLE "I")

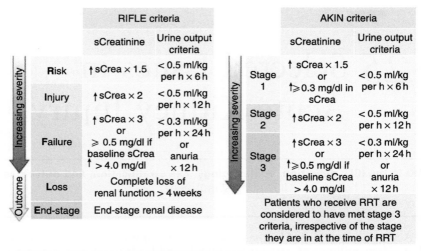

FIGURE 1.—Direct comparison of RIFLE (Risk of renal dysfunction, Injury to the kidney, Failure or Loss of kidney function, and End-stage kidney disease) and Acute Kidney Injury (AKI) Network criteria to classify AKI according to Bellomo et al.[7] and Mehta et al.,[8] respectively. Note that the original RIFLE criteria also listed glomerular filtration rates as reference, but these do not precisely agree with the changes in serum creatinine and were subsequently removed. For AKI Network criteria, the change in serum creatinine from baseline follows RIFLE, but there is also the option to use a 0.3 mg/dl increase if it is observed to occur within a 48-h period. RRT, renal replacement therapy. Editor's Note: Please refer to original journal article for full references. (Reprinted with permission from Macmillan Publishers Ltd: Kidney International, Singbartl K, Kellum JA. AKI in the ICU: definition, epidemiology, risk stratification, and outcomes. Kidney Int. 2012;81:819-825. Copyright 2012.)

occurred in 13.6% of patients and RIFLE F in 6.3% of patients. More significant is that hospital mortality was also independently correlated with the RIFLE category. The other benefit of more standardized AKI classification systems is that they help practitioners realize that the complications of AKI are not limited to fluid status and electrolytes alone. For example, the proinflammatory state associated with AKI can affect pulmonary function, and recent studies provide evidence for a link between AKI, progressive chronic kidney disease, and long-term morbidity and mortality. By better recognizing and defining episodes of AKI, practitioners may be more inclined to seek appropriate inpatient consultation and outpatient referral and follow-up.

R. Garrick, MD

Model to Predict Mortality in Critically Ill Adults with Acute Kidney Injury

Demirjian S, Chertow GM, Zhang JH, et al (Cleveland Clinic, OH; Univ School of Medicine, Palo Alto, CA; VA Connecticut Healthcare System, West Haven; et al)

Clin J Am Soc Nephrol 6:2114-2120, 2011

Background and Objectives.—Acute kidney injury (AKI) requiring dialysis is associated with high mortality. Most prognostic tools used to describe case complexity and to project patient outcome lack predictive accuracy when applied in patients with AKI. In this study, we developed an AKI-specific predictive model for 60-day mortality and compared the model to the performance of two generic (Sequential Organ Failure Assessment [SOFA] and Acute Physiology and Chronic Health Evaluation II [APACHE II]) scores, and a disease specific (Cleveland Clinic [CCF]) score.

Design, Setting, Participants, & Measurements.—Data from 1122 subjects enrolled in the Veterans Affairs/National Institutes of Health Acute Renal Failure Trial Network study; a multicenter randomized trial of intensive *versus* less intensive renal support in critically ill patients with AKI conducted between November 2003 and July 2007 at 27 VA- and university-affiliated centers.

Results.—The 60-day mortality was 53%. Twenty-one independent predictors of 60-day mortality were identified. The logistic regression model exhibited good discrimination, with an area under the receiver operating characteristic (ROC) curve of 0.85 (0.83 to 0.88), and a derived integer risk score yielded a value of 0.80 (0.77 to 0.83). Existing scoring systems, including APACHE II, SOFA, and CCF, when applied to our cohort, showed relatively poor discrimination, reflected by areas under the ROC curve of 0.68 (0.64 to 0.71), 0.69 (0.66 to 0.73), and 0.65 (0.62 to 0.69), respectively.

Conclusions.—Our new risk model outperformed existing generic and disease-specific scoring systems in predicting 60-day mortality in critically ill patients with AKI. The current model requires external validation before it can be applied to other patient populations.

▶ It is clear that the occurrence of acute kidney injury (AKI) confers an increased risk of adverse outcomes in hospitalized patients.[1] The accurate quantification of this risk is something of a holy grail in our evidence-based environment. An accurate model would be useful for testing various avenues for risk adjustment, as well as for providing accurate risk assessment for stratification in clinical trials.

These authors have constructed a risk model that accurately predicts 60-day all-cause mortality in patients with AKI requiring renal replacement therapy. Using data from 1122 subjects in the VA/NIH ATN study,[2] a multicenter randomized trial of intensive versus less intensive renal support in critically ill patients, they calculated the observed coefficient of risk for multiple individual measured parameters. These parameters were then weighted to reflect the relative predictive value of each for all-cause mortality. The most weighty were the use of mechanical ventilation and high fraction of inspired oxygen requirements. The least were the effects of coexisting cardiovascular disease, the presence of ischemic AKI, and hyperphosphatemia. The authors entered these and other parameters into a computerized predictive model that actually demonstrated good calibration with actual mortality (Hosmer—Lemeshow goodness-of-fit; $P = .76$).

Using these same risk coefficients, they then devised an integer risk score designed to facilitate a "paper and pencil" calculation of this risk. The final risk score was calculated as the sum of all the risk integers. This score was then tested against the actual mortality, and it demonstrated a remarkably high predictive value.

Although the nonintegerized computer-based score had a slightly better correlation than the integer risk score, as determined by area under the receiver operating characteristic calculation (0.80 vs 0.85), both performed statistically better than the APACHE II, SOFA, and Cleveland clinic scores (0.68, 0.69, 0.65, respectively).

This lends some predictability of outcome for inpatients with AKI requiring dialysis. This kind of predictability may result in more accurate clinical trials, as well as in more rational care decisions for these critically ill patients.

M. Klein, MD, JD

References

1. Chertow GM, Burdick E, Honour M, Bonventre JV, Bates DW. Acute kidney injury, mortality, length of stay, and costs in hospitalized patients. *J Am Soc Nephrol.* 2005; 16:3365-3370.
2. VA/NIH Acute Renal Failure Trial Network, Palevsky PM, Zhang JH, O'Connor TZ, et al. Intensity of renal support in critically ill patients with acute kidney injury. *N Engl J Med.* 2008;359:7-20.

Urinary Calprotectin and the Distinction between Prerenal and Intrinsic Acute Kidney Injury

Heller F, Frischmann S, Grünbaum M, et al (Charité Campus Benjamin Franklin, Berlin, Germany)
Clin J Am Soc Nephrol 6:2347-2355, 2011

Background and Objectives.—To date there is no reliable marker for the differentiation of prerenal and intrinsic acute kidney injury (AKI). We investigated whether urinary calprotectin, a mediator protein of the innate immune system, may serve as a diagnostic marker in AKI.

Design, Setting, Participants, & Measurements.—This was a cross-sectional study with 101 subjects including 86 patients with AKI (34 prerenal, 52 intrinsic including 23 patients with urinary tract infection) and 15 healthy controls. Assessment of urinary calprotectin concentration was by ELISA and immunohistochemistry of kidney biopsy specimens using a calprotectin antibody. Inclusion criteria were: admission to hospital for AKI stage 1 to 3 (Acute Kidney Injury Network); exclusion criteria were: prior renal transplantation and obstructive uropathy.

Results.—Median urinary calprotectin was 60.7 times higher in intrinsic AKI (1692 ng/ml) than in prerenal AKI (28 ng/ml, $p < 0.01$). Urinary calprotectin in prerenal disease was not significantly different from healthy controls (45 ng/ml, $p = 0.25$). Receiver operating curve curve analysis revealed a high accuracy of calprotectin (area under the curve, 0.97) in predicting intrinsic AKI. A cutoff level of 300 ng/ml provided a sensitivity of 92.3% and a specificity of 97.1%. Calculating urinary calprotectin/creatinine ratios did not lead to a further increase of accuracy. Immunostainings of kidney biopsies were positive for calprotectin in intrinsic AKI and negative in prerenal AKI.

Conclusions.—Accuracy of urinary calprotectin in the differential diagnosis of AKI is high. Whereas calprotectin levels in prerenal disease are comparable with healthy controls, intrinsic AKI leads to highly increased calprotectin concentrations.

▶ The differentiation of acute kidney injury (AKI) (or acute renal failure) from a prerenal etiology versus AKI secondary to intrinsic renal disease remains a challenging clinical problem, especially in the intensive care unit setting. The physical examination assessment of intravascular volume status, hemodynamic measurements, urinary osmolality, and electrolyte composition, including the fractional excretion of sodium, the urea/creatinine ratio, and the fractional excretion of urea, are all used to help differentiate prerenal AKI from intrinsic AKI. Unfortunately, each of these has clinical limitations and none, either alone or in combination, is sensitive or specific enough to provide a clear-cut definitive diagnosis.

These authors sought to determine whether urinary calprotectin, a mediator protein of the innate immune system, can be used to differentiate the etiology of acute kidney injury. The patients were diagnosed as having prerenal or intrinsic AKI based on histological criteria (the gold standard) or based on predefined clinical criteria. Serial urine samples were collected 3 times weekly on 86 patients with AKI for determination of the urinary calprotectin/creatinine and on 15 healthy controls.

The calprotectin concentration and the calprotectin/creatinine ratio did not differ between healthy controls and individuals with prerenal AKI. These levels were significantly higher in patients with intrinsic AKI, and the results remained statistically significant after exclusion of individuals with urinary tract infections. A urinary calprotectin level of 300 ng/mL provided a sensitivity and specificity of 92.3% and 97.1%, respectively. The urinary calprotectin/creatinine ratio did not enhance the diagnostic accuracy.

These results are very promising and may prove to have great clinical applicability. Further investigation is required to determine if or how the presence of specific underlying kidney diseases or systemic diseases affect urinary calprotectin excretion.

R. Garrick, MD

Urinary Biomarkers and Renal Recovery in Critically Ill Patients with Renal Support
Srisawat N, Wen X, Lee M, et al (Univ of Pittsburgh School of Medicine, PA; et al)
Clin J Am Soc Nephrol 6:1815-1823, 2011

Background and Objectives.—Despite significant advances in the epidemiology of acute kidney injury (AKI), prognostication remains a major clinical challenge. Unfortunately, no reliable method to predict renal recovery exists. The discovery of biomarkers to aid in clinical risk prediction for recovery after AKI would represent a significant advance over current practice.

Design, Setting, Participants, & Measurements.—We conducted the Biological Markers of Recovery for the Kidney study as an ancillary to the Acute Renal Failure Trial Network study. Urine samples were collected on days 1, 7, and 14 from 76 patients who developed AKI and received renal replacement therapy (RRT) in the intensive care unit. We explored whether levels of urinary neutrophil gelatinase-associated lipocalin (uNGAL), urinary hepatocyte growth factor (uHGF), urinary cystatin C (uCystatin C), IL-18, neutrophil gelatinase-associated lipocalin/matrix metalloproteinase-9, and urine creatinine could predict subsequent renal recovery.

Results.—We defined renal recovery as alive and free of dialysis at 60 days from the start of RRT. Patients who recovered had higher uCystatin C on day 1 (7.27 *versus* 6.60 ng/mg·creatinine) and lower uHGF on days 7 and 14 (2.97 *versus* 3.48 ng/mg·creatinine; 2.24 *versus* 3.40 ng/mg·creatinine). For predicting recovery, decreasing uNGAL and uHGF in the first 14 days was associated with greater odds of renal recovery. The most predictive model combined relative changes in biomarkers with clinical variables and resulted in an area under the receiver-operator characteristic curve of 0.94.

Conclusions.—We showed that a panel of urine biomarkers can augment clinical risk prediction for recovery after AKI.

▶ The study of Koyner et al[1] suggested that urinary biomarkers can predict the progression of acute kidney injury (AKI) after cardiac surgery. This article evaluates whether biomarkers can be used to predict renal recovery (defined as being dialysis free 60 days from the start of renal replacement therapy) after AKI in critically ill patients. The study was conducted as an ancillary to the Acute Renal Failure Trial Network Study and urine samples were collected from 76 patients who developed AKI requiring renal replacement therapy. As noted, these markers correlate well with renal injury and function, and the authors postulated whether a panel of candidate biomarkers could be used to predict the likelihood of renal recovery following an episode of AKI that was significant enough to require dialysis. The authors constructed a clinical risk prediction model based on age, Charlson Comorbidity Index, and the Acute Physiology and Chronic Health Evaluation II Score. Of these, the best predictors for renal recovery were age and the Charlson Comorbidity Index. When the clinical tool was modeled together with the biomarker data, the authors demonstrated that together they improved the ability to predict recovery (Fig 3 in the original article).

One caveat is that these data may not be generalizable to patients with AKI who did not receive renal replacement therapy. The study strengths are that it was a multicenter prospective trial that collected data over multiple time points. This is the first trial that has demonstrated that biomarkers combined with clinical data may be used to predict renal recovery. The data are very important. Based on clinical judgment alone, it is often extremely difficult for nephrologists to determine which patients with AKI are likely to recover, and this prognostic determinant is obviously critically important for patients and their families. Similar studies in other populations of patients with AKI are certainly warranted.

R. Garrick, MD

Reference

1. Koyner JL, Garg AX, Coca SG, et al. Biomarkers predict progression of acute kidney injury after cardiac Surgery. *J Am Soc Nephrol.* 2012;23:905-914.

Acute-on-chronic kidney injury at hospital discharge is associated with long-term dialysis and mortality

Wu V-C, on behalf of the NSARF Group (Natl Taiwan Univ Hosp, Taipei; et al)
Kidney Int 80:1222-1230, 2011

Existing chronic kidney disease (CKD) is among the most potent predictors of postoperative acute kidney injury (AKI). Here we quantified this risk in a multicenter, observational study of 9425 patients who survived to hospital discharge after major surgery. CKD was defined as a baseline estimated glomerular filtration rate < 45 ml/min per 1.73 m^2. AKI was stratified according to the maximum simplified RIFLE classification at hospitalization and unresolved AKI defined as a persistent increase in serum creatinine of more than half above the baseline or the need for dialysis at discharge. A Cox proportional hazard model showed that patients with AKI-on-CKD during hospitalization had significantly worse long-term survival over a median follow-up of 4.8 years (hazard ratio, 3.3) than patients with AKI but without CKD. The incidence of long-term dialysis was 22.4 and 0.17 per 100 person-years among patients with and without existing CKD, respectively. The adjusted hazard ratio for long-term dialysis in patients with AKI-on-CKD was 19.8 compared to patients who developed AKI without existing CKD. Furthermore, AKI-on-CKD but without kidney recovery at discharge had a worse outcome (hazard ratios of 4.6 and 213, respectively) for mortality and long-term dialysis as compared to patients without CKD or AKI. Thus, in a large cohort of postoperative patients who developed AKI, those with existing CKD were at higher risk for long-term mortality and dialysis after hospital discharge than those without. These outcomes were significantly worse in those with unresolved AKI at discharge (Table 3).

▶ The adverse effects of an episode of postoperative acute kidney injury (AKI) on long-term outcome has been recently demonstrated.[1,2] Although the presence of underlying kidney disease appears to worsen patient and renal outcomes,[3] the long-term effect of an episode of AKI on chronic kidney disease (CKD) has not been well studied. This multicenter observational study of 9425 patients who had undergone major surgery utilized the standardized RIFLE (risk, injury, failure, loss, and end stage) classification system to characterize AKI.[4] The results demonstrated that in patients with underlying CKD, defined as a baseline glomerular filtration rate (GFR) of less than 45 mL/min/1.73 m^2, an episode of AKI superimposed on a CKD resulted in significantly worse long-term survival and a higher incidence of dialysis dependence. The outcomes were even worse for patients who suffered an episode of AKI on CKD and had not recovered renal function at the time of discharge (Table 3). The very high incidence of

TABLE 3.—Hazard Ratio of Long-Term Outcomes Using Cox Proportional Hazard Model Among Subgroups Stratified by CKD and AKI Status[||]

CKD	AKI	Long-Term Mortality, HR (95% CI)[a]				Long-Term Dialysis, HR (95% CI)[a]		
Without prior CKD	Non-AKI	1 (reference)				1 (reference)		
	AKI	1.94 (1.76–2.14)***				4.64 (2.51–8.56)***		
Prior CKD	Non-AKI	1.39 (1.03–1.87)*	1 (reference)			40.86 (20.01–83.50)***	1 (reference)	
	AKI	3.28 (2.66–4.03)***	1.73 (1.42–2.10)***	1.26 (1.09–1.78)*	1 (reference)	91.6 (49.3–170.1)***	8.82 (5.20–14.96)***	1 (reference)
ESRD		4.27 (3.42–5.32)***	2.27 (1.84–2.80)***	1.66 (1.17–2.37)**	1.30 (0.99–1.71)	—	19.8 (13.6–28.7)***	2.24 (1.35–3.72)**

Abbreviations: Af, Atrial fibrillation; AKI, acute kidney disease; CAD, coronary artery disease; CHF, congestive heart failure; CI, confidence interval; CKD–AKI, acute-on-chronic kidney disease; CKD, chronic kidney disease; COPD, chronic obstructive pulmonary disease; DM, diabetes mellitus; ECMO, extracorporeal membrane oxygenation; ESRD, end-stage renal disease; HR, hazard ratio; HTN, hypertension; IABP, intra-aortic balloon pump; ICP, intracranial pressure; TCP, transcutaneous pacemaker.

Note, Table 2 has non-CKD–AKI as three groups and therefore the HR of prior CKD or ESRD come out differently even for other groups in Table 3.

[a]HRs of long-term mortality and dialysis in each group are compared with different reference.

*P < 0.05.

**P < 0.01.

***P < 0.001.

[||]Adjusted hazard ratio (95% CI) estimated from logistic regression model, adjusted for age, gender, admission subgroups, intervention (ECMO, ventilator, IABP, ICP, TCP, Swan–Ganz tube, PiCCO, and Sengstaken–Blakemore tube), comorbidity (HTN, DM, liver cirrhosis, CHF, chronic hepatitis, COPD, CAD, Af, and cancer), admission subgroups (Charlson score) by Cox regression modeling.

postoperative acute kidney injury and the current trend toward using intensivists, rather than nephrologists, to provide postoperative renal support, coupled with prior data showing the difficulty patients with AKI experience in obtaining outpatient referrals to nephrologists,[5] make the results of this study particularly worrisome.

R. Garrick, MD

References

1. Levy EM, Viscoli CM, Horwitz RI. The effect of acute renal failure on mortality. A cohort analysis. *JAMA*. 1996;275:1489-1494.
2. Mangano CM, Diamondstone LS, Ramsay JG, Aggarwal A, Herskowitz A, Mangano DT. Renal dysfunction after myocardial revascularization: risk factors, adverse outcomes, and hospital resource utilization. The Multicenter Study of Perioperative Ischemia Research Group. *Ann Intern Med*. 1998;128:194-203.
3. Hsu CY, Chertow GM, McCulloch CE, Fan D, Ordoñez JD, Go AS. Nonrecovery of kidney function and death after acute on chronic renal failure. *Clin J Am Soc Nephrol*. 2009;4:891-898.
4. Bellomo R, Ronco C, Kellum JA, et al. Acute renal failure - definition, outcome measures, animal models, fluid therapy and information technology needs: the Second International Consensus Conference of the Acute Dialysis Quality Initiative (ADQI) Group. *Crit Care*. 2004;8:R204-R212.
5. Chawla LS, Amdur R, Amodeo S, Kimmel PL, Palant CE. The severity of acute kidney injury predicts progression to chronic kidney disease. *Kidney Int*. 2011; 79:1361-1369.

Referral Patterns and Outcomes in Noncritically Ill Patients with Hospital-Acquired Acute Kidney Injury
Meier P, Bonfils RM, Vogt B, et al (Centre Hospitalier Universitaire Vaudois and Univ of Lausanne, Switzerland; Hôpital du Valais, Sion, Switzerland)
Clin J Am Soc Nephrol 6:2215-2225, 2011

Background and Objectives.—Despite modern treatment, the case fatality rate of hospital-acquired acute kidney injury (HA-AKI) is still high. We retrospectively described the prevalence and the outcome of HA-AKI without nephrology referral (nrHA-AKI) and late referred HA-AKI patients to nephrologists (lrHA-AKI) compared with early referral patients (erHA-AKI) with respect to renal function recovery, renal replacement therapy (RRT) requirement, and in-hospital mortality of HA-AKI.

Design, Setting, Participants, & Measurements.—Noncritically ill patients admitted to the tertiary care academic center of Lausanne, Switzerland, between 2004 and 2008 in the medical and surgical services were included. Acute kidney injury was defined using the Acute Kidney Injury Network (AKIN) classification.

Results.—During 5 years, 4296 patients (4.12% of admissions) experienced 4727 episodes of HA-AKI during their hospital stay. The mean ± SD age of the patients was 61 ± 15 years with a 55% male predominance. There were 958 patients with nrHA-AKI (22.3%) and 2504 patients with lrHA-AKI (58.3%). RRT was required in 31% of the patients with lrHA-AKI compared with 24% of the patients with erHA-AKI. In the multiple

TABLE 4.—Time to Refer HA-AKI Patients and In-Hospital Mortality in Medicine and Surgery Wards

Time to Refer (Days)	Mortality (OR)	95% CI	P
≤5	Reference		
6 to 10	1.81	1.36 to 2.42	<0.01
11 to 15	2.44	1.89 to 3.15	<0.01
>15	3.45	2.68 to 4.43	<0.01

HA-AKI, hospital-acquired acute kidney injury; OR, odds ratio; CI, confidence interval.

risk factor analysis, compared with erHA-AKI, nrHA-AKI and lrHA-AKI were significantly associated with worse renal outcome and higher in-hospital mortality.

Conclusions.—These data suggest that HA-AKI is frequent and the patients with nrHA-AKI or lrHA-AKI are at increased risk for in-hospital morbidity and mortality (Table 4).

▶ An episode of acute kidney injury (AKI) increases a patient's long-term risk of death and chronic kidney disease (CKD) compared with hospitalized patients without an AKI episode.[1] Surprisingly, patients with multiple comorbidities are less likely to be referred,[2] despite the fact that early referral to a nephrologist may even prevent further rise in level of creatinine.[3]

This study (Table 4) showed that earlier referral (within 5 days) decreased mortality and improves the patient's overall renal outcome. These observations are in accord with a delay in nephrology referral and may be associated with a higher intensive care unit mortality.[4,5]

Despite the rising incidence of AKI, referral to nephrologists remains low. Awareness of the risk factors for AKI, including older age and underlying CKD, may be helpful. In addition, a lack of awareness of the definition of AKI could be a cause of late, or nonreferral, and gaining familiarity with new AKI classification systems such as the RIFLE and AKIN may help providers better identify and respond to episodes of AKI.[6]

M. Brogan, MD

References

1. Coca SG, Yusuf B, Shlipak MG, Garg AX, Parikh CR. Long-term risk of mortality and other adverse outcomes after acute kidney injury: a systematic review and meta-analysis. *Am J Kidney Dis.* 2009;53:961-973.
2. Ali T, Tachibana A, Khan I, et al. The changing pattern of referral in acute kidney injury. *QJM.* 2011;104:497-503.
3. Balasubramanian G, Al-Aly Z, Moiz A, et al. Early nephrologist involvement in hospital-acquired acute kidney injury: a pilot study. *Am J Kidney Dis.* 2011;57:228-234.
4. Ponce D, Zorzenon Cde P, dos Santos NY, Balbi AL. Early nephrology consultation can have an impact on outcome of acute kidney injury patients. *Nephrol Dial Transplant.* 2011;26:3202-3206.
5. Mehta RL, McDonald B, Gabbai F, et al. Nephrology consultation in acute renal failure: does timing matter? *Am J Med.* 2002;113:456-461.

6. Mehta RL, Kellum JA, Shah SV, et al. Acute Kidney Injury Network. Acute Kidney Injury Network: report of an initiative to improve outcomes in acute kidney injury. *Crit Care.* 2007;11:R31-R34.

Biomarkers Predict Progression of Acute Kidney Injury after Cardiac Surgery

Koyner JL, for the TRIBE-AKI Consortium (Univ of Chicago, IL; et al)
J Am Soc Nephrol 23:905-914, 2012

Being able to predict whether AKI will progress could improve monitoring and care, guide patient counseling, and assist with enrollment into trials of AKI treatment. Using samples from the Translational Research Investigating Biomarker Endpoints in AKI study (TRIBE-AKI), we evaluated whether kidney injury biomarkers measured at the time of first clinical diagnosis of early AKI after cardiac surgery can forecast AKI severity. Biomarkers included urinary IL-18, urinary albumin to creatinine ratio (ACR), and urinary and plasma neutrophil gelatinase-associated lipocalin (NGAL); each measurement was on the day of AKI diagnosis in 380 patients who developed at least AKI Network (AKIN) stage 1 AKI. The primary end point (progression of AKI defined by worsening AKIN stage) occurred in 45 (11.8%) patients. Using multivariable logistic regression, we determined the risk of AKI progression. After adjustment for clinical predictors, compared with biomarker values in the lowest two quintiles, the highest quintiles of three biomarkers remained associated with AKI progression: IL-18 (odds ratio = 3.0, 95% confidence interval = 1.3—7.3), ACR (odds ratio = 3.4, 95% confidence interval = 1.3—9.1), and plasma NGAL (odds ratio = 7.7, 95% confidence interval = 2.6—22.5). Each biomarker improved risk classification compared with the clinical model alone, with plasma NGAL performing the best (category-free net reclassification improvement of 0.69, $P < 0.0001$). In conclusion, biomarkers measured on the day of AKI diagnosis improve risk stratification and identify patients at higher risk for progression of AKI and worse patient outcomes (Tables 1 and 2).

▶ As demonstrated by other studies, lifelong after-effects can follow an episode of postoperative acute kidney injury (AKI).[1] Preoperative risk stratification tools exist for defining who is at risk for suffering an episode of postoperative AKI. Recent data suggest that urinary biomarkers are potentially useful for demonstrating patients at risk for AKI.[2,3] The current prospective, multicenter observational cohort study evaluated urinary biomarkers in patients who had undergone cardiac surgery and who had early clinical suggestions of AKI as based on a rise in the serum creatinine.

An important caveat of such trials is that to be clinically useful, these markers need to define a population of patients with clinically significant kidney injury who are at risk for progression. As such, in this trial the primary endpoint was progression of AKI, as defined by worsening of the acute kidney injury score. Among 1219 cardiac surgery patients, 426 (34.9%) developed AKI. Biomarkers

TABLE 1.—Clinical Characteristics in Patients with and Without AKI Progression

| | AKI Progressed | | |
	No ($n=335$)	Yes ($n=45$)	P Value
Demographics			
age, years	72.3 (9.4)	71.3 (9.9)	0.39
female	93 (28%)	13 (29%)	0.87
white race	314 (94%)	41 (91%)	0.52
patients with diabetes	144 (43%)	24 (53%)	0.19
congestive heart failure	103 (31%)	20 (44%)	0.07
ejection fraction, mean percent (SD)	49.6 (13.7)	50.5 (10.6)	0.69
preoperative creatinine, mg/dl[a]	1.14 (0.34)	1.26 (0.45)	0.12
preoperative eGFR (CKD-EPI) ml/min	64.3 (18.9)	60.7 (22.7)	0.22
<30	12 (3.6%)	4 (8.9%)	
30–60	126 (38%)	17 (38%)	
60–90	171 (51%)	19 (42%)	
>90	26 (7.8%)	5 (11%)	
preoperative medications			
β-blockers	251 (75%)	34 (77%)	0.78
ACE inhibitors/ARB	231 (69%)	30 (67%)	0.76
aspirin	245 (74%)	36 (82%)	0.24
statins	250 (75%)	28 (64%)	0.11
Preoperative biomarkers			
urine albumin to creatinine ratio (mg/g)	23.2 (10.3, 73.8)	29.6 (11.7, 69.5)	0.66
urine NGAL (ng/ml)	10.1 (5.1, 21.6)	9.8 (6.2, 17.4)	0.78
urine IL-18 (pg/ml)	14.4 (6.9, 31.4)	18.8 (9.2, 32.7)	0.66
plasma NGAL (ng/ml)	64.3 (60.0, 106.1)	67.9 (60.0, 125.1)	0.51
Operative factors			
status of the procedure			0.06
elective	246 (73%)	27 (60%)	
urgent or emergent	89 (27%)	18 (40%)	
Cardiac catheterization in the last 72 hours	31 (9.4%)	4 (8.9%)	0.91
surgery type			0.17
CABG	158 (47%)	17 (38%)	
valve	94 (28%)	11 (24%)	
CABG and valve	83 (25%)	17 (38%)	
IABP	18 (5.4%)	6 (13%)	0.051
repeat cardiac surgery	77 (24%)	8 (18%)	0.38
off CPB surgery	22 (6.6%)	4 (8.9%)	0.57
CPB time (min)[b]	120.9 (58.1)	165.2 (93.3)	<0.001
aortic cross-clamp time (min)[b]	82.4 (44.6)	112.5 (64.1)	<0.001

Mean (SD), median (interquartile range), or number (percent). AKI progression defined by worsening of AKIN stage from original diagnosis of AKI. eGFR, estimated GFR; CKD-EPI, CKD epidemiology collaboration equation; ACE, angiotensin converting enzyme; ARB, angiotensin receptor blockers; CABG, coronary artery bypass grafting; IABP, intra-aortic balloon pump; CPB, cardiopulmonary bypass.
[a]To convert serum creatinine values (to μmol/L), multiply by 88.4.
[b]Perfusion time is reported for the patients who had CPB and cross-clamping.

were available on 380 patients and, of those, 45 patients (11.8% of AKI) progressed to a higher severity of AKI, and 15 (33.3%) required acute dialysis. The clinical characteristics of the patients in whom AKI progressed and those it did not are shown in Table 1. The addition of the biomarkers (albumin creatinine ratio, urinary interleukin-18 levels, urinary and plasma neutrophil gelatinase-associated lipocalin [NGAL]) improved risk classification compared with clinical models alone (based on urine output and serum creatinine). The data suggest that measurement of the albumin creatinine ratio (> 133 mg/g) and plasma NGAL (> 323 ng/mL) may identify populations that are at highest

TABLE 2.—Postoperative Characteristics and Outcomes in Patients with and Without AKI Progression

	No (*n*=335)	AKI Progressed Yes (*n*=45)	*P* Value
Time of AKI			
serum creatinine[a]	1.6 (0.4)	1.9 (0.6)	0.08
percent change in serum creatinine day of AKI	39.5 (18.0)	54.7 (34.7)	0.01
oliguria[b] on day of AKI	13 (4%)	4 (9%)	0.25
Diuretic use			
day before the day of AKI	85 (35%)	6 (30%)	0.63
day of AKI	135 (41%)	15 (33%)	0.35
Outcomes			
repeat cardiac surgery during hospitalization	22 (6.6%)	10 (22%)	0.0018
received RRT	0 (0%)	15 (33%)	<0.0001
length of ICU stay, days	3.8 (8.0)	15.7 (28.8)	<0.0001
length of hospital stay, days	9.5 (10.1)	22.9 (32.2)	<0.0001
in-hospital mortality	7 (2%)	10 (22%)	<0.0001

Mean (SD) or number (percent). AKI progression defined by worsening of AKIN stage from original diagnosis of AKI. RRT, renal replacement therapy.
[a]To convert serum creatinine values (to μmol/L), multiply by 88.4.
[b]Oliguria defined as a patient who had <500 ml in 24 hours.

risk for the most significant adverse renal outcomes. The ultimate hope is that early risk prediction may help guide clinical decision-making and improve outcomes. This is especially important because, as shown in Table 2, the occurrence of clinically significant progressive AKI significantly affects overall hospital outcomes and mortality.

R. Garrick, MD

References

1. Brown JR, Kramer RS, Coca SG, Parikh CR. Duration of acute kidney injury impacts long-term survival after cardiac surgery. *Ann Thorac Surg.* 2010;90:1142-1148.
2. Nickolas TL, O'Rourke MJ, Yang J, et al. Sensitivity and specificity of a single emergency department measurement of urinary neutrophil gelatinase-associated lipocalin for diagnosing acute kidney injury. *Ann Intern Med.* 2008;148:810-819.
3. Parikh CR, Coca SG, Thiessen-Philbrook H; TRIBE-AKI Consortium. Postoperative biomarkers predict acute kidney injury and poor outcomes after adult cardiac surgery. *J Am Soc Nephrol.* 2011;22:1748-1757.

26 Selected Issues in Chronic Renal Failure and Transplantation

Early Changes in Kidney Function Predict Long-Term Chronic Kidney Disease and Mortality in Patients After Liver Transplantation
Cantarovich M, Tchervenkov J, Paraskevas S, et al (McGill Univ Health Ctr, Montréal, Quebec, Canada; et al)
Transplantation 92:1358-1363, 2011

Background.—Chronic kidney disease (CKD) is a well-known complication after liver transplantation (LT) and is associated with increased mortality. The purpose of this study was to determine risk factors of advanced CKD and mortality after LT.

Methods.—Four hundred forty-five adult patients underwent LT between June 1990 and September 2007 and survived more than 1 month. Multivariate Cox regression analyses were performed for time to CKD stage 4 (glomerular filtration rate [GFR] $\leq$30 mL/min), time to chronic dialysis, and all-cause mortality. Several patient and disease characteristics were used as independent pre- and posttransplant variables. We specifically analyzed a drop more than or equal to 30% in the estimated GFR (eGFR) during the first year posttransplant.

Results.—Diabetes mellitus pretransplant and a drop more than or equal to 30% in the eGFR between 3 and 12 months predicted CKD stage 4 (odds ratio [OR] 4.1, 95% confidence interval [CI] 1.9−5.4, $P < 0.001$ and OR 16.1, 95% CI 5.9−44.5, $P < 0.0001$, respectively), the need for chronic dialysis (OR 3.8, 95% CI 1.1−13.2, $P = 0.03$ and OR 14.6, 95% CI 3.0−71.4, $P < 0.001$, respectively), and all-cause mortality (OR 1.9, 95% CI 1.2−2.9, $P = 0.004$ and OR 2.6, 95% CI 1.6−4.4, $P < 0.001$, respectively), more than 1 year after LT.

Conclusions.—Diabetes mellitus pretransplant and a drop more than or equal to 30% in the eGFR within the first year are strong predictors of advanced CKD, chronic dialysis, and death more than 1 year after LT.

These easily determined clinical variables define a population at risk for CKD who should be targeted for renal protection strategies.

▶ In previous studies, these authors demonstrated a marked reduction in survival in liver transplant patients who required chronic dialysis (49.2% vs 26.8%).[1]

This article evaluates the risk factors for the development of advanced chronic kidney disease (CKD) (estimated glomerular filtration rate [eGFR] less than 30 mL/min/1.73 m^2), new onset dialysis, and the mortality risk posthepatic transplantation. The strongest risk factors for stage 4 CKD (eGFR less than 30 mL/min/1.73 m^2), postliver transplantation was an eGFR drop of 30% or more between 3 months and 1 year posttransplant (odds ratio [OR], 16.1; $P < .0001$) and pretransplant diabetes mellitus (OR 4.1; $P < .001$). These same risk factors also most strongly predicted the likelihood of new initiation of dialysis and mortality.

Additional predictors of advanced CKD stage 4 (eGFR less than 30 mL/min/1.73 m^2) included a positive serology for hepatitis C virus (OR 4.0; 95% confidence interval [CI], 2.0-8.2; $P < .001$), new onset diabetes mellitus within the first year posttransplant (OR 5.4; 95% CI, 1.5-20.2; $P = .01$), and total bilirubin at 1 month (OR 3.2; 95% CI, 1.9-5.4; $P < .001$). Among patients with a drop in eGFR of 30% between postoperative months 3 and 12, the cumulative incidence of CKD stage 4 reached approximately 25% by the 5th year posttransplant.

Limitations of the findings include the lack of information on albuminuria throughout the study. In addition, eGFR equations have been shown to be of variable utility when used in patients with liver disease,[2] and other evaluations of renal function would strengthen these observations.

Despite these limitations, the data clearly demonstrate that preventing a drop in renal function during the early posttransplant interval is an important goal. Posttransplant immunosuppressive therapy is no longer the singular risk factor for CKD. Modifiable risk factors such as dyslipidemia, elevated uric acid, insulin dependent diabetes, and hypertension have been associated with late decline in renal function.[3,4] Treatment of these modifiable risk factors, the avoidance of nephrotoxins posttransplant, and the use of calcineurin-sparing agents may help prevent progression of CKD in this population. In addition, pretransplant counseling should include a discussion of the risk and burden of CKD postliver transplantation.[5]

M. Brogan, MD

References

1. Al Riyami D, Alam A, Badovinac K, Ivis F, Trpeski L, Cantarovich M. Decreased survival in liver transplant patients requiring chronic dialysis: a Canadian experience. *Transplantation.* 2008;85:1277-1280.
2. Attia A, Zahran A, Shoker A. Comparison of equations to estimate the glomerular filtration rate in post-renal transplant chronic kidney disease patients. *Saudi J Kidney Dis Transpl.* 2012;23:453-460.
3. Leithead JA, Ferguson JW, Hayes PC. Modifiable patient factors are associated with the late decline in renal function following liver transplantation. *Clin Transplant.* 2012;26:316-323.
4. de Boccardo G, Kim JY, Schiano TD, et al. The burden of chronic kidney disease in long-term liver transplant recipients. *Transplant Proc.* 2008;40:1498-1503.
5. Ojo AO, Held PJ, Port FK, et al. Chronic renal failure after transplantation of a nonrenal organ. *N Engl J Med.* 2003;349:931-940.

Center-Level Factors and Racial Disparities in Living Donor Kidney Transplantation

Hall EC, James NT, Garonzik Wang JM, et al (Johns Hopkins School of Medicine, Baltimore, MD)
Am J Kidney Dis 59:849-857, 2012

Background.—On average, African Americans attain living donor kidney transplantation (LDKT) at decreased rates compared with their non–African American counterparts. However, center-level variations in this disparity or the role of center-level factors is unknown.

Study Design.—Observational cohort study.

Setting & Participants.—247,707 adults registered for first-time kidney transplants from 1995-2007 as reported by the Scientific Registry of Transplant Recipients.

Predictors.—Patient-level factors (age, sex, body mass index, insurance status, education, blood type, and panel-reactive antibody level) were adjusted for in all models. The association of center-level characteristics (number of candidates, transplant volume, LDKT volume, median time to transplant, percentage of African American candidates, percentage of pre-listed candidates, and percentage of LDKT) and degree of racial disparity in LDKT was quantified.

Outcomes.—Hierarchical multivariate logistic regression models were used to derive center-specific estimates of LDKT attainment in African American versus non–African American candidates.

Results.—Racial parity was not seen at any of the 275 transplant centers in the United States. At centers with the least racial disparity, African Americans had 35% lower odds of receiving LDKT; at centers with the most disparity, African Americans had 76% lower odds. Higher percentages of African American candidates (interaction term, 0.86; $P = 0.03$) and prelisted candidates (interaction term, 0.80; $P = 0.001$) at a given center were associated with increased racial disparity at that center. Higher rates of LDKT (interaction term, 1.25; $P < 0.001$) were associated with less racial disparity.

Limitations.—Some patient-level factors are not captured, including a given patient's pool of potential donors. Geographic disparities in deceased donor availability might affect LDKT rates. Center-level policies and practices are not captured.

Conclusions.—Racial disparity in attainment of LDKT exists at every transplant center in the country. Centers with higher rates of LDKT attainment for all races had less disparity; these high-performing centers might provide insights into policies that might help address this disparity.

▶ These are important albeit troubling data. Based on 247 707 adults registered (1995–2007) for first-time kidney transplants, as reported by the Scientific Registry of Transplant Recipients, racial disparities exist regarding living donor transplant candidacy in every dialysis unit in the country, including centers with a large African American population. The findings are based on a hierarchical multivariate logistic regression model that evaluated center-specific estimates of living donor kidney transplants in African American versus non—African American candidates. In the centers with the highest disparity, African Americans had a 76% lower odds ratio of receiving a living donor transplant.

The specific reasons for these findings are unclear. However, it is clear that now that these data are available, there is a need to carefully examine distinct patient-, donor-, and center-specific reasons for this striking disparity. In addition, it is important for all practitioners who care for patients with chronic kidney disease to be aware of these data in order to best help patients achieve appropriate evaluation and, if possible and available, living donor transplantation.

R. Garrick, MD

27 Dialysis

All-cause mortality in hemodialysis patients with heart valve calcification
Raggi P, Bellasi A, Gamboa C, et al (Emory Univ, Atlanta, GA; Univ of Bologna, Italy; Univ of Alabama at Birmingham)
Clin J Am Soc Nephrol 6:1990-1995, 2011

Background and Objectives.—Calcification of the mitral and aortic valves is common in dialysis patients (CKD-5D). However, the prognostic significance of valvular calcification (VC) in CKD is not well established.

Design, Setting, Participants, & Measurements.—144 adult CKD-5D patients underwent bidimensional echocardiography for qualitative assessment of VC and cardiac computed tomography (CT) for quantification of coronary artery calcium (CAC) and VC. The patients were followed for a median of 5.6 years for mortality from all causes.

Results.—Overall, 38.2% of patients had mitral VC and 44.4% had aortic VC on echocardiography. Patients with VC were older and less likely to be African American; all other characteristics were similar between groups. The mortality rate of patients with calcification of either valve was higher than for patients without VC. After adjustment for age, gender, race, diabetes mellitus, and history of atherosclerotic disease, only mitral VC remained independently associated with all-cause mortality (hazard ratio [HR], 1.73; 95% confidence interval [CI], 1.03 to 2.91). Patients with calcification of both valves had a two-fold increased risk of death during follow-up compared with patients without VC (HR, 2.16; 95% CI, 1.14 to 4.08). A combined CT score of VC and CAC was strongly associated with all-cause mortality during follow-up (HR for highest versus lowest tertile, 2.21; 95% CI, 1.08 to 4.54).

Conclusions.—VC is associated with a significantly increased risk for all-cause mortality in CKD-5D patients. These findings support the use of echocardiography for risk stratification in CKD-5D as recently suggested in the Kidney Disease Improving Global Outcomes guidelines.

▶ Although cardiac valve calcification has been associated with a poor prognosis in the general population,[1,2] in patients with end-stage renal disease and advanced chronic kidney disease (CKD), the association remains less clear.[3,4] The study by Raggi and colleagues evaluated the association between valvular calcification (as diagnosed by echocardiogram) and all-cause mortality in dialysis patients recruited from 2 geographically disparate populations (Denver and New Orleans). Including the recruitment period, patients were followed up for a median of 5.6 years, and mortality was verified by searching the Social

233

Security Death Index. Patients with calcified valves were older and less likely to be African American. After adjustment for a number of confounding indicators (age, race, gender, diabetes, atherosclerotic disease), mitral-, but not aortic-valve calcification was independently associated with all-cause mortality.

These data are important. Prior studies suggested a relationship between valvular calcification and mortality in peritoneal dialysis.[4] This prospective observational study is the first to suggest that the presence of mitral-valve calcification is of prognostic significance in patients on hemodialysis. Echocardiography is currently routinely indicated for diabetic patients on hemodialysis. The current findings support the recommendations proposed in the Kidney Disease Improving Global Outcomes (KDIGO) guidelines, that echocardiograms should be obtained in stage 5 CKD. These observations will be strengthened by studies in additional cohorts of dialysis patients, and if confirmed, this simple noninvasive test may be used to help practitioners better direct resources toward the most at-risk patients within the dialysis population.

R. Garrick, MD

References

1. Fox CS, Vasan RS, Parise H, et al. Mitral annular calcification predicts cardiovascular morbidity and mortality: the Framingham Heart Study. *Circulation.* 2003; 107:1492-1496.
2. Volzke H, Haring R, Lorbeer R, et al. Heart valve sclerosis predicts all-cause and cardiovascular mortality. *Atherosclerosis.* 2010;209:606-610.
3. Panuccio V, Tripepi R, Tripepi G, et al. Heart valve calcifications, survival, and cardiovascular risk in hemodialysis patients. *Am J Kidney Dis.* 2004;43:479-484.
4. Wang AY, Wang M, Woo J, et al. Cardiac valve calcification as an important predictor for all-cause mortality and cardiovascular mortality in long term peritoneal dialysis patients: a prospective study. *J Am Soc Nephrol.* 2003;14:159-168.

PART FIVE

PULMONARY DISEASE

JAMES A. BARKER, MD

Introduction

Welcome to the PULMONARY DISEASE section of the 2012 YEAR BOOK OF MEDICINE. 2012 has been another great year for reading articles. We have selected 30 of the best articles from the YEAR BOOK OF PULMONARY DISEASE.

Topical Summaries

ASTHMA

First of all, in ASTHMA many advances continue to be made in the genetic and molecular aspects of asthma. In addition, there are important new improvements in therapy. Our first article shows that 2 days of dexamethasone is just as good as 5 days of prednisone in an acute exacerbation therapy and thus this is a really nice useful article that might make it easier for patients to be compliant.

The second ASTHMA article is definitely worth reading. Many clinicians already use this, namely, using tiotropium as an added therapy to the inhaled beta agonist's steroid. This randomly controlled trial does show that this may indeed be helpful in severe asthma.

The third article will be the most interesting to many people. Many of us have heard of bronchial thermoplasty. Shifren and coauthors have now given us a definitive article about bronchial thermoplasty. This has been done as a point—counterpoint discussion. Over 275 patients are discussed from 3 different studies. They all come down on the point that bronchial thermoplasty does have advantage in the very severely afflicted patient. Please read this great article.

There is also a wonderful article about using the Internet to help do a rational taper for steroids in severe asthma. I think artificial intelligence is going to continue to be a bigger part of our practice in the next 5 to 25 years. This is just a taste of what is to come.

CHRONIC OBSTRUCTIVE PULMONARY DISEASE

Dr Maurer is the chapter editor for CHRONIC OBSTRUCTIVE PULMONARY DISEASE (COPD). She has very nicely put together a number of articles about population health and COPD. These are well represented in the YEAR BOOK OF PULMONARY DISEASE and I would encourage you to read these. Included are some very representative articles. For example, Gershon and coauthors have a great article about developing COPD. In addition, there is a very useful article by deTorres and coauthors in regard to lung cancer risk in patients with COPD. It has long been my observation that the risk is high. This article confirms that. I would encourage everyone to read this article.

Foreman and COPDGene Investigator coauthors again give us very important information to help us understand that there is a precedent for early onset (or low tobacco dose) COPD associated with females and African Americans.

Lung Cancer

Thirdly, Dr Tanoue has put together some excellent regarding the new information around lung cancer. Lung cancer remains the leading cause of death worldwide. Dr Tanoue points out that "In the United States, a projected 156 940 individuals will have succumbed to lung cancer in 2011." This is a staggering number. Lung cancer deaths are more than breast, colorectal, and prostate cancers combined. Lung cancer screening is finally taking off. There is a very nice discussion here about the Prostate, Lung, Colorectal, and Ovarian (PLCO) trial that is nicely summarized. However, of more practical use to us in Pulmonary is probably the low dose CT scan trial which has actually shown efficacy and is truly changing our practice in approaching these patients. These articles are included and are definitely worth reviewing in detail. I have also included some of Dr Tanoue's articles about tobacco cessation strategies and statistics. Clearly, to decrease lung cancer and COPD, we must go to the root of the problem and get more patients to stop smoking.

Pleural, Interstitial Lung, and Pulmonary Vascular Disease

Dr Christopher Spradley has updated information on Pleural, Interstitial Lung, and Pulmonary Vascular Disease. He found a very nice article with a noninvasive algorithm to screen for pulmonary hypertension that may allow us to do fewer right heart catheterizations. In addition, there are articles about using BNP to help with stratification of risk of scleroderma associated with pulmonary hypertension. These are wonderful, exciting articles.

In addition, we have included Rubin and coauthors on the SUPER-2 Study, which showed that sildenafil does indeed have efficacy. Read within for details.

Finally, there is a nice review by du Bois et al about the mortality risk in patients with IPF. This is always a question for those of us caring for these patients.

Sleep Disorders

Dr Shirley Jones did a wonderful job summarizing the new sleep disorder boundaries this year. She is particularly interested in sleep medicine across a lifespan. She selected articles that reflect that. The Sleep Disorder chapter has some very nice state-of-the-art articles about Obstructive Sleep Apnea, Risk and Consequences. One thing that I did not know was that OSA is an independent risk factor for chronic kidney disease.

Kohler et al have an extremely useful article about what happens if you stop CPAP. We all tell patients what we think will happen if they stop CPAP and now we can read this article and tell them that indeed all of their symptoms and signs, including edema and hypertension, will regress rapidly upon withdrawal of CPAP.

Finally she has a nice practical article from Quach et al about doing a brief sleep intervention in elementary school children, which showed marked improvement in functionality and quality of life.

CRITICAL CARE

The CRITICAL CARE chapter has some excellent state-of-the-art information. The lead article for this section was from Drs Schweickert and Cress which shows continued innovation in critical care. This article is about early mobilization and goes over how and why it works, the interaction of mind and body, and the fact that it is the cutting edge of what we need to be doing. Of course, there is a lot involved in early mobilization. Restraint plans will need to be changed, as will traditional roles, since physical therapists can't do this alone. Real team effort will be required to have patients stand or walk. In addition, this has proven to be safe. Obviously, medications would need to be markedly decreased so patients would not be asleep when they need to be walking. As we learn more about ICU delirium, we realize that medications are often part of the problem rather than part of the solution.

Of course, ventilated-assisted pneumonia is always a hot topic, and this year we have a nice article by Dr Yeh and partners from Taiwan showing that dysphagia screening markedly decreases pneumonia in acute stroke patients. There is a very high rate of pneumonia in stroke patients (30%) and anything we can do to decrease this will improve morbidity and mortality.

In addition, there is a nice article about noninvasive versus invasive ventilation for acute respiratory failure in patients with hematologic malignancies. This continues to be debated. It is clear that patients who are not too ill can be treated with noninvasive ventilation early on and may do better.

Nolan and Kelly from the United Kingdom have summarized airway challenges in the ICU from a huge data base. Their findings were very helpful but not very surprising. Read within to see more about this. Ten percent of ICU intubations being extremely difficult certainly seems spot on!

Finally, do read the article about stroke and mortality increasing in patients who develop atrial fibrillation when hospitalized with sepsis. Septic shock is extremely common in our critical care units. Atrial fibrillation is also common. Many of us have not thought to put this together, but we should have. We have always presumed that the atria are irritable in patients who are very ill and that they have catecholamine excess. However, this shows that we do need to take atrial fibrillation seriously and we should be anticoagulating these patients. Patients really do not want to have strokes.

Every one of these articles is worthwhile, and I encourage you to read them all and enjoy.

James A. Barker, MD

28 Asthma, Allergy, and Cystic Fibrosis

Two Days of Dexamethasone Versus 5 Days of Prednisone in the Treatment of Acute Asthma: A Randomized Controlled Trial
Kravitz J, Dominici P, Ufberg J, et al (St Barnabas Health System, Toms River, NJ; Albert Einstein Med Ctr, Philadelphia, PA; Temple Univ, Philadelphia, PA; et al)
Ann Emerg Med 58:200-204, 2011

Study Objective.—Dexamethasone has a longer half-life than prednisone and is well tolerated orally. We compare the time needed to return to normal activity and the frequency of relapse after acute exacerbation in adults receiving either 5 days of prednisone or 2 days of dexamethasone.

Methods.—We randomized adult emergency department patients (aged 18 to 45 years) with acute exacerbations of asthma (peak expiratory flow rate less than 80% of ideal) to receive either 50 mg of daily oral prednisone for 5 days or 16 mg of daily oral dexamethasone for 2 days. Outcomes were assessed by telephone follow-up.

Results.—Ninety-six prednisone and 104 dexamethasone subjects completed the study regimen and follow-up. More patients in the dexamethasone group reported a return to normal activities within 3 days compared with the prednisone group (90% versus 80%; difference 10%; 95% confidence interval 0% to 20%; $P = .049$). Relapse was similar between groups (13% versus 11%; difference 2%; 95% confidence interval -7% to 11%, $P = .67$).

Conclusion.—In acute exacerbations of asthma in adults, 2 days of oral dexamethasone is at least as effective as 5 days of oral prednisone in returning patients to their normal level of activity and preventing relapse (Table 2).

▶ Based on previous pediatric studies, this randomized controlled trial compared 2 days of 16 mg oral dexamethasone (D) to 5 days of 50 mg oral prednisone (P). Table 2 demonstrates that a statistically significant increase in numbers of D subjects returned to baseline activity levels at 3 days versus the group assigned to P. There was no significant difference between relapse rates, exacerbations, or visits to primary care practitioners. Weaknesses identified in the study design include telephone follow-up only and lack of objective scoring systems/pulmonary function outcomes. Several studies have demonstrated that as

TABLE 2.—Outcome Measures

Outcome Measure	Prednisone (%), N = 96	Dexamethasone (%), N = 104	Difference (%)	95% CI*
Days to return to normal, 0−3 days†	72 (80)	91 (90)	10	(0 to 20)
Any hospital admissions	1 (1)	3 (3)	2	(−6 to 2)
Any ED visits since discharge	6 (6)	5 (5)	1	(−5 to 8)
Any primary care provider visits since discharge	5 (5)	3 (3)	2	(−3 to 8)

*$P = .049$.
†Return to normal daily activity information missing for 6 prednisone and 3 dexamethasone patients.

many as 28% of patients leaving an emergency department (ED) following treatment for an acute exacerbation of asthma fail to fill prescriptions.[1,2] This study bears repeating with collection of objective data pre- and postdosing of steroids, assessment of safety parameters including a follow-up visit after the ED visit, and an in-clinic evaluation following treatment. Other useful data would be an objective evaluation of practitioner visits, prescription usage, ED visits, and use of reliever medications post ED visit. Based on this investigation, use of a long-acting, higher-potency, compressed steroid-dosing regimen appears to offer potential advantages, particularly if the first dose of D is administered in the ED and the following day's dose is dispensed to the patient on discharge from the ED. In addition, long-term administration of inhaled corticosteroids should be addressed at the time of ED admission for those patients not receiving controller medications on a regular basis.

S. K. Willsie, DO, MA

References

1. Thomas EJ, Burstin HR, O'Neil AC, Orav EJ, Brennan TA. Patient noncompliance with medical advice after the emergency department visit. *Ann Emerg Med.* 1996; 27:49-55.
2. Saunders CE. Patient compliance in filling prescriptions after discharge from the emergency department. *Am J Emerg Med.* 1987;5:283-286.

Tiotropium improves lung function in patients with severe uncontrolled asthma: A randomized controlled trial
Kerstjens HAM, Disse B, Schröder-Babo W, et al (Univ of Groningen, The Netherlands; Boehringer Ingelheim Pharma GmbH & Co KG, Biberach, Germany; Krankenhaus Gelnhausen, Germany; et al)
J Allergy Clin Immunol 128:308-314, 2011

Background.—Some patients with severe asthma remain symptomatic and obstructed despite maximal recommended treatment. Tiotropium, a long-acting inhaled anticholinergic agent, might be an effective bronchodilator in such patients.

Objective.—We sought to compare the efficacy and safety of 2 doses of tiotropium (5 and 10 μg daily) administered through the Respimat inhaler with placebo as add-on therapy in patients with uncontrolled severe asthma (Asthma Control Questionnaire score, ≥ 1.5; postbronchodilator FEV_1, $\leq 80\%$ of predicted value) despite maintenance treatment with at least a high-dose inhaled corticosteroid plus a long-acting β_2-agonist.

Methods.—This was a randomized, double-blind, crossover study with three 8–week treatment periods. The primary end point was peak FEV_1 at the end of each treatment period.

Results.—Of 107 randomized patients (54% female patients; mean, 55 years of age; postbronchodilator FEV_1, 65% of predicted value), 100 completed all periods. Peak FEV_1 was significantly higher with 5 μg (difference, 139 mL; 95% CI, 96−181 mL) and 10 μg (difference, 170 mL; 95% CI, 128−213 mL) of tiotropium than with placebo (both $P < .0001$). There was no significant difference between the active doses. Trough FEV_1 at the end of the dosing interval was higher with tiotropium (5 μg: 86 mL [95% CI, 41−132 mL]; 10 μg: 113 mL [95% CI, 67−159 mL]; both $P < .0004$). Daily home peak expiratory flow measurements were higher with both tiotropium doses. There were no significant differences in asthma-related health status or symptoms. Adverse events were balanced across groups except for dry mouth, which was more common on 10 μg of tiotropium.

Conclusion.—The addition of once-daily tiotropium to asthma treatment, including a high-dose inhaled corticosteroid plus a long-acting β_2-agonist, significantly improves lung function over 24 hours in patients with inadequately controlled, severe, persistent asthma (Figs 2 and 3).

▶ Symptomatic severe asthmatics already being treated with maximized therapy, including inhaled corticosteroids and long-acting β-agonists, were randomly

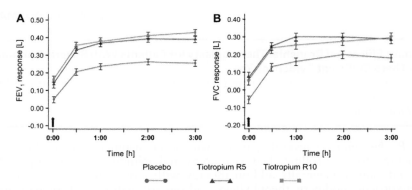

FIGURE 2.—FEV_1 (**A**) and FVC (**B**) responses relative to baseline values within 3 hours after dosing after 8 weeks of treatment. The difference in level at *0:00* h is the trough effect of tiotropium administered 24 hours earlier. The measurement obtained at baseline (visit 2 before any maintenance or study medication) is defined as the baseline value. At the on-treatment visits, this was immediately followed by the usual medication (including ICS plus LABA), and this in turn was followed by the study medication. *Error bars* represent SEMs. *Arrows* indicate the timing of the maintenance medication: ICS plus LABA. *Tiotropium R5,* 5 μg of tiotropium; *Tiotropium R10,* 10 μg of tiotropium. (Reprinted from The Journal of Allergy and Clinical Immunology, Kerstjens HAM, Disse B, Schröder-Babo W, et al. Tiotropium improves lung function in patients with severe uncontrolled asthma: a randomized controlled trial. *J Allergy Clin Immunol.* 2011;128:308-314. Copyright 2011, with permission from Elsevier.)

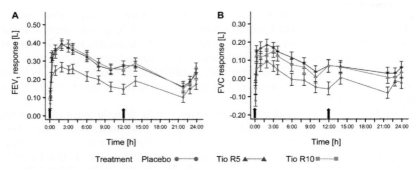

FIGURE 3.—Twenty-four-hour FEV$_1$ (**A**) and FVC (**B**) responses as shown in Fig 2 in the subgroup of patients with 24-hour assessments (n = 67). The baseline value was defined on visit 2 before any maintenance or study medication. At the on-treatment visits, this was immediately followed by the usual medication (including ICS plus LABA), which was followed in turn by the study medication. The afternoon dosing of ICS plus LABA treatment was also taken. *Error bars* represent SEMs. *Arrows* indicate the timing of the maintenance medication: ICS plus LABA. *Tio R5*, 5 µg of tiotropium; *Tio R10*, 10 µg of tiotropium. (Reprinted from The Journal of Allergy and Clinical Immunology, Kerstjens HAM, Disse B, Schröder-Babo W, et al. Tiotropium improves lung function in patients with severe uncontrolled asthma: a randomized controlled trial. *J Allergy Clin Immunol.* 2011;128:308-314. Copyright 2011, with permission from Elsevier.)

assigned to receive placebo, tiotropium 5 µg (T5) or 10 µg (T10) inhaled daily. Figs 2 and 3 show improvement in FEV$_1$, FVC, and peak expiratory flow over time. The only adverse event that was more prominent in the treated group versus placebo was dry mouth, which was most prominent in the T10 group. Improvement in pulmonary function was not statistically different between the T5 and T10 groups. Health care providers should consider adding T5 to their armamentarium for severe asthmatics not responding appropriately to guideline-directed care.

S. K. Willsie, DO, MA

Point: Efficacy of Bronchial Thermoplasty for Patients With Severe Asthma. Is There Sufficient Evidence? Yes

Shifren A, Chen A, Castro M, et al (Washington Univ School of Medicine, St Louis, MO)
Chest 140:573-579, 2011

Background.—Currently patients with severe asthma have no effective therapy for controlling their symptoms and minimizing their impaired health status. Generally add-on therapy with long-acting beta agonists, leukotriene modifiers, theophylline, and omalizumab is used for patients whose asthma is uncontrolled with inhaled corticosteroids. However, studies are showing that this approach tends to be ineffective in many patients, does not improve quality of life, is expensive, carries substantial side effects, and requires strict adherence to daily medications or monthly or biweekly injections. An alternative, more efficacious approach is desirable for these patients.

Alternative Treatment.—The controlled heating of the airway will diminish the amount of airway smooth muscle and reduce the airway's ability to bronchoconstrict in response to agonists such as methacholine. Bronchial thermoplasty is performed with the Alair Bronchial Thermoplasty System, which delivers a specific amount of radiofrequency (thermal) energy through a dedicated catheter. Treatments are delivered in three sessions and include careful preprocedure and postprocedure monitoring of the patient to manage any respiratory complications that may occur. This treatment can be delivered safely and effectively by pulmonologists.

Evidentiary Support.—Three controlled clinical trials of bronchial thermoplasty covering more than 275 patients have been conducted. In the first, patients demonstrated improved asthma symptoms and an encouraging reduction in mild exacerbations after 1 year of bronchial thermoplasty. The second revealed major improvements in various asthma measures, including forced expiratory volume at 1 second, quality of life, asthma control, and use of rescue medications, compared to a control group. A trend toward a greater reduction in the use of oral corticosteroids was noted in the treated group compared with controls after 1 year. The third study showed a significant improvement in asthma quality of life from baseline to 1 year when bronchial thermoplasty was compared with sham bronchoscopy. Treated patients showed a significant decline in severe exacerbations, emergency department visits, and days lost from work or school. The effects extended for over 2 years in patients receiving bronchial thermoplasty.

The most common adverse reactions to bronchial thermoplasty are breathlessness, wheeze, cough, chest discomfort, night awakenings, and productive cough. These generally occur within a day of the procedure and resolve in an average of 7 days with bronchodilators and corticosteroids. Computed tomography scans of the chest have shown no evidence of airway or parenchymal injury related to the procedure after 5 years.

Conclusions.—Patients with resistant asthma should be evaluated systematically to confirm the diagnosis, exclude any alternative diagnosis, identify comorbid conditions, evaluate treatment compliance, and assess treatment-induced side effects. With appropriate patient selection, management, and follow-up, bronchial thermoplasty may be an effective alternative treatment for severe asthma.

▶ This is a point—counterpoint discussing bronchial thermoplasty as an alternative for patients with severe, uncontrolled asthma and nowhere to turn. Summarized are the clinical trials that led to initial Food and Drug Administration approval of this technique in the United States. More than 55 centers worldwide now have clinicians who are reportedly applying this technique. Health care providers considering this technique for specific patients are encouraged to contact referral centers with experience in applying the technology.

S. K. Willsie, DO, MA

Internet-based tapering of oral corticosteroids in severe asthma: a pragmatic randomised controlled trial

Hashimoto S, Ten Brinke A, Roldaan AC, et al (Univ of Amsterdam, The Netherlands; Med Centre Leeuwarden, The Netherlands; Haga Ziekenhuis, Den Haag, The Netherlands; et al)
Thorax 66:514-520, 2011

Background.—In patients with prednisone-dependent asthma the dose of oral corticosteroids should be adjusted to the lowest possible level to reduce long-term adverse effects. However, the optimal strategy for tapering oral corticosteroids is unknown.

Objective.—To investigate whether an internet-based management tool including home monitoring of symptoms, lung function and fraction of exhaled nitric oxide (FE_{NO}) facilitates tapering of oral corticosteroids and leads to reduction of corticosteroid consumption without worsening asthma control or asthma-related quality of life.

Methods.—In a 6-month pragmatic randomised prospective multicentre study, 95 adults with prednisone-dependent asthma from six pulmonary outpatient clinics were allocated to two tapering strategies: according to conventional treatment (n = 43) or guided by a novel internet-based monitoring system (internet strategy) (n = 52). Primary outcomes were cumulative sparing of prednisone, asthma control and asthma-related quality of life. Secondary outcomes were forced expiratory volume in 1 s (FEV_1), exacerbations, hospitalisations and patient's satisfaction with the tapering strategy.

Results.—Median cumulative sparing of prednisone was 205 (25—75th percentile −221 to 777) mg in the Internet strategy group compared with 0 (−497 to 282) mg in the conventional treatment group ($p = 0.02$). Changes in prednisone dose (mixed effect regression model) from baseline were −4.79 mg/day and +1.59 mg/day, respectively ($p < 0.001$). Asthma control, asthma-related quality of life, FEV_1, exacerbations, hospitalisations and satisfaction with the strategy were not different between groups.

Conclusions.—An internet-based management tool including home monitoring of symptoms, lung function and FE_{NO} in severe asthma is superior to conventional treatment in reducing total corticosteroid consumption without compromising asthma control or asthma-related quality of life.

Clinical Trial Registration Number.—Clinical trial registered with http://www.trialregister.nl (Netherlands Trial Register number 1146).

▶ This is a novel and sophisticated instrument- and technology-laden approach compared with usual care (UC) in tapering prednisone dose in severe uncontrolled steroid-dependent asthmatics over 6 months. There have been successful efforts with reduction in prednisone (−4.79 mg/d vs +1.59 mg/d—usual care; $P < .001$). Drawbacks to this program appear to be individual use of sophisticated equipment (spirometry, fractional excretion of nitric oxide), required computers, required computer skills of subjects, and intensive nursing interventions. Despite this, the treatment algorithm appears to have potential merit, and further studies appear warranted with an evaluation of alternate delivery techniques that may be more cost effective.

S. K. Willsie, DO, MA

A CFTR Potentiator in Patients with Cystic Fibrosis and the *G551D* Mutation

Ramsey BW, for the VX08-770-102 Study Group (Seattle Children's Hosp and Univ of Washington School of Medicine; et al)
N Engl J Med 365:1663-1672, 2011

Background.—Increasing the activity of defective cystic fibrosis transmembrane conductance regulator (CFTR) protein is a potential treatment for cystic fibrosis.

Methods.—We conducted a randomized, double-blind, placebo-controlled trial to evaluate ivacaftor (VX-770), a CFTR potentiator, in subjects 12 years of age or older with cystic fibrosis and at least one *G551D-CFTR* mutation. Subjects were randomly assigned to receive 150 mg of ivacaftor every 12 hours (84 subjects, of whom 83 received at least one dose) or placebo (83, of whom 78 received at least one dose) for 48 weeks. The primary end point was the estimated mean change from baseline through week 24 in the percent of predicted forced expiratory volume in 1 second (FEV_1).

Results.—The change from baseline through week 24 in the percent of predicted FEV_1 was greater by 10.6 percentage points in the ivacaftor group than in the placebo group ($P < 0.001$). Effects on pulmonary function were noted by 2 weeks, and a significant treatment effect was maintained through week 48. Subjects receiving ivacaftor were 55% less likely to have a pulmonary exacerbation than were patients receiving placebo, through week 48 ($P < 0.001$). In addition, through week 48, subjects in the ivacaftor group scored 8.6 points higher than did subjects in the placebo group on the respiratory-symptoms domain of the Cystic Fibrosis Questionnaire—revised instrument (a 100-point scale, with higher numbers indicating a lower effect of symptoms on the patient's quality of life) ($P < 0.001$). By 48 weeks, patients treated with ivacaftor had gained, on average, 2.7 kg more weight than had patients receiving placebo ($P < 0.001$). The change from baseline through week 48 in the concentration of sweat chloride, a measure of CFTR activity, with ivacaftor as compared with placebo was -48.1 mmol per liter ($P < 0.001$). The incidence of adverse events was similar with ivacaftor and placebo, with a lower proportion of serious adverse events with ivacaftor than with placebo (24% vs. 42%).

Conclusions.—Ivacaftor was associated with improvements in lung function at 2 weeks that were sustained through 48 weeks. Substantial improvements were also observed in the risk of pulmonary exacerbations, patient-reported respiratory symptoms, weight, and concentration of sweat chloride. (Funded by Vertex Pharmaceuticals and others; VX08-770-102 ClinicalTrials.gov number, NCT00909532.)

▶ *Late Breaking Development in Cystic Fibrosis: January 31, 2012: New drug approved for use in Cystic Fibrosis.* Ivacaftor was approved by the US Food and Drug Administration (FDA) on January 31, 2012, for use in cystic fibrosis patients aged 6 and older who have at least 1 copy of the G551D mutation in the cystic fibrosis transmembrane conductance regulator (*CFTR*) gene. This investigation, published in the *New England Journal of Medicine*, was part of the research considered by the FDA in making its decision to approve this drug for use in the United States. Fig 1 in the original article depicts changes from baseline in percentage of predicted forced expiratory volume in 1 second, respiratory symptoms, and weight, and time to the first pulmonary exacerbation, according to the study group. The estimated annual cost of twice-daily dosing for ivacaftor is nearly $300 000; however, Vertex has announced plans to provide the drug for free to patients without insurance and who make less than $150 000 annually. FDA approval of this drug represents expedited approval of a genetic-based approach to disease management. The biggest winners in 2012 are the patients who will benefit from this new drug.

S. K. Willsie, DO, MA

29 Chronic Obstructive Pulmonary Disease

Lifetime risk of developing chronic obstructive pulmonary disease: a longitudinal population study

Gershon AS, Warner L, Cascagnette P, et al (Inst for Clinical Evaluative Sciences, Toronto, Ontario, Canada; et al)

Lancet 378:991-996, 2011

Background.—Although chronic obstructive pulmonary disease (COPD) is one of the most deadly, prevalent, and costly chronic diseases, no comprehensive estimates of the risk of developing COPD in the general population have been published. We aimed to quantify the lifetime risk of developing physician-diagnosed COPD in a large, multicultural North American population.

Methods.—We did a retrospective longitudinal cohort study using population-based health administrative data from Ontario, Canada (total population roughly 13 million). All individuals free of COPD in 1996 were monitored for up to 14 years for three possible outcomes; diagnosis of COPD by a physician, reached 80 years of age, or death. COPD was identified with a previously validated case definition based on COPD health services claims. The cumulative incidence of physician-diagnosed COPD over a lifetime adjusted for the competing risk of death was calculated by a modified survival analysis technique. Results were stratified by sex, socioeconomic status, and whether individuals lived in a rural or urban setting.

Findings.—A total of 579 466 individuals were diagnosed with COPD by a physician over the study period. The overall lifetime risk of physician-diagnosed COPD at age 80 years was 27·6%. Lifetime risk was higher in men than in women (29·7% vs 25·6%), individuals of lower socioeconomic status than in those of higher socioeconomic status (32·1% vs 23·0%), and individuals who lived in a rural setting than in those who lived in an urban setting (32·4% vs 26·7%).

Interpretation.—About one in four individuals are likely to be diagnosed and receive medical attention for COPD during their lifetime. Clinical evidence-based approaches, public health action, and more research

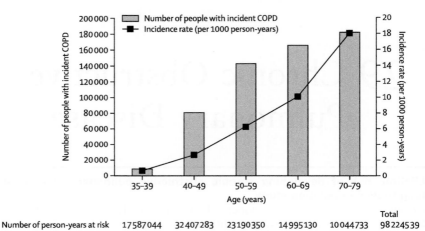

| Number of person-years at risk | 17 587 044 | 32 407 283 | 23 190 350 | 14 995 130 | 10 044 733 | Total 98 224 539 |

FIGURE 1.—Number of people with incident COPD, number of person-years at risk, and COPD incidence rate per 1000 person-years by age. COPD=chronic obstructive pulmonary disease. (Reprinted from The Lancet, Gershon AS, Warner L, Cascagnette P, et al. Lifetime risk of developing chronic obstructive pulmonary disease: a longitudinal population study. *Lancet.* 2011;378:991-996. © 2011, with permission from Elsevier.)

are needed to identify effective strategies to prevent COPD and ensure that those with the disease have the highest quality of life possible (Fig 1).

▶ Despite increased attention to chronic obstructive pulmonary disease (COPD) in recent years, it remains both an underfunded and underrecognized disease.[1] Gershon et al note that although it is currently the fourth most common cause of death worldwide and expected by the World Health Organization to be the third most common cause by 2030, there is a general paucity of public knowledge about the disease. That, they speculate, is because the average person believes that this is a disease people "bring on themselves" through unhealthy behaviors such as smoking. Although smoking-related disease is a common cause of the disease, biofuel use is increasingly recognized as a causative factor, and it is increasingly recognized that among the general public, there is a significant rate of COPD that does not (at present) have a specific known cause. The authors believe that increased public awareness through articles such as this showing a general population risk of disease will help to funnel more funding to better understand the causes and impact of chronic pulmonary disease. The strength of this study is that it covers the lifetime risk of physician-diagnosed COPD (Fig 1) in a complete population of a specific region (Ontario, Canada); however, that the study uses physician diagnoses and not confirmatory spirometry is also its greatest limitation. Physicians frequently assign a diagnosis of COPD to symptomatology (eg, shortness of breath) and record a diagnosis without objective confirmation. On the other hand, it is estimated that many people with actual COPD never have objective confirmation because the clinician does not order it. Which of these is most prevalent is unknown. At any rate, the study is thought-provoking and likely to achieve the authors' goal of increasing awareness.

J. R. Maurer, MD, MBA

Reference

1. Wise RA, Tashkin DP. Preventing chronic obstructive pulmonary disease: what is known and what needs to be done to make a difference to the patient? *Am J Med.* 2007;120:S14-S22.

Lung Cancer in Patients with Chronic Obstructive Pulmonary Disease: Incidence and Predicting Factors

de Torres JP, Marín JM, Casanova C, et al (Clínica Universidad de Navarra, Pamplona, Spain; Hospital Universitario Miguel Servet, Zaragoza, Spain; Hospital Nuestra Sra de Candelaria, Tenerife, Spain; et al)
Am J Respir Crit Care Med 184:913-919, 2011

Rationale.—Little is known about the clinical factors associated with the development of lung cancer in patients with chronic obstructive pulmonary disease (COPD), although airway obstruction and emphysema have been identified as possible risk factors.

Objectives.—To explore incidence, histologic type, and factors associated with development of lung cancer diagnosis in a cohort of outpatients with COPD attending a pulmonary clinic.

Methods.—A cohort of 2,507 patients without initial clinical or radiologic evidence of lung cancer was followed a median of 60 months (30—90). At baseline, anthropometrics, smoking history, lung function, and body composition were recorded. Time to diagnosis and histologic type of lung cancer was then registered. Cox analysis was used to explore factors associated with lung cancer diagnosis.

Measurements and Main Results.—A total of 215 of the 2,507 patients with COPD developed lung cancer (incidence density of 16.7 cases per 1,000 person-years). The most frequent type was squamous cell carcinoma (44%). Lung cancer incidence was lower in patients with worse severity of airflow obstruction. Global Initiative for Chronic Obstructive Lung Disease Stages I and II, older age, lower body mass index, and lung diffusion capacity of carbon monoxide less than 80% were associated with lung cancer diagnosis.

Conclusions.—Incidence density of lung cancer is high in outpatients with COPD and occurs more frequently in older patients with milder airflow obstruction (Global Initiative for Chronic Obstructive Lung Disease Stages I and II) and lower body mass index. A lung diffusion capacity of carbon monoxide less than 80% is associated with cancer diagnosis. Squamous cell carcinoma is the most frequent histologic type. Knowledge of these factors may help direct efforts for early detection of lung cancer and disease management.

▶ It seems intuitively obvious that there would be a high likelihood that patients with more severe chronic obstructive pulmonary disease (COPD) are also particularly susceptible to lung cancer since tobacco is the primary risk factor in both diseases. Yet the data linking these diseases are often not very detailed and somewhat contradictory.[1,2] One of the larger studies reported from registry data gave an incidence estimate in the population with moderate and severe obstruction followed over a median of 17.9 years but did not identify people with milder degrees of airway obstruction and therefore may underestimate the correlation between mild COPD and lung cancer.[3] The exclusion of patients with milder obstruction may be important, because other studies, including this one, identify a higher incidence of cancers in patients with milder obstructive disease, a seemingly paradoxical finding.[4,5] The authors provide speculation as to why this might be. The most intriguing reason hinges on immune function. The authors speculate that possibly smokers with mild disease that get cancer are relatively immune-suppressed by their smoking and therefore have less immune-related lung destruction but also have a higher susceptibility to cancer because of immunosuppression. This study provides several valuable insights in addition to confirming the inverse relationship between airflow obstruction and development of lung cancer. In particular, because it was a study in which the patients were followed up clinically for a median of 5 years, other risk factors for lung cancer were observed: older age, lower body mass index, and diffusing capacity of the lung < 80%. Knowing the risk factors allows easier and less expensive monitoring of a specific subgroup and the potential for early diagnosis and improved outcomes.

J. R. Maurer, MD, MBA

References

1. Tockman MS, Anthonisen NR, Wright EC, Donithan MG. Airways obstruction and the risk for lung cancer. *Ann Intern Med.* 1987;106:512-518.
2. Van den Eeden SK, Friedman GD. Forced expiratory volume (1 second) and lung cancer incidence and mortality. *Epidemiology.* 1992;3:253-257.
3. Mannino DM, Aguayo SM, Petty TL, Redd SC. Low lung function and incident lung cancer in the United States: data from the First National Health and Nutrition Examination Survey follow-up. *Arch Intern Med.* 2003;163:1475-1480.
4. Caplin M, Festenstein F. Relation between lung cancer, chronic bronchitis, and airways obstruction. *Br Med J.* 1975;3:678-680.
5. Wilson DO, Weissfeld JL, Balkan A, et al. Association of radiographic emphysema and airflow obstruction with lung cancer. *Am J Respir Crit Care Med.* 2008;178:738-744.

Early-Onset Chronic Obstructive Pulmonary Disease Is Associated with Female Sex, Maternal Factors, and African American Race in the COPDGene Study

Foreman MG, the COPDGene Investigators (Morehouse School of Medicine, Atlanta, GA; et al)

Am J Respir Crit Care Med 184:414-420, 2011

Rationale.—The characterization of young adults who develop late-onset diseases may augment the detection of novel genes and promote new pathogenic insights.

Methods.—We analyzed data from 2,500 individuals of African and European ancestry in the COPDGene Study. Subjects with severe, early-onset chronic obstructive pulmonary disease (COPD) (n = 70, age < 55 yr, FEV_1 < 50% predicted) were compared with older subjects with COPD (n = 306, age > 64 yr, FEV_1 < 50% predicted).

Measurements and Main Results.—Subjects with severe, early-onset COPD were predominantly females (66%), $P = 0.0004$. Proportionally, early-onset COPD was seen in 42% (25 of 59) of African Americans versus 14% (45 of 317) of non-Hispanic whites, $P < 0.0001$. Other risk factors included current smoking (56 vs. 17%, $P < 0.0001$) and self-report of asthma (39 vs. 25%, $P = 0.008$). Maternal smoking (70 vs. 44%, $P = 0.0001$) and maternal COPD (23 vs. 12%, $P = 0.03$) were reported more commonly in subjects with early-onset COPD. Multivariable regression analysis found association with African American race, odds ratio (OR), 7.5 (95% confidence interval [CI], 2.3—24; $P = 0.0007$); maternal COPD, OR, 4.7 (95% CI, 1.3—17; $P = 0.02$); female sex, OR, 3.1 (95% CI, 1.1—8.7; $P = 0.03$); and each pack-year of smoking, OR, 0.98 (95% CI, 0.96—1.0; $P = 0.03$).

Conclusions.—These observations support the hypothesis that severe, early-onset COPD is prevalent in females and is influenced by maternal factors. Future genetic studies should evaluate (*1*) gene-by-sex interactions to address sex-specific genetic contributions and (*2*) gene-by-race interactions.

▶ Chronic obstructive pulmonary disease (COPD) is well recognized in most cases as a primarily tobacco-caused disease with a loose dose-related relationship to the amount of tobacco used. Genetic studies are starting to identify innate susceptibilities to the effects of smoking. In recent years, the first large studies of populations with obstructive disease along with the collections of patients with advanced obstructive pathology in transplant centers and lung volume reduction programs have led to a better understanding of a complex array of disease features. One observation was that there exists a cohort of patients with early-onset disease. A report of a particular family cohort that did not have evidence of known hereditary alpha-1 antitrypsin disease but appeared to have onset of disease before the age of 52 noted that a large number of the family members with disease were women.[1] Another report from analysis of the database of the National Emphysema Treatment Trial (NETT) showed that the African-American participants appeared to have more severe and earlier-onset disease compared with whites with similar amounts of smoking.[2] With that background, Foreman et al looked at the first 2500 entrants into the COPDGene study in an attempt to more systematically confirm or disprove these findings. In addition to the propensity of women and African Americans to be victims of this disease, the authors found that maternal smoking and COPD were also influential. The "why" remains unknown. The good news is that the early-onset disease is a relatively rare phenotype of COPD in that only 70 participants were identified. However, those with early-onset disease had significantly lower levels of smoking than the general population of patients with COPD, suggesting that a dose response is not the primary factor in development of their disease. There is a significant limitation to this disease: it is not population based but rather a subanalysis of 2500 patients with COPD who voluntarily participate in a COPD database. This is, therefore, a self-selected population. Nevertheless, the description of this phenotype of COPD should help direct future genetic and molecular studies with, as the authors note, particular attention "to maternally inherited factors such as mitochondrial and X- chromosome genes as well as gene-by-sex and gene-by-race interactions." Only when we have the results of such studies will we be better able to understand the "why."

J. R. Maurer, MD, MBA

References

1. Silverman EK, Chapman HA, Drazen JM, et al. Genetic epidemiology of severe, early-onset chronic obstructive pulmonary disease. Risk to relatives for airflow obstruction and chronic bronchitis. *Am J Respir Crit Care Med.* 1998;157: 1770-1778.
2. Chatila WM, Hoffman EA, Gaughan J, Robinswood GB, Criner GJ. Advanced emphysema in African-American and white patients: do differences exist? *Chest.* 2006;130:108-118.

The Progression of Chronic Obstructive Pulmonary Disease Is Heterogeneous: The Experience of the BODE Cohort

Casanova C, de Torres JP, Aguirre-Jaíme A, et al (Hospital Universitario La Candelaria, Tenerife, Spain; Clínica Universitaria de Navarra, Pamplona, Spain; et al)
Am J Respir Crit Care Med 184:1015-1021, 2011

Rationale.—Chronic obstructive pulmonary disease (COPD) is thought to result in rapid and progressive loss of lung function usually expressed as mean values for whole cohorts.

Objectives.—Longitudinal studies evaluating individual lung function loss and other domains of COPD progression are needed.

Methods.—We evaluated 1,198 stable, well-characterized patients with COPD (1,100 males) recruited in two centers (Florida and Tenerife, Spain) and annually monitored their multidomain progression from 1997 to 2009. Patients were followed for a median of 64 months and up to 10 years. Their individual FEV_1 (L) and BODE index slopes, expressed as annual change, were evaluated using regression models for repeated measures. A total of 751 patients with at least three measurements were used for the analyses.

Measurements and Main Results.—Eighteen percent of patients had a statistically significant FEV_1 slope decline (-86 ml/yr; 95% confidence interval [CI], -32 to -278 ml/yr). Higher baseline FEV_1 (relative risk, 1.857; 95% CI, 1.322$-$2.610; $P < 0.001$) and low body mass index (relative risk, 1.071; 95% CI, 1.035$-$1.106; $P < 0.001$) were independently associated with FEV_1 decline. The BODE index had a statistically significant increase (0.55, 0.20$-$1.37 point/yr) in only 14% of patients and these had more severe baseline obstruction. Concordance between FEV_1 and BODE change was low (κ Cohen, 16%). Interestingly, 73% of patients had no significant slope change in FEV_1 or BODE. Only the BODE change was associated with mortality in patients without FEV_1 progression.

Conclusions.—The progression of COPD is very heterogeneous. Most patients show no statistically significant decline of FEV_1 or increase in BODE. The multidimensional evaluation of COPD should offer insight into response to COPD management (Fig 2).

▶ The progression of chronic obstructive pulmonary disease (COPD) was initially documented by Fletcher and Peto in the 1970s.[1] Surprisingly, few longitudinal studies of patients with COPD have been done since that description of the natural history of airway obstruction, yet it has become very clear that COPD is a heterogeneous disease with many phenotypes. The studies that have been done have usually been in the context of drug treatment trials and included patients with specific characteristics that met the inclusion criteria of the study, which potentially limits the ability to capture varying courses of different phenotypes.[2,3] Clinical experience suggests that some patients may remain stable for long periods, whereas others may appear to progress rapidly. It would be natural to assume that different phenotypes behave differently and that progression may also be different. The study by Casanova et al sheds some light on this. The study

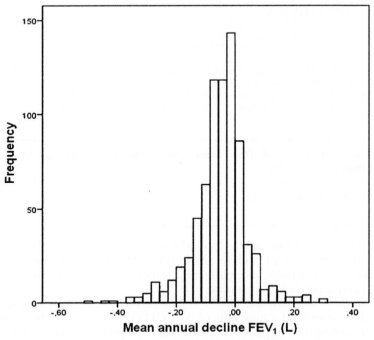

FIGURE 2.—Histogram of the mean annual FEV_1 decline (L) for the whole group. (Reprinted from Casanova C, de Torres JP, Aguirre-Jaíme A, et al. The progression of chronic obstructive pulmonary disease is heterogeneous: the experience of the BODE cohort. *Am J Respir Crit Care Med.* 2011;184:1015-1021. Official Journal of the American Thoracic Society © American Thoracic Society.)

reports follow up on a group of nearly 1200, mostly male, patients with COPD for a median of more than 5 years and up to 10 years. Progression was defined not only by change in FEV_1, but also by changes in the other parameters of the BODE index. During the follow-up period, most patients had neither a significant decrease in FEV_1 (Fig 2), or increase in BODE score. There was a small group that had a rapid progression of disease as measured by the BODE index but without a significant change in FEV_1. A third group had significant decreases in FEV_1 that was not related to their baseline level of obstruction. Vestbo et al,[4] reporting data from the ECLIPSE (Evaluation of COPD Longitudinally to Identify Predictive Surrogate Endpoints) trial, also noted large variability in the rate of decrease of FEV_1 and noted that the rate of decrease in smokers was greater than in nonsmokers and in patients with emphysema than those without.

These findings by Casanova et al led the authors to suggest that COPD should be thought of as having domains of both severity and activity. As COPD phenotype characteristics are better defined, categorizing by severity and activity—or using some other approach—may be helpful in tailoring therapy that is specific to the individual's needs.

J. R. Maurer, MD, MBA

References

1. Fletcher C, Peto R. The natural history of chronic airflow obstruction. *Br Med J.* 1977;1:1645-1648.
2. Anthonisen NR, Connett JE, Kiley JP, et al. Effects of smoking intervention and the use of an inhaled anticholinergic bronchodilator on the rate of decline of FEV1. The Lung Health Study. *JAMA.* 1994;272:1497-1505.
3. Celli BR, Thomas NE, Anderson JA, et al. Effect of pharmacotherapy on rate of decline of lung function in chronic obstructive pulmonary disease: results from the TORCH study. *Am J Respir Crit Care Med.* 2008;178:332-338.
4. Vestbo J, Edwards LD, Scanlon PD, et al. ECLIPSE investigators. Changes in forced expiratory volume in 1 second over time in COPD. *N Engl J Med.* 2011; 365:1184-1192.

Validation of a Novel Risk Score for Severity of Illness in Acute Exacerbations of COPD

Shorr AF, Sun X, Johannes RS, et al (Washington Hosp Ctr, DC; MedMined Services, Marlborough, MA)
Chest 140:1177-1183, 2011

Background.—Clinicians lack a validated tool for risk stratification in acute exacerbations of COPD (AECOPD). We sought to validate the BAP-65 (elevated BUN, altered mental status, pulse >109 beats/min, age > 65 years) score for this purpose.

Methods.—We analyzed 34,699 admissions to 177 US hospitals (2007) with either a principal diagnosis of AECOPD or acute respiratory failure with a secondary diagnosis of AECOPD. Hospital mortality and need for mechanical ventilation (MV) served as co-primary end points. Length of stay (LOS) and costs represented secondary end points. We assessed the accuracy of BAP-65 via the area under the receiver operating characteristic curve (AUROC).

Results.—Nearly 4% of subjects died while hospitalized and approximately 9% required MV. Mortality increased with increasing BAP-65 class, ranging from < 1% in subjects in class I (score of 0) to >25% in those meeting all BAP-65 criteria (Cochran-Armitage trend test $z = -38.48$, $P < .001$). The need for MV also increased with escalating score (2% in the lowest risk cohort vs 55% in the highest risk group, Cochran-Armitage trend test $z = -58.89$, $P < .001$). The AUROC for BAP-65 for hospital mortality and/or need for MV measured 0.79 (95% CI, 0.78—0.80). The median LOS was 4 days, and mean hospital costs equaled $5,357. These also varied linearly with increasing BAP-65 score.

Conclusions.—The BAP-65 system captures severity of illness and represents a simple tool to categorize patients with AECOPD as to their risk for adverse outcomes. BAP-65 also correlates with measures of resource use. BAP-65 may represent a useful adjunct in the initial assessment of AECOPDs.

▶ Acute exacerbations of chronic obstructive pulmonary disease (COPD) contribute disproportionately to the morbidity and mortality of the disease. Despite the high rate of exacerbations in the disease, especially in moderately severe and severe disease, clinicians do not have a validated, easy-to-use tool to stratify exacerbation events according to severity or prognosis. Such a tool could improve treatment by assisting in making appropriate decisions early as well as providing much needed information about the epidemiology of COPD exacerbations. Similar tools have been useful to clinicians in the early management of community-acquired pneumonia[1,2] and pulmonary embolism.[3,4] In fact, clinicians may not even agree on what constitutes an exacerbation. Trappenburg et al[5] recently reviewed more than 50 articles assessing existing symptom-based algorithms to identify exacerbations. Most of the existing algorithms use a scoring system based on pulmonary symptoms. The authors found that not only were there "large inconsistencies in definitions, methods and accuracy to define symptom-based COPD exacerbations," they also found that minor changes in symptom criteria had large impacts on incidence and other features of exacerbations. Some investigators continue to pursue this approach; however, Jones et al[6] reported a possibly more sophisticated approach to pulmonary symptom assessment that tries to quantify symptoms to better characterize exacerbations. Unfortunately, this does not seem to meet the need for a useful tool to provide information on severity and prognosis. Shorr et al[7] have taken a different tack that is promising. They used an approach similar to that used in community-acquired pneumonia that relies on easily objectively measured systemic features of illness rather than specific qualitative or quantitative features of pulmonary symptoms. In this article, they validate retrospectively their previously reported scoring system in a very large cohort of patients who presented with COPD exacerbations. Of course, the patient requires a diagnosis of acute exacerbation before the tool can be applied. But the precise clinical changes an individual clinician uses to define an acute exacerbation may not be so important if this new tool can provide useful prognostic information once a diagnosis is made. The tool now requires validation prospectively over a large cohort of patients.

J. R. Maurer, MD, MBA

References

1. Fine MJ, Auble TE, Yealy DM, et al. A prediction rule to identify low-risk patients with community-acquired pneumonia. *N Engl J Med.* 1997;336:243-250.
2. Lim WS, van der Eerden MM, Laing R, et al. Defining community acquired pneumonia severity on presentation to hospital: an international derivation and validation study. *Thorax.* 2003;58:377-382.
3. Aujesky D, Obrosky DS, Stone RA, et al. Derivation and validation of a prognostic model for pulmonary embolism. *Am J Respir Crit Care Med.* 2005;172:1041-1046.
4. Sanchez O, Trinquart L, Caille V, et al. Prognostic factors for pulmonary embolism: the prep study, a prospective multicenter cohort study. *Am J Respir Crit Care Med.* 2010;181:168-173.
5. Trappenburg JC, van Deventer AC, Troosters T, et al. The impact of using different symptom-based exacerbation algorithms in patients with COPD. *Eur Respir J.* 2011;37:1260-1268.
6. Jones PW, Chen WH, Wilcox TK, Sethi S, Leidy NK; EXACT-PRO Study Group. Characterizing and quantifying the symptomatic features of COPD exacerbations. *Chest.* 2011;139:1388-1394.
7. Tabak YP, Sun X, Johannes RS, Gupta V, Shorr AF. Mortality and need for mechanical ventilation in acute exacerbations of chronic obstructive pulmonary disease: development and validation of a simple risk score. *Arch Intern Med.* 2009;169:1595-1602.

30 Lung Cancer

Reduced Lung-Cancer Mortality with Low-Dose Computed Tomographic Screening
The National Lung Screening Trial Research Team (Univ of California at Los Angeles; Brown Univ, Providence, RI; Natl Cancer Inst, Bethesda, MD; et al)
N Engl J Med 365:395-409, 2011

Background.—The aggressive and heterogeneous nature of lung cancer has thwarted efforts to reduce mortality from this cancer through the use of screening. The advent of low-dose helical computed tomography (CT) altered the landscape of lung-cancer screening, with studies indicating that low-dose CT detects many tumors at early stages. The National Lung Screening Trial (NLST) was conducted to determine whether screening with low-dose CT could reduce mortality from lung cancer.

Methods.—From August 2002 through April 2004, we enrolled 53,454 persons at high risk for lung cancer at 33 U.S. medical centers. Participants were randomly assigned to undergo three annual screenings with either low-dose CT (26,722 participants) or single-view posteroanterior chest radiography (26,732). Data were collected on cases of lung cancer and deaths from lung cancer that occurred through December 31, 2009.

Results.—The rate of adherence to screening was more than 90%. The rate of positive screening tests was 24.2% with low-dose CT and 6.9% with radiography over all three rounds. A total of 96.4% of the positive screening results in the low-dose CT group and 94.5% in the radiography group were false positive results. The incidence of lung cancer was 645 cases per 100,000 person-years (1060 cancers) in the low-dose CT group, as compared with 572 cases per 100,000 person-years (941 cancers) in the radiography group (rate ratio, 1.13; 95% confidence interval [CI], 1.03 to 1.23). There were 247 deaths from lung cancer per 100,000 person-years in the low-dose CT group and 309 deaths per 100,000 person-years in the radiography group, representing a relative reduction in mortality from lung cancer with low-dose CT screening of 20.0% (95% CI, 6.8 to 26.7; $P = 0.004$). The rate of death from any cause was reduced in the low-dose CT group, as compared with the radiography group, by 6.7% (95% CI, 1.2 to 13.6; $P = 0.02$).

Conclusions.—Screening with the use of low-dose CT reduces mortality from lung cancer. (Funded by the National Cancer Institute; National Lung Screening Trial ClinicalTrials.gov number, NCT00047385.)

▶ The results of the National Lung Screening Trial presented in this report demonstrate that screening for lung cancer with low-dose CT scanning reduces mortality from lung cancer. This is a landmark study. No prior study of lung cancer screening by any modality has ever demonstrated a mortality benefit. As shown in Fig 1 in the original article, low-dose CT screening resulted in an increase in the number of lung cancers diagnosed as well as a decrease in the number of deaths from lung cancer when compared with screening with chest radiography. The Prostate, Lung, Colorectal, and Ovarian (PLCO) Cancer Randomized Trial demonstrated that chest radiography as a lung cancer screening intervention is no better than usual care (ie, no systematic screening).[1] Although no direct comparison of low-dose CT versus usual care is available, the negative finding of the PLCO is integral to the interpretation and application of the NLST.

Several key points should be noted regarding application of the results of the NLST. First, the study population was clearly defined and included only individuals aged 55 to 74 with relatively heavy smoking history (> 30 pack-years, currently smoking, or if former smokers, having quit within the previous 15 years). Generalizing the NLST results to other populations is problematic. Specifically, the NLST does not address individuals with other lung cancer risk factors, such as positive family history, domestic or occupational carcinogen exposure, underlying pulmonary diseases such as chronic obstructive pulmonary disease, interstitial lung disease, for example, or individuals who smoked less than 30 pack-years. The question of whether screening would be of benefit in these other populations remains unanswered. Second, as with prior studies of low-dose CT screening, the NLST had a very high rate of false-positive findings.[2,3] Approximately 25% of all subjects had an abnormality identified on screening each year of the study, of which 96% were false positives. The health care and emotional costs of these false-positive findings have as yet to be measured but will undoubtedly be substantial. Third, the issue of overdiagnosis, specifically cancers diagnosed by screening that are not destined to cause death, is still a concern, as it has been with prior studies evaluating screening with either chest radiography or low-dose CT.[4] Fourth, both the medical and lay communities are increasingly aware of the potential carcinogenic risks associated with diagnostic radiation. The NLST investigators estimated that the radiation incurred from serial screening studies in 55-year-old smokers would result in 1 to 3 new lung cancer deaths per 10 000 screened and 0.3 new breast cancers deaths per 10 000 screened. Strict adherence to radiation dosing protocols at sites providing screening CT studies will be necessary and should be monitored. Fifth, the population who would potentially be screening candidates is large, even by the strict criteria of the NLST, consisting of an estimated 7 million Americans. An even larger number, 94 million American adults, are either current or former smokers. The costs of a broadly applied screening program would be staggering. Publication of a health care cost analysis of the NLST is anticipated soon.

Despite the many questions that remain, the NLST demonstrates that screening for lung cancer with low-dose CT saves lives. The current 5-year survival rate for lung cancer is a dismal 16%.[5] The need for an intervention that will improve our ability to detect lung cancer early is clearly pressing. Although many advances have been made in treatment for lung cancer, the fact remains that the majority of patients are diagnosed at advanced stage, when cure is unlikely and improvements in survival related to treatment are measured in months, not years. Further work of the NLST investigators is anticipated regarding cost-effectiveness of screening and the increases in heath care utilization that seem inevitable, as well as the impact of screening on smoking behavior and quality of life. The results of these studies are likely to inform any major changes in health care policy on a national level.

L. T. Tanoue, MD

References

1. Oken MM, Hocking WG, Kvale PA, et al. Screening by chest radiograph and lung cancer mortality: the Prostate, Lung, Colorectal, and Ovarian (PLCO) randomized trial. *JAMA.* 2011;306:1865-1873.
2. Swensen SJ, Jett JR, Hartman TE, et al. CT screening for lung cancer: five-year prospective experience. *Radiology.* 2005;235:259-265.
3. Henschke CI, Naidich DP, Yankelevitz DF, et al. Early lung cancer action project: initial findings on repeat screenings. *Cancer.* 2001;92:153-159.
4. Marcus PM, Bergstralh EJ, Zweig MH, Harris A, Offord KP, Fontana RS. Extended lung cancer incidence follow-up in the Mayo Lung Project and overdiagnosis. *J Natl Cancer Inst.* 2006;98:748-756.
5. Siegel R, Ward E, Brawley O, Jemal A. Cancer statistics, 2011: the impact of eliminating socioeconomic and racial disparities on premature cancer deaths. *CA Cancer J Clin.* 2011;61:212-236.

Screening by Chest Radiograph and Lung Cancer Mortality: The Prostate, Lung, Colorectal, and Ovarian (PLCO) Randomized Trial

Oken MM, for the PLCO Project Team (Univ of Minnesota, Minneapolis; et al)
JAMA 306:1865-1873, 2011

Context.—The effect on mortality of screening for lung cancer with modern chest radiographs is unknown.

Objective.—To evaluate the effect on mortality of screening for lung cancer using radiographs in the Prostate, Lung, Colorectal, and Ovarian (PLCO) Cancer Screening Trial.

Design, Setting, and Participants.—Randomized controlled trial that involved 154 901 participants aged 55 through 74 years, 77 445 of whom were assigned to annual screenings and 77 456 to usual care at 1 of 10 screening centers across the United States between November 1993 and July 2001. The data from a subset of eligible participants for the National Lung Screening Trial (NLST), which compared chest radiograph with spiral computed tomographic (CT) screening, were analyzed.

Intervention.—Participants in the intervention group were offered annual posteroanterior view chest radiograph for 4 years. Diagnostic follow-up of positive screening results was determined by participants and their health care practitioners. Participants in the usual care group were offered no interventions and received their usual medical care. All diagnosed cancers, deaths, and causes of death were ascertained through the earlier of 13 years of follow-up or until December 31, 2009.

Main Outcome Measures.—Mortality from lung cancer. Secondary outcomes included lung cancer incidence, complications associated with diagnostic procedures, and all-cause mortality.

Results.—Screening adherence was 86.6% at baseline and 79% to 84% at years 1 through 3; the rate of screening use in the usual care group was 11%. Cumulative lung cancer incidence rates through 13 years of follow-up were 20.1 per 10 000 person-years in the intervention group and 19.2 per 10 000 person-years in the usual care group (rate ratio [RR]; 1.05, 95% CI, 0.98-1.12). A total of 1213 lung cancer deaths were observed in the intervention group compared with 1230 in usual care group through 13 years (mortality RR, 0.99; 95% CI, 0.87-1.22). Stage and histology were similar between the 2 groups. The RR of mortality for the subset of participants eligible for the NLST, over the same 6-year follow-up period, was 0.94 (95% CI, 0.81-1.10).

Conclusion.—Annual screening with chest radiograph did not reduce lung cancer mortality compared with usual care.

Trial Registration.—clinicaltrials.gov Identifier: NCT00002540.

▶ The Prostate, Lung, Colorectal, and Ovarian (PLCO) Cancer Screening Trial was initiated in 1993, eventually enrolling more than 154 000 subjects aged 55 to 74 years in the United States. The intent of the PLCO trial was to evaluate the effect of a package of screening interventions on prevention of death from 4 cancers. The PLCO participants were enrolled from 10 centers across the country, representing a geographically and ethnically diverse population. There was no eligibility requirement for smoking. Subjects in the lung cancer arm were randomized to either usual care (ie, no screening) or to a lung cancer screening intervention, which consisted of a baseline chest radiograph with 3 annual follow-up studies. Subjects were then monitored over 13 years. As demonstrated in Fig 2 in the original article, there was no difference in cumulative lung cancer incidence in the usual care group compared with the intervention group (19.2 per 10 000 person-years in the usual care group vs 20.1 per 10 000 person-years in the intervention group). As demonstrated in Fig 3 in the original article, there was also no difference in lung cancer mortality (relative risk of mortality in the usual care vs intervention group 0.99; 95% confidence interval, 0.87−1.22). Similar negative results were reported more than 20 years ago in several lung cancer screening trials evaluating chest radiography as a screening intervention.[1,2] The PLCO trial robustly confirms that lung cancer screening with chest radiography is not effective.

The PLCO trial results are of great significance in the context of the National Lung Screening Trial (NLST), which did not include an arm with chest radiography as a screening intervention. Of note, approximately 21% of subjects in the PLCO trial met the more than 30 pack-year smoking entry requirement for the NLST.[3] It is particularly pertinent to note that, in a subset analysis, this group also did not demonstrate any decrease in lung cancer mortality with chest radiography as the screening intervention compared with the benefit in mortality demonstrated with low-dose chest CT scanning in the NLST. The findings of the PLCO are thus fundamentally important to the interpretation of the NLST and to health policy recommendations that should inevitably evolve from the results of the 2 trials.

L. T. Tanoue, MD

References

1. Melamed MR, Flehinger BJ, Zaman MB, Heelan RT, Perchick WA, Martini N. Screening for early lung cancer. Results of the Memorial Sloan-Kettering study in New York. *Chest.* 1984;86:44-53.
2. Fontana RS, Sanderson DR, Woolner LB, Taylor WF, Miller WE, Muhm JR. Lung cancer screening: the Mayo program. *J Occup Med.* 1986;28:746-750.
3. Aberle DR, Adams AM, Berg CD, et al. Reduced lung-cancer mortality with low-dose computed tomographic screening. *N Engl J Med.* 2011;365:395-409.

Seventh Edition of the Cancer Staging Manual and Stage Grouping of Lung Cancer: Quick Reference Chart and Diagrams

Lababede O, Meziane M, Rice T (Cleveland Clinic, OH)
Chest 139:183-189, 2011

Lung cancer remains the most common cause of cancer-related death in the United States. TNM staging, which is an important guide to the prognosis and treatment of lung cancer, has been revised recently. In this article, we propose a quick reference chart and diagrams that consolidate TNM staging information in a simple format. The current classification of lymph node stations and zones is illustrated as well (Fig 1).

▶ The TNM cancer staging system provides an anatomic framework for consistent and reproducible descriptions of solid tumors, including lung cancer. The current 7th edition of the TNM staging classification for lung cancer reflects a remarkable decade of work by the International Association for the Study of Lung Cancer (IASLC), culminating in endorsement by the International Union Against Cancer and the American Joint Committee on Cancer in 2009, and subsequent implementation into clinical practice.[1-4] The IASLC also adopted a new international lymph node map, resolving differences between previous mapping strategies.[5] The descriptors for the primary tumor (T), lymph node involvement (N), and distant metastasis (M) contain a great deal of detail that can be challenging to remember. Lababede and colleagues offer a user-friendly staging chart for clinicians, which concisely incorporates much of this detail (Fig 1). The accompanying tables and diagrams should serve as useful references in the office or bronchoscopy suite.

L. T. Tanoue, MD

References

1. Goldstraw P, Crowley J, Chansky K, et al; International Association for the Study of Lung Cancer International Staging Committee, Participating Institutions. The IASLC Lung Cancer Staging Project: proposals for the revision of the TNM stage groupings in the forthcoming (seventh) edition of the TNM classification of malignant tumours. *J Thorac Oncol.* 2007;2:706-714.
2. Postmus PE, Brambilla E, Chansky K, et al; International Association for the Study of Lung Cancer International Staging Committee, Cancer Research and Biostatistics, Observers to the Committee, Participating Institutions. The IASLC Lung Cancer Staging Project: proposals for revision of the M descriptors in the forthcoming

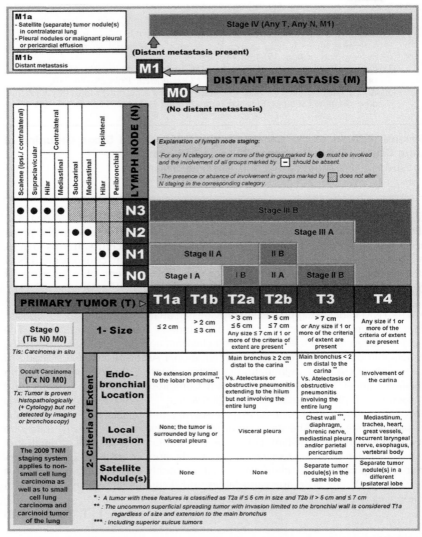

FIGURE 1.—Reference chart for 2009 TNM staging system of lung cancer. M = metastases; N = regional lymph node involvement; T = tumor. (Reprinted from Lababede O, Meziane M, Rice T. Seventh edition of the cancer staging manual and stage grouping of lung cancer: quick reference chart and diagrams. *Chest.* 2011;139:183-189. © American College of Chest Physicians.)

(seventh) edition of the TNM classification of lung cancer. *J Thorac Oncol.* 2007;2: 686-693.

3. Rusch VW, Crowley J, Giroux DJ, et al; International Association for the Study of Lung Cancer International Staging Committee, Cancer Research and Biostatistics, Observers to the Committee, Participating Institutions. The IASLC Lung Cancer Staging Project: proposals for the revision of the N descriptors in the forthcoming

seventh edition of the TNM classification for lung cancer. *J Thorac Oncol.* 2007;2: 603-612.

4. Rami-Porta R, Ball D, Crowley J, et al; International Association for the Study of Lung Cancer International Staging Committee, Cancer Research and Biostatistics, Observers to the Committee, Participating Institutions. The IASLC Lung Cancer Staging Project: proposals for the revision of the T descriptors in the forthcoming (seventh) edition of the TNM classification for lung cancer. *J Thorac Oncol.* 2007; 2:593-602.

5. Rusch VW, Asamura H, Watanabe H, Giroux DJ, Rami-Porta R, Goldstraw P; Members of IASLC Staging Committee. The IASLC lung cancer staging project: a proposal for a new international lymph node map in the forthcoming seventh edition of the TNM classification for lung cancer. *J Thorac Oncol.* 2009;4:568-577.

Quitting Smoking Among Adults — United States, 2001—2010

Centers for Disease Control and Prevention (CDC)
MMWR Morb Mortal Wkly Rep 60:1513-1519, 2011

Quitting smoking is beneficial to health at any age, and cigarette smokers who quit before age 35 years have mortality rates similar to those who never smoked. From 1965 to 2010, the prevalence of cigarette smoking among adults in the United States decreased from 42.4% to 19.3%, in part because of an increase in the number who quit smoking. Since 2002, the number of former U.S. smokers has exceeded the number of current smokers. Mass media campaigns, increases in the prices of tobacco products, and smoke-free policies have been shown to increase smoking cessation. In addition, brief cessation advice by health-care providers; individual, group, and telephone counseling; and cessation medications are effective cessation treatments. To determine the prevalence of 1) current interest in quitting smoking, 2) successful recent smoking cessation, 3) recent use of cessation treatments, and 4) trends in quit attempts over a 10-year period, CDC analyzed data from the 2001—2010 National Health Interview Surveys (NHIS). This report summarizes the results of that analysis, which found that, in 2010, 68.8% of adult smokers wanted to stop smoking, 52.4% had made a quit attempt in the past year, 6.2% had recently quit, 48.3% had been advised by a health professional to quit, and 31.7% had used counseling and/or medications when they tried to quit. The prevalence of quit attempts increased during 2001—2010 among smokers aged 25—64 years, but not among other age groups. Health-care providers should identify smokers and offer them brief cessation advice at each visit; counseling and medication should be offered to patients willing to make a quit attempt.

▶ Tobacco control is hailed as one of the 10 great public health achievements in the United States over the last decade.[1] Despite significant gains, it is estimated that cigarette smoking and second-hand smoke exposure still result in approximately 443 000 premature deaths and $193 billion in health care costs and productivity losses annually.[2] This report from the Centers for Disease Control and its accompanying editorial provide a comprehensive look at the various aspects of smoking cessation, both its successes and its continued challenges, in the United States from 2001 to 2010. Data were obtained from the National Health Interview Surveys (NHIS) over that period of time. Overall, approximately 61% of surveyed individuals responded to the NHIS questionnaire. In 2010, 68.8% of current cigarette smokers said they would like to completely quit. A total of 52.4% had tried to quit within the previous year, but only 31.7% had used medications and/or received counseling. Only 48.3% of those who had visited a health care provider within that year reported receiving smoking cessation counseling.

Smoking cessation counseling by a health professional and the use of pharmacotherapy are individually effective in increasing the likelihood of smoking cessation and are more effective when used together. Clinical guidelines for treating tobacco use and dependence are available through the US Department of Health and Human Services at http://www.surgeongeneral.gov/tobacco/treating_tobacco_use08.pdf.[3] Medicare now compensates health care providers for time spent in tobacco cessation counseling. Effective pharmacotherapies as well as a number of nicotine replacement therapies are readily available. Every state now has a cessation quitline (national toll-free number 1-800-QUIT NOW). Since approximately 20% of all adult Americans continue to be habitual tobacco users, all of these resources should be used to help enable our patients to quit smoking.

L. T. Tanoue, MD

References

1. Centers for Disease Control and Prevention (CDC). Ten great public health achievements—United States, 2001—2010. *MMWR Morb Mortal Wkly Rep.* 2011;60: 619-623.
2. Centers for Disease Control and Prevention (CDC). Smoking-attributable mortality, years of potential life lost, and productivity losses—United States, 2000—2004. *MMWR Morb Mortal Wkly Rep.* 2008;57:1226-1228.
3. Fiore M, Jaen C, Baker T, et al. *Treating Tobacco Use and Dependence: 2008 Update. Clinical Practice Guideline.* Rockville, MD: US Department of Health and Human Services, Public Health Service; 2008, http://www.surgeongeneral.gov/tobacco/treating_tobacco_use08.pdf. Accessed January 2, 2012.

Treating Smokers in the Health Care Setting

Fiore MC, Baker TB (Univ of Wisconsin School of Medicine and Public Health, Madison)
N Engl J Med 365:1222-1231, 2011

Background.—Smoking prevalence has fallen dramatically in the United States, but recently prevalence rates have been concentrated among persons with low incomes, low educational levels, and psychiatric conditions. However, these persons benefit from the same treatments that help other smokers, so clinicians should be vigilant about offering help and guidance for smoking cessation.

Clinical Effects of Smoking.—Within 10 seconds of each inhalation, nicotine is carried by tar particles into lung alveoli, then to the brain. It binds to nicotinic cholinergic receptors in the brain and triggers the release of neurotransmitters that augment the attractiveness of smoking and reinforce smoking cues. Tolerance develops with long-term smoking, leading to the proliferation of nicotinic receptors and higher levels of self-administered nicotine. If nicotine is unavailable to bind to receptors, through reduced smoking or smoking cessation, withdrawal symptoms such as craving, negative moods, and restlessness develop. These symptoms prompt the person to return to smoking. About half of phenotypic variance in tobacco dependence is the result of genetic influences.

Challenges to Clinical Treatment.—Many clinicians fail to consistently offer smoking cessation treatments to smokers. Only about 20% of smokers are ready to quit at any given time, and smokers often choose unaided methods of quitting, which fail in 95% of cases. The success of smoking cessation is less likely with nonadherence to medications and counseling, but this nonadherence is common. Typically, patients take about half of the recommended doses of medication and attend fewer than half of their counseling appointments.

Evidence-Based Treatments and Strategies.—At every health care visit, smokers should be encouraged to quit and asked if they are willing to do so. Patients who are initially unwilling can be approached using motivational interviewing, which involves the use of nonconfrontational counseling to resolve the patient's ambivalence and encourages choices consistent with the patient's long-term goals. Motivational interviewing increases 6-month cessation rates, especially if smokers receive two or more sessions that last at least 20 minutes. "Five R's" counseling focuses on personally relevant reasons to quit, risks associated with continued smoking, rewards for quitting, and roadblocks to successful quitting, with repetition of the counseling at each clinic visit. Counseling using these approaches plus the offer of nicotine-replacement therapy is associated with a higher quit rate among smokers. Patients unwilling to quit can be encouraged to reduce their smoking and use nicotine-replacement therapy for at least several months. Patients who are willing to quit should be provided with practical advice on avoiding smoking triggers and encouraged to use available resources for smoking cessation. These include adjuvant counseling, online resources, or both. Clinicians should explain the benefits and risks associated with medications and clarify any misconceptions the patient may have.

Conclusions.—The use of motivational interviewing, counseling, and smoking reduction is in line with the clinical practice guidelines of the US Public Health Service. Nicotine-replacement therapy is a useful alternative for smokers reluctant to take on smoking cessation. Adhering to the use of these medications shows a strong link to successful outcomes (Table 3).

▶ Smoking rates have decreased dramatically in the United States since the publication of the first Surgeon General's report on the health consequences of smoking in 1964. However, smoking rates over the last decade among the adult American population have plateaued at approximately 20%, still unacceptably

TABLE 3.—Medications for Smoking Cessation

Medication	Dose	Instructions	Cautions and Warnings	Side Effects	Availability
Sustained-release bupropion	Days 1–3: 150 mg each morning; day 4 –end: 150 mg twice daily	Start 1–2 wk before quit date; use for 2 –6 mo	Do not use with monoamine oxidase inhibitors or bupropion in any other form or in patients with a history of seizures or eating disorders; see FDA black-box warning on serious mental health events: www.fda.gov/News Events/Newsroom/PressAnnounce ments/ucm170100.htm	Insomnia, dry mouth, vivid or abnormal dreams	Prescription only; generic or brandname drugs (Zyban, Wellbutrin SR)
Nicotine gum	1 piece every 1–2 hr initially, then taper; up to 24 pieces/day; 2 mg if patient smokes ≤24 cigarettes/day and 4 mg if patient smokes ≥25 cigarettes/day	Use up to 12 weeks	Patients with dentures should use with caution; patients should not eat or drink 15 min before or during use	Mouth soreness, heartburn	Over-the-counter only; generic or brand-name drug (Nicorette)
Nicotine inhaler	6–16 cartridges/day; inhale 80 times/ cartridge	Use up to 6 mo; taper at end	May irritate mouth and throat	Mouth and throat irritation	Prescription only (Nicotrol inhaler)
Nicotine lozenges	1 piece every 1–2 hr initially, then taper; 2 mg if patient smokes 30 min or more after waking and 4 mg if patient smokes <30 min after waking	Use 3–6 mo	Patients should not eat or drink 15 min before or during use	Hiccups, cough, heartburn	Over-the-counter only; generic or brand-name drug (Commit)
Nicotine nasal spray	1 dose is 1 squirt/nostril; 1–2 doses/ hr; up to 40 doses/day	Use 3–6 mo	Not for patients with asthma; may irritate nose; may cause dependence	Nasal irritation	Prescription only (Nicotrol NS)
Nicotine patch	If patient smokes ≥10 cigarettes/day, 21 mg/day for 4 wk, then 14 mg/day for 2 wk, then 7 mg/day for 2 wk; if patient smokes <10 cigarettes/day, start with 14 mg/day for 6 wk, then 7 mg/day for 2 wk	Use new patch every morning for 8 –12 wks	Do not use if patient has severe eczema or psoriasis; patch can be removed at night if sleep is disrupted	Local skin reaction, insomnia	Over-the-counter or prescription; generic or brand-name drugs (Nicoderm CQ, Nicotrol)

Varenicline	Days 1–3: 0.5 mg every morning; days 4–7: 0.5 mg twice daily; days 8–end: 1 mg twice daily	Start 1 wk before quit date; use 3–6 mo	Use with caution in patients with clinically significant renal impairment, patients undergoing dialysis, and patients with serious psychiatric illness; see FDA Web sites for black-box warning on serious mental health events and statement on risk of cardiovascular adverse events among patients with cardiovascular disease: www.fda.gov/NewsEvents/Newsroom/Press Announcements/ucm170100.htm and www.fda.gov/Drugs/DrugSafety/ucm259161.htm	Nausea, insomnia, vivid or abnormal dreams	Prescription only (Chantix)
Combination therapies*					
Patch plus bupropion	Follow instructions for individual medications above	Follow instructions for individual medications above	See information for individual medications above	See information for individual medications above	See above
Patch plus gum, inhalers, or lozenges	Follow instructions for individual medications above	Follow instructions for individual medications above	See information for individual medications above	See information for individual medications above	See above

*Only the nicotine patch plus bupropion is currently approved by the Food and Drug Administration.

high. This concise and practical review by Fiore and Baker summarizes many of the points of the clinical practice guideline of the US Public Health Service, "Treating Tobacco Use and Dependence."[1] On average, smokers incur $1600 more in annual health care costs than nonsmokers.[2] From the perspectives of both disease prevention and health economics, smoking cessation must be a priority. Strong and positive interventions can be highly effective in the health care setting. Seventy percent of smokers in the United States see a primary care physician each year, providing substantial opportunity for intervention. While higher smoking prevalence correlates with lower income, lower levels of education, and the presence of psychiatric illness, smoking cessation interventions that are effective in general have been demonstrated to be of benefit in these populations. Fiore and Baker clearly and succinctly describe the interventions that can and should be made by health care providers, particularly motivational interviewing and counseling for the patient willing to quit as well as the patient unwilling to quit, and outlines strategies for nicotine replacement and pharmacotherapy (Table 3). This useful and practical reference should be a must read for all physicians.

L. T. Tanoue, MD

References

1. Fiore M, Jaen C, Baker T, et al. *Treating Tobacco Use and Dependence: 2008 Update. Clinical Practice Guideline.* Rockville, MD: US Department of Health and Human Services, Public Health Service; 2008, http://www.surgeongeneral.gov/tobacco/treating_tobacco_use08.pdf. Accessed January 2, 2012.
2. Centers for Disease Control and Prevention (CDC). Annual smoking-attributable mortality, years of potential life lost, and economic costs—United States, 1995–1999. *MMWR Morb Mortal Wkly Rep.* 2002;51:300-303.

31 Pleural, Interstitial Lung, and Pulmonary Vascular Disease

A noninvasive algorithm to exclude pre-capillary pulmonary hypertension
Bonderman D, Wexberg P, Martischnig AM, et al (Med Univ of Vienna, Austria)
Eur Respir J 37:1096-1103, 2011

Current guidelines recommend right heart catheterisation (RHC) in symptomatic patients at risk of pre-capillary pulmonary hypertension (PH) with echocardiographic systolic pulmonary artery pressures ≥36 mmHg. Growing awareness for PH, a high prevalence of post-capillary PH and the inability to distinguish between pre- and post-capillary PH by echocardiography have led to unnecessary RHCs. The aim of our study was to assess whether standard noninvasive diagnostic procedures are able to safely exclude pre-capillary PH.

Data from 251 patients referred for suspicion of pre-capillary PH were used to develop a noninvasive diagnostic decision tree. A prospectively collected data set of 121 consecutive patients was utilised for temporal validation.

According to the decision tree, patients were stratified by the presence or absence of an electrocardiographic right ventricular strain pattern (RVS) and serum N-terminal brain natriuretic peptide (NT-proBNP) levels below and above 80 pg·mL^{-1}. In the absence of RVS and elevated NT-proBNP, none of the patients in the prospective validation cohort were diagnosed with pre-capillary PH by RHC. Combining echocardiography with the diagnostic algorithm increased specificity to 19.3% ($p = 0.0009$), while sensitivity remained at 100%.

Employing ECG and NT-proBNP on top of echocardiography helps recognise one false positive case per five patients referred with dyspnoea and echocardiographic suspicion of PH, while not missing true pre-capillary PH.

► The traditional teaching concerning right heart failure is that the most common cause is left heart failure. Awareness in the health care and the lay public has shifted the focus to pulmonary arterial hypertension (PAH). Indeed, current guidelines advocate the gold standard study, right heart catheterization, for all patients with echocardiographic evidence of pulmonary artery systolic pressure ≥36 mm Hg. In this setting, 55% of patients sent to pulmonary hypertension referral centers are found to have Dana Point group 2 disease (owing to left ventricular dysfunction).

Right heart catheterization is a relatively benign test, but it is invasive. Procedural risks include, but are not limited to, infection, bleeding, pneumothorax (depending on the approach), dysrhythmia, and the dreaded and potentially deadly pulmonary artery rupture. Bonderman and colleagues devised a simple noninvasive approach to rule out precapillary pulmonary hypertension by analyzing data from 251 consecutive patients referred for suspicion of PAH. They then validated their findings using a prospective pool of 121 patients.

The algorithm presented identified a significant percentage of referred patients who could be ruled out for PAH without subjecting them to right heart catheterization. No patient with precapillary PAH was excluded. Interestingly, electrocardiogram is recommended in the initial evaluation of presumed PAH by current guidelines. In addition, N-terminal brain natriuretic peptide at baseline has prognostic implications for patients with PAH.

Application of this simple approach may reduce cost and exposure to a potentially harmful invasive test.

C. D. Spradley, MD

Usefulness of Serial N-Terminal Pro–B-Type Natriuretic Peptide Measurements for Determining Prognosis in Patients With Pulmonary Arterial Hypertension

Mauritz G-J, Rizopoulos D, Groepenhoff H, et al (Inst for Cardiovascular Res and VU Univ Med Ctr, Amsterdam, The Netherlands; Erasmus Univ Med Ctr, Rotterdam, The Netherlands)

Am J Cardiol 108:1645-1650, 2011

Previous studies have shown the prognostic benefit of N-terminal pro–brain natriuretic peptide (NT–pro-BNP) in pulmonary arterial hypertension (PAH) at time of diagnosis. However, there are only limited data on the clinical utility of serial measurements of the inactive peptide NT–pro-BNP in PAH. This study examined the value of serial NT–pro-BNP measurements in predicting prognosis PAH. We retrospectively analyzed all available NT–pro-BNP plasma samples in 198 patients who were diagnosed with World Health Organization group I PAH from January 2002 through January 2009. At time of diagnosis median NT–pro-BNP levels were significantly different between survivors (610 pg/ml, range 6 to 8,714) and nonsurvivors (2,609 pg/ml, range 28 to 9,828, p <0.001). In addition, NT–pro-BNP was significantly associated (p <0.001) with other parameters of disease severity (6-minute walking distance, functional class). Receiver operating curve analysis identified ≥1,256 pg/ml as the optimal NT–pro-BNP cutoff for predicting mortality at time of diagnosis. Serial measurements allowed calculation of baseline NT–pro-BNP (i.e., intercept obtained by back-extrapolation of concentration time graph), providing a better discrimination between survivors and nonsurvivors

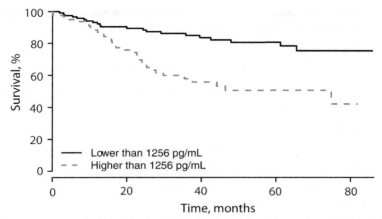

FIGURE 5.—Kaplan—Meier estimate for time to death for low (<1,256 pg/ml) and high (>1,256 pg/ml) values of baseline N-terminal pro—B-type natriuretic peptide. (Reprinted from the American Journal of Cardiology, Mauritz G-J, Rizopoulos D, Groepenhoff H, et al. Usefulness of serial N-terminal Pro—B-type natriuretic peptide measurements for determining prognosis in patients with pulmonary arterial hypertension. *Am J Cardiol*. 2011;108:1645-1650. Copyright 2011, with permission from Elsevier.)

than NT—pro-BNP at time of diagnosis alone ($p = 0.010$). Furthermore, a decrease of NT—pro-BNP of >15%/year was associated with survival. In conclusion, a serum NT—pro-BNP level <1,256 pg/ml at time of diagnosis identifies poor outcome in patients with PAH. In addition, a decrease in NT—pro-BNP of >15%/year is associated with survival in PAH (Fig 5).

▶ Mauritz and colleagues have asked a compelling question. We know that N-terminal pro-brain natriuretic peptide (NT—pro-BNP) levels can be used to predict outcome in pulmonary arterial hypertension (PAH) at baseline based on multiple studies. Can the marker be followed over time as well? The precedent does exist in the realm of left-sided heart failure.

The team identified a level of greater than 1256 pg/mL (Fig 5) as a predictor of mortality at baseline in close agreement with prior work. The team also found that a reduction of NT—pro-BNP of greater than 15% per year predicts long-term survival. This applied even in early diagnosis. In light of these findings, the authors conclude that simply maintaining a low threshold may not be an appropriate therapeutic goal.

Issues with the study centered around its retrospective design and wide bio-variability between measurements. The latter necessitated linear regression for extrapolation. This will limit practical application. That said, the finding is compelling and may add a new tool to the pulmonary hypertension disease monitoring process. As is frequently the case in this field, a well-designed prospective study may shed more light on the applicability of these findings.

C. D. Spradley, MD

Race and Sex Differences in Response to Endothelin Receptor Antagonists for Pulmonary Arterial Hypertension

Gabler NB, French B, Strom BL, et al (Univ of Pennsylvania, Philadelphia; et al)
Chest 141:20-26, 2012

Background.—Recently studied therapies for pulmonary arterial hypertension (PAH) have improved outcomes among populations of patients, but little is known about which patients are most likely to respond to specific treatments. Differences in endothelin-1 biology between sexes and between whites and blacks may lead to differences in patients' responses to treatment with endothelin receptor antagonists (ERAs).

Methods.—We conducted pooled analyses of deidentified, patient-level data from six randomized placebo-controlled trials of ERAs submitted to the US Food and Drug Administration to elucidate heterogeneity in treatment response. We estimated the interaction between treatment assignment (ERA vs placebo) and sex and between treatment and white or black race in terms of the change in 6-min walk distance from baseline to 12 weeks.

Results.—Trials included 1,130 participants with a mean age of 49 years; 21% were men, 74% were white, and 6% were black. The placebo-adjusted response to ERAs was 29.7 m (95% CI, 3.7–55.7 m) greater in women than in men ($P = .03$). The placebo-adjusted response was 42.2 m for whites and −1.4 m for blacks, a difference of 43.6 m (95% CI, −3.5–90.7 m) ($P = .07$). Similar results were found in sensitivity analyses and in secondary analyses using the outcome of absolute distance walked.

Conclusions.—Women with PAH obtain greater responses to ERAs than do men, and whites may experience a greater treatment benefit than do blacks. This heterogeneity in treatment-response may reflect pathophysiologic differences between sexes and races or distinct disease phenotypes.

▶ The BREATH and ARIES trials[1,2] demonstrated the efficacy of endothelin receptor antagonist (ERA) therapy in the treatment of pulmonary arterial hypertension (PAH). The authors of this study ask the question, "Does race and sex difference impact response to specific therapy for PAH?" This is a worthy question given the known difference in response to therapy for systemic hypertension found in different ethnic groups. In PAH, this may be particularly important in light of the fact that most PAH patients are female.

Interestingly, men are known to have higher levels of circulating ET-1 than women, and black patients have higher circulating levels than whites.

The study retrospectively reviewed data from randomized placebo-controlled trials of ERAs in the treatment of PAH. Women in these studies demonstrated a 29.7 m greater improvement in 6-minute walk distance than men, and a 43.6 m greater response was noted in whites compared with blacks. The first observation was statistically significant. The second was hampered by small sample size.

This study dispels the myth of one-size-fits-all adherence to guidelines in PAH therapy. Unfortunately, given the small numbers of patients affected by this disease, the likelihood of efficacious targeted therapy for specific populations may be a fantasy. That said, in light of these findings, response to therapy in men and minorities may need to be monitored closely. Unfortunately, tailored alternatives have not been identified. Future studies are definitely needed.

C. D. Spradley, MD

References

1. Rubin LJ, Badesch DB, Barst RJ, et al. Bosentan therapy for pulmonary arterial hypertension. *N Engl J Med.* 2002;346:896-903.
2. Galiè N, Olschewski H, Oudiz RJ, et al; Ambrisentan in Pulmonary Arterial Hypertension, Randomized, Double-Blind, Placebo-Controlled, Multicenter, Efficacy Studies (ARIES) Group. Ambrisentan for the treatment of pulmonary arterial hypertension: results of the ambrisentan in pulmonary arterial hypertension, randomized, double-blind, placebo-controlled, multicenter, efficacy (ARIES) study 1 and 2. *Circulation.* 2008;117:3010-3019.

Long-term effects of inhaled treprostinil in patients with pulmonary arterial hypertension: The TReprostinil sodium Inhalation Used in the Management of Pulmonary arterial Hypertension (TRIUMPH) study open-label extension
Benza RL, Seeger W, McLaughlin VV, et al (Allegheny General Hosp, Pittsburgh, PA; Univ of Giessen Lung Ctr, Germany; Univ of Michigan Health System, Ann Arbor; et al)
J Heart Lung Transplant 30:1327-1333, 2011

Background.—Inhaled treprostinil improved functional capacity as add-on therapy in the short-term management of patients with pulmonary arterial hypertension (PAH). This study investigated the long-term effects of inhaled treprostinil in patients concurrently receiving oral background therapy.

Methods.—A total of 206 patients (81% women) completing the 12-week double-blind phase of the Treprostinil Sodium Inhalation Used in the Management of Pulmonary Arterial Hypertension (TRIUMPH) study transitioned into an open-label extension. Patients were assessed every 3 months for changes in 6-minute walk distance (6MWD), Borg dyspnea score, New York Heart Association (NYHA) functional class, quality of life (QOL) scores, and signs and symptoms of PAH.

Results.—Patients were primarily NYHA class III (86%), with a mean baseline 6MWD of 349 ± 81 meters. A median change in 6MWD of 28, 31, 32, and 18 meters in patients continuing therapy was observed at 6, 12, 18, and 24 months, respectively. This effect was more prominent in those patients originally allocated to active therapy in the double-blind phase. Survival rates for patients remaining on therapy were 97%, 94%, and 91% at 12, 18, and 24 months, respectively. In addition, 82%, 74%, and 69% of patients maintained treatment benefit as evidenced by lack of clinical worsening at 12, 18, and 24 months. The most common adverse events were known effects of prostanoid therapy (headache [34%], nausea [21%], and vomiting [10%]) or were due to the route of administration (cough [53%], pharyngolaryngeal pain [13%], and chest pain [13%]).

Conclusions.—Long-term therapy with inhaled treprostinil demonstrated persistent benefit for PAH patients who remained on therapy for up to 24 months.

▶ A total of 4 open-label extension studies in pharmacologic therapy for pulmonary arterial hypertension are reviewed in this text. This particular study is unique in that it evaluates the efficacy of add-on inhaled prostacyclin to established oral therapy.

The TRIUMPH study showed the efficacy of inhaled treprostinil in improving 6-minute walking distance in patients on stable background therapy with sildenafil or bosentan. The question of whether the median 20 M gained with the addition of the therapy would be maintained or improved upon was answered by this open-label extension study.

The study found statistically significant increase in 6-minute walk distance from baseline at all time points in the study. Additionally, survival of the cohort that began the study in New York Heart Association class III was 90% after 2 years.

The study suffers from the typical issues associated with open-label extension studies, in that it represents a population heavily influenced by the inclusion of a large cohort of responders. That said, inhaled treprostinil is an attractive option for additional therapy in patients who do not have robust response to monotherapy with oral agents, especially when there are contraindications or patient resistance to subcutaneous or intravenous therapy. Indeed, percentage of patients reporting improvement from baseline at 24 months was 36%. A total of 90% demonstrated improvement or no change in classification. When confronted with the dismal natural history of pulmonary hypertension, these findings should be viewed in a positive light.[1]

C. D. Spradley, MD

Reference

1. Channick RN, Olschewski H, Seeger W, Staub T, Voswinckel R, Rubin LJ. Safety and efficacy of inhaled treprostinil as add-on therapy to bosentan in pulmonary arterial hypertension. *J Am Coll Cardiol.* 2006;48:1433-1437.

Ascertainment of Individual Risk of Mortality for Patients with Idiopathic Pulmonary Fibrosis

du Bois RM, Weycker D, Albera C, et al (Imperial College, London, UK; Policy Analysis Inc, Brookline, MA; Univ of Turin, Italy; et al)
Am J Respir Crit Care Med 184:459-466, 2011

Rationale.—Several predictors of mortality in patients with idiopathic pulmonary fibrosis have been described; however, there is a need for a practical and accurate method of quantifying the prognosis of individual patients.

Objectives.—Develop a practical mortality risk scoring system for patients with idiopathic pulmonary fibrosis.

Methods.—We used a Cox proportional hazards model and data from two clinical trials (n = 1,099) to identify independent predictors of 1-year mortality among patients with idiopathic pulmonary fibrosis. From the comprehensive model, an abbreviated clinical model comprised of only those predictors that are readily and reliably ascertained by clinicians was derived. Beta coefficients for each predictor were then used to develop a practical mortality risk scoring system.

Measurements and Main Results.—Independent predictors of mortality included age, respiratory hospitalization, percent predicted FVC, 24-week change in FVC, percent predicted carbon monoxide diffusing capacity, 24-week change in percent predicted carbon monoxide diffusing capacity, and 24-week change in health-related quality of life. An abbreviated clinical model comprising only four predictors (age, respiratory hospitalization, percent predicted FVC, and 24-wk change in FVC), and the corresponding risk scoring system produced estimates of 1-year mortality risk consistent with observed data (9.9% vs. 9.7%; C statistic = 0.75; 95% confidence interval, 0.71—0.79).

Conclusions.—The prognosis for patients with idiopathic pulmonary fibrosis may be accurately determined using four readily ascertainable predictors. Our simplified scoring system may be a valuable tool for determining prognosis and guiding clinical management. Additional research is needed to validate the applicability and accuracy of the scoring system (Table 4).

▶ Treatment options for patients with idiopathic pulmonary fibrosis (IPF) are severely limited. Multiple recent multicenter randomized placebo controlled trials have failed to demonstrate clinical benefit of pharmacotherapy. Given

---

TABLE 4.—Mortality Risk Scoring System for Patients With Idiopathic Pulmonary Fibrosis

(1) Sum Individual Scores Corresponding to Level of Each Risk Factor for a Given Patient*		(2) Find Expected 1-Year Probability of Death Corresponding to Total Risk Score	
Risk Factors	Score	Total Risk Score	Expected 1-Year Risk of Death
Age			
≥70	8		
60—69	4	0—4	<2%
<60	0	8—14	2—5%
History of respiratory hospitalization		16—21	5—10%
Yes	14	22—29	10—20%
No	0	30—33	20—30%
% Predicted FVC		34—37	30—40%
≤50	18	38—40	40—50%
51—65	13	41—43	50—60%
66—79	8	44—45	60—70%
≥80	0	47—49	70—80%
24-Week change in % predicted FVC		>50	>80%
≤ −10	21		
−5 to −9.9	10		
> −4.9	0		

*For example: total score for a patient aged 70 years, with no history of respiratory hospitalization, a % predicted FVC of 51—65, and a 24-week change in % predicted FVC of −5 to −9.9, is 31 (8 + 0 + 13 + 10) and predicted 1-year probability of death, 20—30%.

the progressive and fatal nature of the disease, mortality prediction tools would prove valuable in a clinical setting to assist in decision making. Participate in a clinical trial? Proceed with transplant evaluation and listing? Reevaluate code status?

The authors of this study applied multiple known independent predictors of mortality to data derived from 2 of the large clinical trials in IPF; 1099 subjects were included. The authors found that age, respiratory hospitalization, percentage predicted forced vital capacity (FVC), and 24-week change in FVC used in a scoring system (Table 4) were strongly predictive of mortality at 1 year. Impressively, change in FVC of only 5% in 24 weeks was associated with a greater than 2-fold risk of death. Strikingly, this change in FVC is within the accepted variability of the test.

The study is limited by the fact that the patient pool consisted of primarily patients with mild and moderate disease at assumed low risk of death, and validation is needed; however, this prediction tool may prove valuable in the future when counseling patients with IPF concerning treatment options and goals of therapy.

C. D. Spradley, MD

32 Sleep Disorders

An Integrated Health-Economic Analysis of Diagnostic and Therapeutic Strategies in the Treatment of Moderate-to-Severe Obstructive Sleep Apnea
Pietzsch JB, Garner A, Cipriano LE, et al (Wing Tech Inc, CA; Stanford Univ, CA)
Sleep 34:695-709, 2011

Study Objectives.—Obstructive sleep apnea (OSA) is a common disorder associated with substantially increased cardiovascular risks, reduced quality of life, and increased risk of motor vehicle collisions due to daytime sleepiness. This study evaluates the cost-effectiveness of three commonly used diagnostic strategies (full-night polysomnography, split-night polysomnography, unattended portable home-monitoring) in conjunction with continuous positive airway pressure (CPAP) therapy in patients with moderate-to-severe OSA.

Design.—A Markov model was created to compare costs and effectiveness of different diagnostic and therapeutic strategies over a 10-year interval and the expected lifetime of the patient. The primary measure of cost-effectiveness was incremental cost per quality-adjusted life year (QALY) gained.

Patients or Participants.—Baseline computations were performed for a hypothetical average cohort of 50-year-old males with a 50% pretest probability of having moderate-to-severe OSA (apnea-hypopnea index [AHI] ≥15 events per hour).

Measurements and Results.—For a patient with moderate-to-severe OSA, CPAP therapy has an incremental cost-effectiveness ratio (ICER) of $15,915 per QALY gained for the lifetime horizon. Over the lifetime horizon in a population with 50% prevalence of OSA, full-night polysomnography in conjunction with CPAP therapy is the most economically efficient strategy at any willingness-to-pay greater than $17,131 per-QALY gained because it dominates all other strategies in comparative analysis.

Conclusions.—Full-night polysomnography (PSG) is cost-effective and is the preferred diagnostic strategy for adults suspected to have moderate-to-severe OSA when all diagnostic options are available. Split-night PSG and unattended home monitoring can be considered cost-effective alternatives when full-night PSG is not available.

▶ The cost of health care is climbing. Management of chronic medical diseases such as obstructive sleep apnea (OSA) and its related comorbidities of cardiovascular disease, hypertension, and stoke will consume a significant portion of health care dollars. So studies examining both the cost-effectiveness and the comparative effectiveness of therapies are important. This study evaluated the cost-effectiveness of full-night polysomnogram, split-night polysomnogram, and unattended portable home monitoring plus continuous positive airway pressure (CPAP) therapy in patients with moderate to severe OSA. A variety of scenarios were considered and accounted for in a Markov model. This is a detailed and comprehensive study for which the investigators should receive accolades.

Pietzsch et al report that use of CPAP has an incremental cost-effective ratio (ICER) of $15 915 per quality-adjusted life years (QALY), which falls well below $100 000 per QALY and thus is good value.[1] Estimates include that use of CPAP would result in an overall per-person risk of a fatal motor vehicle collision by approximately 48% and that nearly 670 motor vehicle collisions could be prevented per 100 000 persons.

I was very surprised by the results of this cost-effectiveness analysis between full-night polysomnogram, split-night polysomnogram, and unattended portable home monitoring (Fig 4 in the original article). Full-night polysomnography was determined to be the most cost-effective and preferred diagnostic strategy. How could this be, you ask? As with any economic model, certain assumptions need to be made, accurate or not. Although these assumptions are supported by the medical literature (ie, impact of OSA and treatment on quality of life), the literature itself is limited. A number of other assumptions are made, including the number of no-shows for in-laboratory studies, for example. In the end, it is the high number of false diagnoses in the unattended portable home monitoring that accounts for its higher ICER. False diagnosis leads to cost of therapy when it is not needed or, in contrast, cost of health care when OSA is not treated.

Am I going to stop using unattended portable home monitoring? No, I am not, but I have realized that it is not just the cost of the technology itself that makes something cost-effective. It is important to note that the cost-effectiveness analysis is modeled based on a population cohort of 50-year-old male patients with a prevalence of moderate to severe OSA of 50%. In situations in which the pretest probability of OSA is high, unattended portable home monitoring and split-night polysomnogram are both cost-effective. Furthermore, the authors do say that unattended portable home monitoring is cost-effective in situations where a full polysomnogram is not possible (limited availability, patient refusal to attend). I believe this a good article to facilitate discussion within your own practice settings.

S. F. Jones, MD, FCCP, DABSM

Reference

1. Weinstein MC, Skinner JA. Comparative effectiveness and heath care spending—implications for reform. *N Engl J Med.* 2010;362:460-465.

Cheyne–Stokes respiration and obstructive sleep apnoea are independent risk factors for malignant ventricular arrhythmias requiring appropriate cardioverter-defibrillator therapies in patients with congestive heart failure
Bitter T, Westerheide N, Prinz C, et al (Ruhr Univ Bochum, Georgstasse, Bad Oeynhausen, Germany; Univ of Bielefeld, Germany)
Eur Heart J 32:61-74, 2011

Aims.—The aim of this first large-scale long-term study was to investigate whether obstructive sleep apnoea (OSA) and/or central sleep apnoea (CSA) are associated with an increased risk of malignant cardiac arrhythmias in patients with congestive heart failure (CHF).

Methods and Results.—Of 472 CHF patients who were screened for sleep disordered breathing (SDB) 6 months after implantation of a cardiac resynchronization device with cardioverter-defibrillator, 283 remained untreated [170 with mild or no sleep disordered breathing (mnSDB) and 113 patients declined ventilation therapy] and were included into this study. During follow-up (48 months), data on appropriately monitored ventricular arrhythmias as well as appropriate cardioverter-defibrillator therapies were obtained from 255 of these patients (90.1%). Time period to first monitored ventricular arrhythmias and to first appropriate cardioverter-defibrillator therapy were significantly shorter in patients with either CSA or OSA. Forward stepwise Cox models revealed an independent correlation for CSA and OSA regarding monitored ventricular arrhythmias [apnoea–hypopnoea index (AHI) $\geq 5\ h^{-1}$: CSA HR 2.15, 95% CI 1.40–3.30, $P < 0.001$; OSA HR 1.69, 95% CI 1.64–1.75, $P = 0.001$; AHI $\geq 15\ h^{-1}$: CSA HR 2.06, 95% CI 1.40–3.05, $P < 0.001$; OSA HR 1.69, 95% CI 1.14–2.51, $P = 0.02$] and appropriate cardioverter-defibrillator therapies (AHI $\geq 5\ h^{-1}$: CSA HR 3.24, 95% CI 1.86–5.64, $P < 0.001$; OSA HR 2.07, 95% CI 1.14–3.77, $P = 0.02$; AHI $\geq 15\ h^{-1}$: CSA HR 3.41, 95% CI 2.10–5.54, $P < 0.001$; OSA HR 2.10, 95% CI 1.17–3.78, $P = 0.01$).

Conclusion.—In patients with CHF, CSA and OSA are independently associated with an increased risk for ventricular arrhythmias and appropriate cardioverter-defibrillator therapies.

▶ Sleep-disordered breathing is common in patients with congestive heart failure. It is important to recognize the significance of this comorbidity, particularly its associated negative outcomes. In patients with congestive heart failure, sleep-disordered breathing is an independent predictor for life-threatening arrhythmias.[1] This study reveals patients with both central and obstructive sleep apnea were more likely to need pacing or defibrillation to treat ventricular arrhythmia than patients with no or minimal sleep disordered breathing. Both central and obstructive sleep apnea are independently associated with ventricular arrhythmias and appropriate therapies delivered by the device. This study is different in that the author examined the association of central and obstructive sleep apnea, separately, on arrhythmias and need for device therapy. Although the study does not explore causation, the authors hypothesized that hypoxemia and recurrent arousals from sleep may incite sympathetic activation. Future studies examining the effect of continuous positive airway pressure on mitigating the degree of arrhythmogenic potential are needed.

S. F. Jones, MD, FCCP, DABSM

Reference

1. Serizawa N, Yumino D, Kajimoto K, et al. Impact of sleep-disordered breathing on life-threatening ventricular arrhythmia in heart failure patients with implantable cardioverter-defibrillator. *Am J Cardiol.* 2008;102:1064-1068.

Obstructive sleep apnoea: a stand-alone risk factor for chronic kidney disease
Chou Y-T, Lee P-H, Yang C-T, et al (Chang Gung Memorial Hosp, Chiayi, Taiwan; Chang Gung Inst of Technology, Taoyuan, Taiwan; et al)
Nephrol Dial Transplant 26:2244-2250, 2011

Background.—Previous studies have found an association between obstructive sleep apnea (OSA) and chronic kidney disease (CKD). However, subjects with confounding factors such as diabetes and hypertension were not excluded. The purpose of the present study was to determine whether patients with OSA without meeting criteria for diabetes or hypertension would also show increased likelihood of CKD.

Methods.—We prospectively enrolled adult patients with a chief complaint of habitual snoring. Overnight polysomnography, fasting blood triglyceride, cholesterol, glucose, insulin, creatinine, albumin and hemoglobin A1c, and first voiding urine albumin and creatinine were examined. Estimated glomerular filtration rate (eGFR), urine albumin-to-creatinine ratio (UACR), homeostatic model assessment—insulin resistance and percentage of CKD were calculated.

Results.—The final analyses involved 40 patients who were middle-aged [44.8 (8.6) years] predominantly male (83%), obese [body mass index, 28.2 (5.1) kg/m^2] and more severe OSA, with an apnea—hypopnea index (AHI) of 51.6 (39.2)/h. The mean eGFR and UACR were 85.4 (18.3) mL/min/1.73m^2 and 13.4 (23.4) mg/g, respectively. The prevalence of CKD in severe OSA subjects is 18%. With stepwise multivariate linear regression analysis, AHI and desaturation index were the only independent predictor of UACR ($\beta = 0.26$, $P = 0.01$, $R^2 = 0.17$) and eGFR ($\beta = 0.32$, $P < 0.01$, $R^2 = 0.32$), respectively.

Conclusions.—High prevalence of CKD is present in severe OSA patients without hypertension or diabetes. Significantly positive correlations were found between severity of OSA and renal function impairment.

▶ Previous literature supporting an association between chronic kidney disease and obstructive sleep apnea included patients with diabetes and hypertension, both confounders. In this prospective study of 40 snorers conducted in a Taiwanese population, subjects were free of diabetes and hypertension. Apnea and hypopnea index and desaturation index were the only independent predictors of kidney urine albumin to creatinine ratio and estimated glomerular filtration rate. Of the patients in the sample, 14% to 18% had evidence of chronic kidney disease, with higher rates in those with severe obstructive sleep apnea. A possible mechanism for the finding is hyperfiltration induced by obstructive sleep apnea. Furthermore, the degree of microalbuminuria may be reversible.[1]

The study population is Southeast Asian, so the study should be replicated in other populations with different ethnicities. Assessment of estimated glomerular filtration rate should be considered in those with severe obstructive sleep apnea.

S. F. Jones, MD, FCCP, DABSM

Reference

1. Mauer M, Fioretto P, Woredekal Y, et al. Diabetic nephropathy. In: Schrier RW, ed. *Diseases of the Kidney and Urinary Tract.* 7th ed. Philadelphia, PA: Lippincott Williams and Wilkins; 2001:2083-2127.

Effects of Continuous Positive Airway Pressure Therapy Withdrawal in Patients with Obstructive Sleep Apnea: A Randomized Controlled Trial
Kohler M, Stoewhas A-C, Ayers L, et al (Univ of Zurich, Switzerland; Churchill Hosp, Oxford, UK)
Am J Respir Crit Care Med 184:1192-1199, 2011

Rationale.—To establish a new approach to investigate the physiological effects of obstructive sleep apnea (OSA), and to evaluate novel treatments, during a period of continuous positive airway pressure (CPAP) withdrawal.

Objectives.—To determine the effects of CPAP withdrawal.

Methods.—Forty-one patients with OSA and receiving CPAP were randomized to either CPAP withdrawal (subtherapeutic CPAP), or continued CPAP, for 2 weeks. Polysomnography, sleepiness, psychomotor performance, endothelial function, blood pressure (BP), heart rate (HR), urinary catecholamines, blood markers of systemic inflammation, and metabolism were assessed.

Measurements and Main Results.—CPAP withdrawal led to a recurrence of OSA within a few days and a return of subjective sleepiness, but was not associated with significant deterioration of psychomotor performance within 2 weeks. Endothelial function, assessed by flow-mediated dilatation, decreased significantly in the CPAP withdrawal group compared with therapeutic CPAP (mean difference in change, -3.2%; 95% confidence interval [CI], -4.5, -1.9%; $P < 0.001$). Compared with continuing CPAP, 2 weeks of CPAP withdrawal was associated with a significant increase in morning systolic BP (mean difference in change, $+8.5$ mm Hg; 95% CI, $+1.7$, $+15.3$ mm Hg; $P = 0.016$), morning diastolic BP (mean difference in change, $+6.9$ mm Hg; 95% CI, $+1.9$, $+11.9$ mm Hg; $P = 0.008$), and morning HR (mean difference in change, $+6.3$ bpm, 95% CI, $+0.4$, $+12.2$ bpm; $P = 0.035$). CPAP withdrawal was associated with an increase in urinary catecholamines but did not lead to an increase in markers of systemic inflammation, insulin resistance, or blood lipids.

Conclusions.—CPAP withdrawal usually leads to a rapid recurrence of OSA, a return of subjective sleepiness, and is associated with impaired endothelial function, increased urinary catecholamines, blood pressure, and heart rate. Thus the proposed study model appears to be suitable to evaluate physiological and therapeutic effects in OSA. Clinical trial registered with www.controlled-trials.com (ISRCTN93153804).

▶ In my practice, patients ask, "What will happen to me if I don't wear continuous positive airway pressure (CPAP) for 1 night? What will happen to me if I don't take my CPAP machine with me on my 2-week vacation?" I think this study is interesting in that physiologic parameters were measured in patients who had discontinued CPAP for 2 weeks and were compared with controls (patients who continued to wear CPAP). There are both research-related and patient care implications to this study. The protocol implemented by the investigators has created a new model of the effects of untreated obstructive sleep apnea (OSA) that could be used in future studies to examine effects of new interventions. Withdrawal of CPAP led to an increase in number of apneas and hypopneas as early as the first night with no further increase in apnea-hypopnea index after a week of withdrawal (Fig 2 in the original article). Increases in Epworth sleepiness score were significant following withdrawal. The most impressive finding is the increase in morning systolic and diastolic blood pressure and morning heart rate (Fig 4 in the original article). This is something that I have observed in the laboratory, but these investigators have quantified these observations. Furthermore, with the observation of increase in urinary catecholamines, a surge in sympathetic activity is a possible etiology to these findings.

S. F. Jones, MD, FCCP, DABSM

A Brief Sleep Intervention Improves Outcomes in the School Entry Year: A Randomized Controlled Trial

Quach J, Hiscock H, Ukoumunne OC, et al (Univ of Melbourne, Australia; Univ of Exeter, UK)
Pediatrics 128:692-701, 2011

Objective.—To determine the feasibility of screening for child sleep problems and the efficacy of a behavioral sleep intervention in improving child and parent outcomes in the first year of schooling.

Methods.—A randomized controlled trial was nested in a population survey performed at 22 elementary schools in Melbourne, Australia. Intervention involved 2 to 3 consultations that covered behavioral sleep strategies for children whose screening results were positive for a moderate/severe sleep problem. Outcomes were parent-reported child sleep problem (primary outcome), sleep habits, psychosocial health-related quality of life, behavior, and parent mental health (all at 3, 6, and 12 months) and blinded, face-to-face learning assessment (at 6 months).

Results.—The screening survey was completed by 1512 parents; 161 (10.8%) reported a moderate/severe child sleep problem, and 108 of 136 (79.2% of those eligible) entered the trial. Sleep problems tended to resolve more rapidly in intervention children. Sleep problems affected 33% of 54 intervention children versus 43% of 54 control children at 3 months (*P* =.3), 25.5% vs 46.8% at 6 months (*P* =.03), and 32% vs 33% at 12 months (*P* =.8). Sustained sleep-habit improvements were evident at 3, 6, and 12 months (effect sizes: 0.33 [*P* =.03]; 0.51 [*P* =.003]; and 0.40 [*P* =.02]; respectively), and there were initial marked improvements in psychosocial scores that diminished over time (effect sizes: 0.47 [*P* =.02]; 0.41 [*P* =.09]; and 0.26 [*P* =.3]; respectively). Better prosocial behavior was evident at 12 months (effect size: 0.35; *P* =.03), and learning and parent outcomes were similar between groups.

Conclusions.—School-based screening for sleep problems followed by a targeted, brief behavioral sleep intervention is feasible and has benefits relevant to school transition.

▶ Data from the Longtitudinal Study of Australian Children show that sleep problems are common in children aged 4 to 5 years. Poor sleep is associated with negative outcomes, such as health-related quality of life, behavior, language, and learning scores.[1] Quach et al have taken this one step further in this article by examining the effect of a behavioral intervention that included 1 individual session and 2 follow-up phone calls. In this work, screening surveys were sent to 22 schools in Australia, with completion by 1512 parents. The strengths of the study are notable. Seventy-one percent of surveys were completed, and of those children identified with moderate to severe sleep problems, 79% took part in the study. This study had a high retention rate, even 12 months afterward. Improvements in sleep were notable at 6 months. The improvement in psychosocial scores shows that a brief intervention could be effective. Although these improvements diminished over time, the true effect of the intervention on the psychosocial scores is likely dampened by the number of subjects (n = 47). This study should be expanded to include a more diverse population. This work is significant and is a true example of population health research.

S. F. Jones, MD, FCCP, DABSM

Reference

1. Quach J, Hiscock H, Canterford L, Wake M. Outcomes of child sleep problems over the school-transition period: Australian population longitudinal study. *Pediatrics.* 2009;123:1287-1292.

33 Critical Care Medicine

Implementing Early Mobilization Interventions in Mechanically Ventilated Patients in the ICU
Schweickert WD, Kress JP (Univ of Pennsylvania, Philadelphia; Univ of Chicago, IL)
Chest 140:1612-1617, 2011

As ICU survival continues to improve, clinicians are faced with short- and long-term consequences of critical illness. Deconditioning and weakness have become common problems in survivors of critical illness requiring mechanical ventilation. Recent literature, mostly from a medical population of patients in the ICU, has challenged the patient care model of prolonged bed rest. Instead, the feasibility, safety, and benefits of early mobilization of mechanically ventilated ICU patients have been reported in recent publications. The benefits of early mobilization include reductions in length of stay in the ICU and hospital as well as improvements in strength and functional status. Such benefits can be accomplished with a remarkably acceptable patient safety profile. The importance of interactions between mind and body are highlighted by these studies, with improvements in patient awareness and reductions in ICU delirium being noted. Future research to address the benefits of early mobilization in other patient populations is needed. In addition, the potential for early mobilization to impact long-term outcomes in ICU survivors requires further study.

▶ There are many potential pitfalls and roadblocks to ambulating ill patients. Certainly, connection to high-tech devices is one of them. Nonetheless, early mobilization of ventilator patients is rapidly becoming state-of-the-art practice. It makes sense. Truncal stability and strengthening has to improve cough and ventilator weaning. Patients must be awake and interactive to walk. And mental outlook will certainly be improved in patients who are awake and alert and can see some new scenery.

This article is a combination how-to and state of the art. It is nicely written and informative.

J. A. Barker, MD, FACP, FCCP

Dysphagia screening decreases pneumonia in acute stroke patients admitted to the stroke intensive care unit

Yeh S-J, Huang K-Y, Wang T-G, et al (Yun-Lin Branch of Natl Taiwan Univ Hosp, Douliu City, Yunlin County, Taiwan; Natl Taiwan Univ Hosp, Taipei City; et al)
J Neurol Sci 306:38-41, 2011

Dysphagia increases the risk of pneumonia in stroke patients. This study aimed to evaluate bedside swallowing screening for prevention of stroke-associated pneumonia (SAP) in acute stroke patients admitted to the intensive care unit (ICU). Consecutive acute stroke patients admitted to the stroke ICU from May 2006 to March 2007 were included. Patients were excluded if they were intubated on the first day of admission or had a transient ischemic attack. A 3-Step Swallowing Screen was introduced since October 2006 and therefore patients were divided into pre-screen and post-screen groups. A binary logistic regression model was used to determine independent risk factors for SAP and in-hospital death. There were 74 and 102 patients included in the pre- and post-screen groups, respectively. Pneumonia was associated with higher National Institutes of Health Stroke Scale (NIHSS) score, older age, nasogastric and endotracheal tube placement. After adjusting for age, gender, NIHSS score and nasogastric and endotracheal tube insertion, dysphagia screening was associated with a borderline decrease in SAP in all stroke patients (odds ratio, 0.42; 95% CI, 0.18–1.00; $p = 0.05$). However, dysphagia screening was not associated with reduction of in-hospital deaths. Systematic bedside swallowing screening is helpful for prevention of SAP in acute stroke patients admitted to the ICU.

▶ Pneumonia occurs in 30% of patients admitted with new stroke. This simple intervention looks promising for reducing this incidence. I doubt that it will eliminate all pneumonia in these patients, however, because probably a significant number aspirate near the time of the stroke. This nicely done study should change our practice for the better.

J. A. Barker, MD, FACP, FCCP

Noninvasive versus invasive ventilation for acute respiratory failure in patients with hematologic malignancies: A 5-year multicenter observational survey

Gristina GR, on behalf of the GiViTI (Italian Group for the Evaluation of Interventions in Intensive Care Medicine) (San Camillo-Forlanini Hosp, Rome, Italy; et al)
Crit Care Med 39:2232-2239, 2011

Background.—Mortality is high among patients with hematologic malignancies admitted to intensive care units for acute respiratory failure. Early noninvasive mechanical ventilation seems to improve outcomes.

Objective.—To characterize noninvasive mechanical ventilation use in Italian intensive care units for acute respiratory failure patients with hematologic malignancies and its impact on outcomes vs. invasive mechanical ventilation.

Design, Setting, Participants.—Retrospective analysis of observational data prospectively collected in 2002—2006 on 1,302 patients with hematologic malignancies admitted with acute respiratory failure to 158 Italian intensive care units.

Measurements.—Mortality (intensive care unit and hospital) was assessed in patients treated initially with noninvasive mechanical ventilation vs. invasive mechanical ventilation and in those treated with invasive mechanical ventilation *ab initio* vs. after noninvasive mechanical ventilation failure. Findings were adjusted for propensity scores reflecting the probability of initial treatment with noninvasive mechanical ventilation.

Results.—Few patients (21%) initially received noninvasive mechanical ventilation; 46% of these later required invasive mechanical ventilation. Better outcomes were associated with successful noninvasive mechanical ventilation (vs. invasive mechanical ventilation *ab initio* and vs. invasive mechanical ventilation after noninvasive mechanical ventilation failure), particularly in patients with acute lung injury/adult respiratory distress syndrome (mortality: 42% vs. 69% and 77%, respectively). Delayed vs. immediate invasive mechanical ventilation was associated with slightly but not significantly higher hospital mortality (65% vs. 58%, $p = .12$). After propensity-score adjustment, noninvasive mechanical ventilation was associated with significantly lower mortality than invasive mechanical ventilation.

Limitations.—The population could not be stratified according to specific hematologic diagnoses. Furthermore, the study was observational, and treatment groups may have included unaccounted for differences in covariates although the risk of this bias was minimized with propensity score regression adjustment.

Conclusions.—In patients with hematologic malignancies, acute respiratory failure should probably be managed initially with noninvasive mechanical ventilation. Further study is needed to determine whether immediate invasive mechanical ventilation might offer some benefits for those with acute lung injury/adult respiratory distress syndrome.

▶ This is clearly a controversial area because there are previous studies with results falling on both sides of the question. Once again, it appears that noninvasive ventilation not only yields better outcomes but is preferred. Probably those patients who meet acute respiratory distress syndrome criteria (low peak flow ratios) should be the only ones intubated first.

J. A. Barker, MD, FACP, FCCP

Airway challenges in critical care

Nolan JP, Kelly FE (Royal United Hosp, Bath, UK)
Anaesthesia 66:81-92, 2011

Airway management in the intensive care unit is more problematic than during anaesthesia. In general, critically ill patients have less physiological reserve and complications are more common, both during the initial airway intervention (which includes risks associated with induction of anaesthesia), and later once the airway has been secured. Despite these known risks, those managing the airway of a critically ill patient, particularly out of hours, may be relatively inexperienced. Solutions to these challenging airway problems include: recognition of those patients with a potential airway problem; implementation of a plan to deal with their airway; immediate availability of a difficult airway trolley; use of capnography for every airway intervention and continuously in all ventilator-dependent patients; and appropriate training of all intensive care unit staff including use of simulation.

▶ This is a thoughtful, comprehensive discussion of an important everyday problem in the intensive care unit (ICU). The estimation of 10% ICU intubations as being difficult airways is accurate. The off-hours timing, inexperience of operators, and human factors are all important. The risks, of course, are tremendous: death or significant morbidity.

The solutions suggested again are appropriate and reasonable:

1. Plan for difficult airways. Have equipment available and access to experienced operators.

2. Have equipment at the ready.

3. Plan, plan, plan. This includes standardized anesthetics such as ketamine and etomidate.

4. Given the poor results of cricothyrotomy, standardized training in this technique should be included in all advanced airway courses.

5. Have protocols for displaced tracheotomy tubes. I totally agree with this. This seems to be an area that is frequently overlooked in airway management planning.

6. Use simulators and repetition to control for human factors.

I think all trainees and program directors should read this article.

J. A. Barker, MD, FACP, FCCP

Accuracy of a continuous noninvasive hemoglobin monitor in intensive care unit patients

Frasca D, Dahyot-Fizelier C, Catherine K, et al (Centre Hospitalier Universitaire de Poitiers, France)
Crit Care Med 39:2277-2282, 2011

Objective.—To determine whether noninvasive hemoglobin measurement by Pulse CO-Oximetry could provide clinically acceptable absolute and trend accuracy in critically ill patients, compared to other invasive methods of hemoglobin assessment available at bedside and the gold standard, the laboratory analyzer.

Design.—Prospective study.

Setting.—Surgical intensive care unit of a university teaching hospital.

Patients.—Sixty-two patients continuously monitored with Pulse CO-Oximetry (Masimo Radical-7).

Interventions.—None.

Measurements and Results.—Four hundred seventy-one blood samples were analyzed by a point-of-care device (HemoCue 301), a satellite lab CO-Oximeter (Siemens RapidPoint 405), and a laboratory hematology analyzer (Sysmex XT-2000i), which was considered the reference device. Hemoglobin values reported from the invasive methods were compared to the values reported by the Pulse CO-Oximeter at the time of blood draw. When the case-to-case variation was assessed, the bias and limits of agreement were 0.0 ± 1.0 g/dL for the Pulse CO-Oximeter, 0.3 ± 1.3 g/dL for the point-of-care device, and 0.9 ± 0.6 g/dL for the satellite lab CO-Oximeter compared to the reference method. Pulse CO-Oximetry showed similar trend accuracy as satellite lab CO-Oximetry, whereas the point-of-care device did not appear to follow the trend of the laboratory analyzer as well as the other test devices.

Conclusion.—When compared to laboratory reference values, hemoglobin measurement with Pulse CO-Oximetry has absolute accuracy and trending accuracy similar to widely used, invasive methods of hemoglobin measurement at bedside. Hemoglobin measurement with pulse CO-Oximetry has the additional advantages of providing continuous measurements, noninvasively, which may facilitate hemoglobin monitoring in the intensive care unit.

▶ It would seem that this technology has many important advantages. Because this study now independently verifies that it is indeed accurate technology, we will have to assess how our care will change. For example, do we still wait for equilibration effect in gastrointestinal bleeding patients while we give blood and saline, or will we react differently if we know actual hemoglobin trends? I think we will adjust and change practice patterns.

J. A. Barker, MD, FACP, FCCP

PART SIX

HEART AND CARDIOVASCULAR DISEASE

BERNARD J. GERSH, MB, CHB, D.PHIL, FRCP

Introduction

It continues to be an exciting time in cardiology on multiple fronts. Technological innovations have been a boon to interventionalists in diverse areas such as acute and chronic coronary artery disease, congestive heart failure, arrhythmias, hypertension, congenital heart disease, and hypertrophic cardiomyopathy. These innovations and advances also apply to the science of genetics and the goal of personalized medicine. Nonetheless, progress has been tempered by concerns regarding the appropriate use of invasive and diagnostic procedures, which has in turn stimulated an emphasis upon guidelines and appropriateness criteria.

The 30 articles selected are simply a snapshot of a large and exciting area that has been chosen given general interest and clinical application. Hopefully, these will be of interest to our readers.

Bernard J. Gersh, MB, ChB, DPhil, FRCP

34 Cardiac Arrhythmias, Conduction Disturbances, and Electrophysiology

Apixaban versus Warfarin in Patients with Atrial Fibrillation
Granger CB, for the ARISTOTLE Committees and Investigators (Duke Univ Med Ctr, Durham, NC; et al)
N Engl J Med 365:981-992, 2011

Background.—Vitamin K antagonists are highly effective in preventing stroke in patients with atrial fibrillation but have several limitations. Apixaban is a novel oral direct factor Xa inhibitor that has been shown to reduce the risk of stroke in a similar population in comparison with aspirin.

Methods.—In this randomized, double-blind trial, we compared apixaban (at a dose of 5 mg twice daily) with warfarin (target international normalized ratio, 2.0 to 3.0) in 18,201 patients with atrial fibrillation and at least one additional risk factor for stroke. The primary outcome was ischemic or hemorrhagic stroke or systemic embolism. The trial was designed to test for noninferiority, with key secondary objectives of testing for superiority with respect to the primary outcome and to the rates of major bleeding and death from any cause.

Results.—The median duration of follow-up was 1.8 years. The rate of the primary outcome was 1.27% per year in the apixaban group, as compared with 1.60% per year in the warfarin group (hazard ratio with apixaban, 0.79; 95% confidence interval [CI], 0.66 to 0.95; $P < 0.001$ for noninferiority; $P = 0.01$ for superiority). The rate of major bleeding was 2.13% per year in the apixaban group, as compared with 3.09% per year in the warfarin group (hazard ratio, 0.69; 95% CI, 0.60 to 0.80; $P < 0.001$), and the rates of death from any cause were 3.52% and 3.94%, respectively (hazard ratio, 0.89; 95% CI, 0.80 to 0.99; $P = 0.047$). The rate of hemorrhagic stroke was 0.24% per year in the apixaban group, as compared with 0.47% per year in the warfarin group (hazard ratio, 0.51; 95% CI, 0.35 to 0.75; $P < 0.001$), and the rate of ischemic or uncertain type of stroke was 0.97% per year in the apixaban group and 1.05% per year in the warfarin group (hazard ratio, 0.92; 95% CI, 0.74 to 1.13; $P = 0.42$).

Conclusions.—In patients with atrial fibrillation, apixaban was superior to warfarin in preventing stroke or systemic embolism, caused less bleeding, and resulted in lower mortality. (Funded by Bristol-Myers Squibb and Pfizer; ARISTOTLE ClinicalTrials.gov number, NCT00412984.)

▶ Prevention of thromboembolism is an important component of the treatment for patients with atrial fibrillation (AF). Stable therapeutic anticoagulation with warfarin requires strict diet control and frequent laboratory monitoring and can be difficult to manage in even the most closely monitored patients, such as those in clinical trials. Such challenges have led to multiple efforts to develop oral anticoagulants that can effectively prevent stroke and limit bleeding complications without requiring strict diet control or laboratory monitoring. One such agent was tested in the ARISTOTLE trial, which compares a novel oral anticoagulant, apixaban, to warfarin in high-risk patients with AF. ARISTOTLE was a randomized, double-blind trial in 18 201 patients with AF comparing apixaban 5 mg twice daily to dose-adjusted warfarin with a target international normalized ratio of 2 to 3. The primary outcome was ischemic or hemorrhagic stroke or systemic embolism. The trial had a noninferiority design with respect to the primary outcome. Secondary endpoints included superiority with respect to the primary endpoint and to the rates of major bleeding and death. Over a median follow-up period of 1.8 years, the rate of the primary outcome was 1.27% per year in the apixaban group, compared with 1.6% per year in the warfarin group (hazard ratio [HR] 0.79; 95% confidence interval [CI] 0.66−0.95; P < .001 for noninferiority and P = .01 for superiority). The rate of major bleeding was 2.13% per year in the apixaban group compared with 3.09% per year in the warfarin group (HR, 0.69; 95% CI, 0.60−0.80; P < .001). The rate of death from any cause was 3.52% in the apixaban group compared with 3.94% in the warfarin group (HR, 0.89; 95% CI, 0.80−0.99; P = .047). This trial demonstrated the ability of apixaban to reduce the risk of stroke while also reducing the risk of major bleeding (Fig 1 in the original article). The twice-daily dosing schedule is similar to dabigatran, another recently developed warfarin alternative. However, although the currently approved dose of dabigatran was shown in the RE-LY trial to be superior to warfarin in stroke prevention, it had a similar bleeding risk. Therefore, apixaban may have the added advantage of simultaneously improving efficacy while decreasing bleeding. However, such comparisons between studies should be done with caution because entry criteria, study design, and the groups studied had some differences. Although other factors such as cost and drug intolerance will affect the distribution and use of these new anticoagulants, apixaban appears to be a safe and effective alternative to warfarin.

C. P. Rowley, MD

Prevention of stroke and systemic embolism with rivaroxaban compared with warfarin in patients with non-valvular atrial fibrillation and moderate renal impairment

Fox KAA, Piccini JP, Wojdyla D, et al (Univ of Edinburgh, UK)
Eur Heart J 32:2387-2394, 2011

Aims.—Patients with non-valvular atrial fibrillation (AF) and renal insufficiency are at increased risk for ischaemic stroke and bleeding during anticoagulation. Rivaroxaban, an oral, direct factor Xa inhibitor metabolized predominantly by the liver, preserves the benefit of warfarin for stroke prevention while causing fewer intracranial and fatal haemorrhages.

Methods and Results.—We randomized 14 264 patients with AF in a double-blind trial to rivaroxaban 20 mg/day [15 mg/day if creatinine clearance (CrCl) 30–49 mL/min] or dose-adjusted warfarin (target international normalized ratio 2.0–3.0). Compared with patients with CrCl > 50 mL/min (mean age 73 years), the 2950 (20.7%) patients with CrCl 30–49 mL/min were older (79 years) and had higher event rates irrespective of study treatment. Among those with CrCl 30–49 mL/min, the primary endpoint of stroke or systemic embolism occurred in 2.32 per 100 patient-years with rivaroxaban 15 mg/day vs. 2.77 per 100 patient-years with warfarin [hazard ratio (HR) 0.84; 95% confidence interval (CI) 0.57–1.23] in the per-protocol population. Intention-to-treat analysis yielded similar results (HR 0.86; 95% CI 0.63–1.17) to the per-protocol results. Rates of the principal safety endpoint (major and clinically relevant non-major bleeding: 17.82 vs. 18.28 per 100 patient-years; $P = 0.76$) and intracranial bleeding (0.71 vs. 0.88 per 100 patient-years; $P = 0.54$) were similar with rivaroxaban or warfarin. Fatal bleeding (0.28 vs. 0.74% per 100 patient-years; $P = 0.047$) occurred less often with rivaroxaban.

Conclusion.—Patients with AF and moderate renal insufficiency have higher rates of stroke and bleeding than those with normal renal function. There was no evidence of heterogeneity in treatment effect across dosing groups. Dose adjustment in ROCKET-AF yielded results consistent with

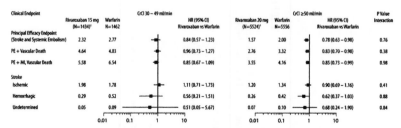

Clinical Endpoint			CrCl 30 – 49 ml/min			CrCl ≥50 ml/min			P Value
	Rivaroxaban 15 mg (N=1434)'	Warfarin N=1462		HR (95% CI) Rivaroxaban vs Warfarin	Rivaroxaban 20 mg (N=5524)'	Warfarin N=5556		HR (95% CI) Rivaroxaban vs Warfarin	Interaction
Principal Efficacy Endpoint (Stroke and Systemic Embolism)	2.32	2.77		0.84 (0.57 – 1.23)	1.57	2.00		0.78 (0.63 – 0.98)	0.76
PE + Vascular Death	4.64	4.83		0.96 (0.73 – 1.27)	2.76	3.32		0.83 (0.70 – 0.98)	0.38
PE + MI, Vascular Death	5.58	6.54		0.85 (0.67 – 1.09)	3.55	4.16		0.85 (0.73 – 0.99)	0.98
Stroke									
Ischemic	1.98	1.78		1.11 (0.71 – 1.73)	1.20	1.34		0.90 (0.69 – 1.16)	0.41
Hemorrhagic	0.29	0.52		0.56 (0.21 – 1.51)	0.26	0.42		0.62 (0.37 – 1.03)	0.88
Undetermined	0.05	0.09		0.51 (0.05 – 5.67)	0.07	0.10		0.68 (0.24 – 1.90)	0.84

* The primary analysis was pre-specified to be performed in the per-protocol population on treatment, which included all patients who received at least 1 dose of study drug, did not have major protocol violations, and were followed for events while on study drug or within 2 days of last dose.
' Event rates per 100 pt/yrs of follow-up

FIGURE 1.—Efficacy events in the per-protocol (on-treatment) population. (Reprinted from Fox KAA, Piccini JP, Wojdyla D, et al. Prevention of stroke and systemic embolism with rivaroxaban compared with warfarin in patients with non-valvular atrial fibrillation and moderate renal impairment. *Eur Heart J.* 2011;32:2387-2394, by permission of The European Society of Cardiology.)

TABLE 3.—Bleeding Rates by Treatment Group Rivaroxaban vs. Warfarin

Clinical Endpoint	Rivaroxaban 15 mg (n = 1474)[a]	CrCl 30–49 mL/min Warfarin (n = 1476)[a]	Hazard Ratio (95% CI), Rivaroxaban vs. Warfarin	Rivaroxaban 20 mg (n = 5637)[a]	CrCl ≥50 mL/min Warfarin (n = 5640)[a]	Hazard Ratio (95% CI), Rivaroxaban vs. Warfarin	P-Value for Interaction
Primary safety endpoint	17.82	18.28	0.98 (0.84–1.14)	14.24	13.67	1.04 (0.96–1.13)	0.4496
Major bleeding	4.49	4.70	0.95 (0.72–1.26)	3.39	3.17	1.07 (0.91–1.26)	0.4800
Hb drop	3.76	3.28	1.14 (0.83–1.58)	2.54	2.03	1.25 (1.03–1.52)	0.6456
Transfusion	2.34	2.00	1.17 (0.77–1.76)	1.49	1.16	1.28 (0.99–1.65)	0.7066
Clinical organ	0.76	1.39	0.55 (0.30–1.00)	0.83	1.13	0.74 (0.55–0.99)	0.3866
Fatal bleeding	0.28	0.74	0.39 (0.15–0.99)	0.23	0.43	0.55 (0.32–0.93)	0.5302
Intracranial haemorrhage	0.71	0.88	0.81 (0.41–1.60)	0.44	0.71	0.62 (0.42–0.92)	0.5065

[a]Event rates per 100 patient-years of follow-up.

the overall trial in comparison with dose-adjusted warfarin (Fig 1, Table 3).

▶ Rivaroxaban is a novel oral direct factor Xa inhibitor that has been shown in the Rivaroxaban Once-daily, oral, direct factor Xa inhibition compared with vitamin K antagonism for prevention of stroke and Embolism Trial in Atrial Fibrillation (ROCKET-AF) to be noninferior to warfarin with respect to stroke prevention in high-risk patients with AF. Due to the pharmocokinetic properties of rivaroxaban, there is a 25% to 30% increase in maximal serum concentration in patients with moderate renal dysfunction (CrCl 30—49 mL/min). Accordingly, such patients in ROCKET-AF were given dose-reduced rivaroxaban 15 mg daily rather than the standard 20-mg daily dose. In this analysis, the authors sought to determine whether dose-reduced rivaroxaban was effective for stroke reduction in patients with renal impairment. Of the 14 264 patients with AF randomized in ROCKET-AF there were 2950 (20.7%) patients with CrCl 30 to 49 mL/min. Of those 2950 patients, 1474 received dose-reduced rivaroxaban, and 1476 received dose-adjusted warfarin with target international normalized ratio 2 to 3. In the per-protocol analysis, the primary endpoint of stroke or systemic embolism occurred in 2.32 per 100 patient-years in the rivaroxaban group compared with 2.77 per 100 patient-years in the warfarin group (hazard ratio, 0.84; 95% confidence interval, 0.57—1.23, Fig 1). Results were similar in the intention-to-treat analysis. The primary safety endpoint of major and clinically relevant nonmajor bleeding occurred in 17.82 versus 18.28 per 100 patient-years in the rivaroxaban and warfarin groups, respectively (Table 3). Fatal bleeding occurred in fewer patients in the rivaroxaban group compared with the warfarin group (0.28% vs 0.74% per 100 patient-years, respectively, $P = .047$). This substudy indicates that patients with impaired renal function had a higher risk of stroke as well as bleeding compared with patients with normal renal function, an observation that is consistent with those of prior studies. Additionally, it provides clinical evidence for safe and effective use of renally adjusted rivaroxaban for stroke prevention in patients with moderate renal impairment.

C. P. Rowley, MD

The Effect of Rate Control on Quality of Life in Patients With Permanent Atrial Fibrillation: Data From the RACE II (Rate Control Efficacy in Permanent Atrial Fibrillation II) Study
Groenveld HF, for the RACE II Investigators (Univ of Groningen, the Netherlands; et al)
J Am Coll Cardiol 58:1795-1803, 2011

Objectives.—The aim of this study was to investigate the influence of rate control on quality of life (QOL).

Background.—The RACE II (Rate Control Efficacy in Permanent Atrial Fibrillation II) trial showed that lenient rate control is not inferior to strict rate control in terms of cardiovascular morbidity and mortality. The influence of stringency of rate control on QOL is unknown.

Methods.—In RACE II, a total of 614 patients with permanent atrial fibrillation (AF) were randomized to lenient (resting heart rate [HR] < 110 beats/min) or strict (resting HR <80 beats/min, HR during moderate exercise < 110 beats/min) rate control. QOL was assessed in 437 patients using the Medical Outcomes Study 36-item Short-Form Health Survey (SF-36) questionnaire, AF severity scale, and Multidimensional Fatigue Inventory-20 (MFI-20) at baseline, 1 year, and end of study. QOL changes were related to patient characteristics.

Results.—Median follow-up was 3 years. Mean age was 68 ± 8 years, and 66% were males. At the end of follow-up, all SF-36 subscales were comparable between both groups. The AF severity scale was similar at baseline and end of study. At baseline and at end of study there were no differences in the MFI-20 subscales between the 2 groups. Symptoms at baseline, younger age, and less severe underlying disease, rather than assigned therapy or heart rate, were associated with QOL improvements. Female sex and cardiovascular endpoints during the study were associated with worsening of QOL.

Conclusions.—Stringency of heart rate control does not influence QOL. Instead, symptoms, sex, age, and severity of the underlying disease influence QOL (Fig 1).

▶ Several studies have shown that rhythm control with antiarrhythmic drugs is not superior to rate control in asymptomatic or mildly symptomatic patients. When a rate control strategy is adopted, the optimal heart rate goal remains

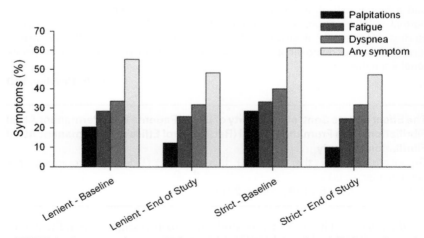

FIGURE 1.—Percentage of Patients With Any Symptom. Symptoms of atrial fibrillation during the study, displayed by randomization strategy at baseline and end of study. (Reprinted from the Journal of the American College of Cardiology, Groenveld HF, for the RACE II Investigators, The effect of rate control on quality of life in patients with permanent atrial fibrillation: data from the RACE II (Rate Control Efficacy in Permanent Atrial Fibrillation II) study. *J Am Coll Cardiol*. 2011;58:1795-1803. Copyright 2011, with permission from the American College of Cardiology.)

controversial. In the Rate Control Efficacy in Permanent Atrial Fibrillation II study (RACE II), mortality and morbidity were not influenced by strict versus lenient rate control in long-standing persistent atrial fibrillation patients. This substudy of RACE II addressed the effects of rate control strategies on quality of life (QOL). Using the SF-36 AF severity scale and MFI-20 metrics at baseline, 1 year, and at the end of the study, there was no demonstrated difference in QOL in strict and lenient rate control groups (Fig 1). Age, female sex, symptom severity, and comorbid conditions were associated with worse QOL. Side effects of rate control agents were speculated to offset the benefit of better rate control. Additionally, more than 40% of patients were asymptomatic, which may have masked the outcome. Those with strict rate control experienced slightly more symptoms compared with lenient control. This report suggests that strict rate control has no measurable benefit in QOL for patients with long-standing persistent atrial fibrillation.

M. L. Bernard, MD, PhD

Driving restrictions after implantable cardioverter defibrillator implantation: an evidence-based approach
Thijssen J, Borleffs CJW, van Rees JB, et al (Leiden Univ Med Ctr, The Netherlands)
Eur Heart J 32:2678-2687, 2011

Aims.—Little evidence is available regarding restrictions from driving following implantable cardioverter defibrillator (ICD) implantation or following first appropriate or inappropriate shock. The purpose of the current analysis was to provide evidence for driving restrictions based on real-world incidences of shocks (appropriate and inappropriate).

Methods and Results.—A total of 2786 primary and secondary prevention ICD patients were included. The occurrence of shocks was noted during a median follow-up of 996 days (inter-quartile range, 428–1833 days). With the risk of harm (RH) formula, using the incidence of sudden cardiac incapacitation, the annual RH to others posed by a driver with an ICD was calculated. Based on Canadian data, the annual RH to others of 5 in 100 000 (0.005) was used as a cut-off value. In both primary and secondary prevention ICD patients with private driving habits, no restrictions to drive directly following implantation, or an inappropriate shock are warranted. However, following an appropriate shock, these patients are at an increased risk to cause harm to other road users and therefore should be restricted to drive for a period of 2 and 4 months, respectively. In addition, all ICD patients with professional driving habits have a substantial elevated risk to cause harm to other road users during the complete follow-up after both implantation and shock and should therefore be restricted to drive permanently.

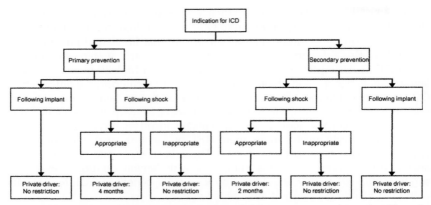

FIGURE 5.—Flowchart demonstrating the recommended driving restrictions for implantable cardioverter defibrillator patients with private driving habits. Based on the current analysis, implantable cardioverter defibrillator patients with professional driving habits should be restricted to drive in all circumstances and therefore are not in the figure. (Reprinted from Thijssen J, Borleffs CJW, van Rees JB, et al. Driving restrictions after implantable cardioverter defibrillator implantation: an evidence-based approach. *Eur Heart J.* 2011;32:2678-2687, by permission of The European Society of Cardiology.)

Conclusion.—The current analysis provides a clinically applicable tool for guideline committees to establish evidence-based driving restrictions (Fig 5).

▶ Guidelines are lacking for driving motor vehicles following implantable cardioverter defibrillator (ICD) placement. This study included 2786 patients following ICD. The median time for follow-up in primary prevention (1718) patients was 2 years and was 4 years for secondary prevention (1068) patients. A risk of harm formula was used based on Canadian data to try to determine whether restrictions for driving should be obtained for appropriate and inappropriate shocks. Only first and second shocks were used in the data. Assessment of risk of harm was developed from a formula to quantify the risk of people driving with ICDs based on the Canadian Cardiovascular Society Consensus Conference. It was assumed that 31% of the patients may experience syncope or near syncope during an appropriate shock. The assumption was that inappropriate shocks had the same instance of syncope and would overestimate the need to limit driving in this population, but they did not. The true incidence of syncope while driving is unknown. It is assumed that injury to others at ≤ 5 in 100 000 would be acceptable to allow people to drive. By using risk assessment guidance, the group developed (Fig 5) a flow chart to determine when driving restrictions should be applied. As expected, those with primary prevention had fewer initial shocks (10%) than those in secondary prevention (17%). Surprisingly, the mean time for initial shock in primary prevention was shorter (417 days) than for secondary prevention patients (509 days). An earlier resumption of driving for secondary prevention would be indicated by this study. The limitations of this study are the changes in device therapy since 1996, lack of antitachycardia pacing therapy, and the assumption of true syncope or near syncope as a percentage of both appropriate and inappropriate shocks. Nevertheless, this study comes to a reasonable mathematical conclusion on these observational data (Fig 5) and adds important data to formulate future guidelines for driving.

B. Leman, MD

Colchicine Reduces Postoperative Atrial Fibrillation: Results of the Colchicine for the Prevention of the Postpericardiotomy Syndrome (COPPS) Atrial Fibrillation Substudy
Imazio M, for the COPPS Investigators (Maria Vittoria Hosp, Torino, Italy; et al)
Circulation 124:2290-2295, 2011

Background.—Inflammation and pericarditis may be contributing factors for postoperative atrial fibrillation (POAF), and both are potentially affected by antiinflammatory drugs and colchicine, which has been shown to be safe and efficacious for the prevention of pericarditis and the postpericardiotomy syndrome (PPS). The aim of the Colchicine for the Prevention of the Post-Pericardiotomy Syndrome (COPPS) POAF substudy was to test the efficacy and safety of colchicine for the prevention of POAF after cardiac surgery.

Methods and Results.—The COPPS POAF substudy included 336 patients (mean age, 65.7 ± 12.3 years; 69% male) of the COPPS trial, a multicenter, double-blind, randomized trial. Substudy patients were in sinus rhythm before starting the intervention (placebo/colchicine 1.0 mg twice daily starting on postoperative day 3 followed by a maintenance dose of 0.5 mg twice daily for 1 month in patients ≥ 70 kg, halved doses for patients < 70 kg or intolerant to the highest dose). The substudy primary end point was the incidence of POAF on intervention at 1 month. Despite well-balanced baseline characteristics, patients on colchicine had a reduced incidence of POAF (12.0% versus 22.0%, respectively; $P = 0.021$; relative risk reduction, 45%; number needed to treat, 11) with a shorter in-hospital stay (9.4 ± 3.7 versus 10.3 ± 4.3 days; $P = 0.040$) and rehabilitation stay (12.1 ± 6.1 versus 13.9 ± 6.5 days; $P = 0.009$). Side effects were similar in the study groups.

Conclusion.—Colchicine seems safe and efficacious in the reduction of POAF with the potentiality of halving the complication and reducing the hospital stay.

Clinical Trial Registration.—URL: http://www.clinicaltrials.gov. Unique identifier: NCT00128427 (Fig 2).

▶ Atrial fibrillation (AF) is very common following cardiac surgery. In contrast to AF in the general population, which is typically due to enhanced automaticity from the pulmonary veins, postoperative AF is more commonly associated with inflammation. Accordingly, this study was part of a prospective, multicenter, randomized trial of colchicine following cardiac surgery in 6 Italian centers. The authors show that colchicine was well tolerated and associated with about a 45% relative reduction in postoperative AF (Fig 2). Hospitalization

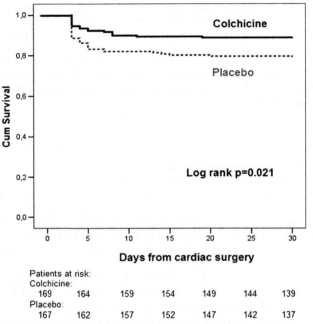

FIGURE 2.—Kaplan-Meier postoperative atrial fibrillation—free survival after postoperative day 3 according to treatment groups. Intervention with placebo/colchicine was started on postoperative day 3. (Reprinted from Imazio M, for the COPPS Investigators, Colchicine reduces postoperative atrial fibrillation: results of the Colchicine for the Prevention of the Postpericardiotomy Syndrome (COPPS) atrial fibrillation substudy. *Circulation*. 2011;124:2290-2295. © American Heart Association, Inc.)

was also shortened in the colchicine group, although hospital durations were long in both groups compared with US standards. Beta-blockers are well documented to reduce postoperative AF and were underused in this trial. However, colchicine remains an independent predictor of AF of similar magnitude to β-blockers. These findings indicate that colchicine may be a safe and important additional agent to reduce postoperative AF. Further study is needed to confirm these results and to identify the role of colchicine in combination with other pharmacologic agents in this population.

M. R. Gold, MD, PhD

35 Cardiac Surgery

2011 ACCF/AHA guideline for coronary artery bypass graft surgery: Executive summary: A report of the American College of Cardiology Foundation/American Heart Association Task Force on Practice Guidelines
Hillis LD, Smith PK, Anderson JL, et al
J Thorac Cardiovasc Surg 143:4-34, 2012

Background.—Guidelines were developed by the American College of Cardiology Foundation/American Heart Association Task Force on Practice Guidelines regarding the use of coronary artery bypass graft (CABG) surgery. These were designed to provide for the safe, appropriate, and efficacious performance of CABG. Included were procedural areas, coronary artery disease (CAD) revascularization, perioperative management, CABG-associated morbidity and mortality, and treatment of special patient subsets.

Procedural Issues.—Anesthetic management is directed at early postoperative extubation and accelerated recovery for patients at low to medium risk who are having uncomplicated CABG. Volatile anesthetic-based regimens are useful, but high thoracic epidural anesthesia/analgesia is not well supported. Cyclooxygenase-2 inhibitors are not recommended for pain relief postoperatively.

The left internal mammary artery is preferred for bypass of the left anterior descending artery when required. Other options for bypass grafting include the right internal mammary artery and a second internal mammary artery to graft the left circumflex or right coronary artery. Complete arterial revascularization may help in patients age 60 years or younger with few or no comorbidities. With critical stenosis, a right coronary artery or radial artery graft may be needed.

When acute, persistent, and life-threatening hemodynamic disturbances do not respond to treatment and when valvular surgery is done concomitantly, intraoperative transesophageal echocardiography is indicated. This helps to monitor hemodynamic status, ventricular function, regional wall motion, and valvular function. To reduce the risk of perioperative myocardial ischemia and infarction, the determinants of coronary arterial perfusion should optimized. However, prophylactic pharmacologic therapies or controlled reperfusion strategies as well as postconditioning strategies have uncertain value. Mechanical preconditioning may reduce the risk of myocardial ischemia and infarction in patients having off-pump CABG. Remote ischemic preconditioning strategies (peripheral extremity occlusion/reperfusion) may attenuate the adverse effects of myocardial reperfusion injury. Specific recommendations vary with clinical status.

CAD Revascularization.—Revascularization is done in patients with CAD to relieve symptoms and improve survival. A Heart Team approach is recommended for patients with unprotected left main or complex CAD. Patients with significant left main coronary artery stenosis should undergo CABG. Selected stable patients with significant unprotected left main CAD and anatomic and clinical characteristics predicting a significantly higher risk of adverse surgical outcomes and those who have unstable acute ST-elevation myocardial infarction (UA/STEMI) can be managed by percutaneous coronary intervention (PCI). Either CABG or PCI is useful in patients with one or more significant coronary artery stenoses amenable to revascularization and unacceptable angina unresponsive to guideline-directed medical therapy (GDMT). Certain conditions are best approached using hybrid coronary revascularization procedures.

Perioperative Management.—Preoperative antiplatelet therapy with aspirin is used for all CABG patients. Patients having elective CABG must discontinue clopidogrel and ticagrelor at least 5 days preoperatively and prasugrel at least 7 days preoperatively. In urgent CABG, clopidogrel and ticagrelor should be suspended for at least 24 hours before surgery. Short-acting intravenous glycoprotein inhibitors should be discontinued at least 2 to 4 hours preoperatively. Aspirin is initiated within 6 hours of surgery and continued indefinitely. Clopidogrel can be given to patients intolerant of or allergic to aspirin.

All patients having CABG should receive statin therapy unless contraindicated. The statin dose should reduce low-density lipoprotein (LDL) cholesterol to less than 100 mg/dL and lower LDL cholesterol by at least 30%. Very high-risk patients should receive statins to lower LDL cholesterol to less than 70 mg/dL. For urgent or emergency CABG in patients not taking statins, high-dose statin therapy is initiated immediately.

Intravenous insulin is administered continuously to achieve and maintain an early postoperative blood glucose concentration of 180 mg/dL or less. Women undergoing CABG should not be receiving postmenopausal hormone therapy. Beta blockers are given to all patients (unless contraindicated) for at least 24 hours before CABG and continued postoperatively. Similar guidelines apply to angiotensin-converting enzyme inhibitors and angiotensin-receptor blockers.

All smokers should be given in-hospital counseling and offered smoking cessation therapy during their stay. Patients with depression should also receive cognitive behavioral therapy or collaborative care. In addition, all eligible patients should undergo cardiac rehabilitation after CABG. Perioperatively patients have central nervous system monitoring, electrocardiographic monitoring, and pulmonary artery catheter placement.

CABG-Associated Morbidity and Mortality.—Epiaortic ultrasound imaging allows assessment of the presence, location, and severity of plaque in the ascending aorta, reducing the incidence of atheroembolic complications. Patients with clinically significant carotid artery disease should be managed via a multidisciplinary team approach. Possible approaches include carotid artery duplex scanning and carotid revascularization in conjunction with CABG.

All patients should receive prophylactic antibiotics preoperatively, usually a first- or second-generation cephalosporin for patients without methicillin-resistant *Staphylococcus aureus* colonization and vancomycin alone or with other antibiotics to cover patients with proved or suspected methicillin-resistant *S aureus* colonization. Leukocyte-filtered blood is recommended for all transfusions.

Patients with preexisting renal dysfunction may benefit from off-pump CABG. Perioperative hematocrit is maintained over 19% and mean arterial pressure over 60 mm Hg. Surgery may be delayed after coronary angiography to assess the effect of contrast material on the kidney.

Patients at high risk for myocardial dysfunction perioperatively can be managed by inserting an intra-aortic balloon. Biomarkers of myonecrosis are monitored for the first 24 hours after CABG. Blood conservation measures are advised.

Special Patients.—Some patients need special handling. Included are those with anomalous coronary arteries, chronic obstructive pulmonary disease and/or respiratory insufficiency, end-stage renal disease who are undergoing dialysis, concomitant valvular disease, and previous cardiac surgery.

Conclusions.—The practice guidelines are designed to help healthcare providers make clinical decisions by providing generally acceptable approaches to the diagnosis, management, and prevention of specific diseases or conditions. The practices described meet the needs of most patients in most situations. Ultimately, however, the care of a specific patient will be determined by the health care provider and patient considering all the circumstances present.

▶ This latest report from American College of Cardiology (ACC) and American Heart Association (AHA) task force on clinical guidelines for management of coronary artery disease (CAD) includes strong participation from the Society of Thoracic Surgeons (STS) and American Association for Thoracic Surgery (AATS). Of note, the Society of Cardiovascular Anesthesiologists also participated in the task force. These comprehensive guidelines cover a broad range of issues related to CAD, from preoperative assessment, intraoperative management, and options of management, to postoperative care, as well as measurement of outcomes. This document is a must-read for those participating in the treatment of patients with coronary disease. One key area of focus is the emphasis on development of the "heart team approach" to revascularization decisions. The task force recognizes the current assessment, management, and treatment of CAD predominantly by cardiology is suboptimal and encourages increased collaboration between cardiology and cardiac surgery. The development of these heart teams will likely improve quality of care for cardiac patients. Another noteworthy contribution of this report is its stance that hybrid revascularization is reasonable if there are poor targets for coronary artery bypass graft, lack of suitable grafts, or unfavorable left anterior descending artery for percutaneous coronary intervention. These guidelines are the product of an effort by a large task force after thorough review of the literature, current methodology, and techniques. As such, they form the cornerstone for effective medical practice.

S. R. Neravetla, MD

V. H. Thourani, MD

Coronary-Artery Bypass Surgery in Patients with Left Ventricular Dysfunction

Velazquez EJ, for the STICH Investigators (Duke Univ Med Ctr, Durham, NC; et al)
N Engl J Med 364:1607-1616, 2011

Background.—The role of coronary-artery bypass grafting (CABG) in the treatment of patients with coronary artery disease and heart failure has not been clearly established.

Methods.—Between July 2002 and May 2007, a total of 1212 patients with an ejection fraction of 35% or less and coronary artery disease amenable to CABG were randomly assigned to medical therapy alone (602 patients) or medical therapy plus CABG (610 patients). The primary outcome was the rate of death from any cause. Major secondary outcomes included the rates of death from cardiovascular causes and of death from any cause or hospitalization for cardiovascular causes.

Results.—The primary outcome occurred in 244 patients (41%) in the medical-therapy group and 218 (36%) in the CABG group (hazard ratio with CABG, 0.86; 95% confidence interval [CI], 0.72 to 1.04; $P = 0.12$). A total of 201 patients (33%) in the medicaltherapy group and 168 (28%) in the CABG group died from an adjudicated cardiovascular cause (hazard ratio with CABG, 0.81; 95% CI, 0.66 to 1.00; $P = 0.05$). Death from any cause or hospitalization for cardiovascular causes occurred in 411 patients (68%) in the medical-therapy group and 351 (58%) in the CABG group (hazard ratio with CABG, 0.74; 95% CI, 0.64 to 0.85; $P < 0.001$). By the end of the followup period (median, 56 months), 100 patients in the medical-therapy group (17%) underwent CABG, and 555 patients in the CABG group (91%) underwent CABG.

Conclusions.—In this randomized trial, there was no significant difference between medical therapy alone and medical therapy plus CABG with respect to the primary end point of death from any cause. Patients assigned to CABG, as compared with those assigned to medical therapy alone, had lower rates of death from cardiovascular causes and of death from any cause or hospitalization for cardiovascular causes. (Funded by the National Heart, Lung, and Blood Institute and Abbott Laboratories; STICH ClinicalTrials.gov number, NCT00023595.)

▶ The role of coronary artery bypass grafting (CABG) in patients with coronary artery disease and heart failure remains unclear. This particular portion of the

Surgical Treatment for Ischemic Heart Failure (STICH) trial reports the results of medical therapy plus CABG versus medical therapy alone in patients with left ventricular systolic dysfunction. This was an international, multicenter, randomized study across 127 clinical sites. Because of enrollment difficulty, the study design was modified by increasing follow-up time to allow smaller enrollment. Overall, 1212 patients were enrolled in this arm of the study. Six hundred ten patients were assigned to CABG and 602 patients were assigned to medical therapy alone. One hundred patients (17%) of the medical therapy group underwent CABG before the end of the follow-up. Although not statistically significant, overall mortality in the medical therapy group was 41% and 36% in the CABG group. With as-treated analysis, the hazard ratio of the CABG arm was 0.70 ($P < .001$). Patients in the medical therapy alone arm did have statistically significant higher rates of cardiovascular deaths and death from any cause or hospitalization for cardiovascular cause. It is not surprising to note that early deaths were higher in the surgical arm. After the first 2 years, however, survival in the surgical arm improved, and the question arises whether the surgical therapy group would have had statistically significant all-cause mortality reduction if the study had continued longer. This was a large study that attempted to elucidate a complex disease. Other reports from the STICH trial expound further on the algorithm for coronary artery disease and heart failure, including defining the impact of myocardial viability on treatment outcomes. Further studies will need to be performed to more definitely define the role of CABG in patients with heart failure. However, long-term follow-up will have to be a critical component of this study, because these data appear to show an increasing trend in benefit of CABG with time.

S. R. Neravetla, MD
V. H. Thourani, MD

Bypass Versus Drug-Eluting Stents at Three Years in SYNTAX Patients With Diabetes Mellitus or Metabolic Syndrome

Mack MJ, Banning AP, Serruys PW, et al (Heart Hosp Baylor Plano, Dallas, TX; John Radcliffe Hosp, Oxford, UK; Erasmus Univ Med Ctr Rotterdam, The Netherlands; et al)

Ann Thorac Surg 92:2140-2146, 2011

Background.—Diabetes mellitus increases adverse outcomes after coronary revascularization; however, the impact of metabolic syndrome is unclear. We examined the impact of diabetes and metabolic syndrome on coronary artery bypass graft surgery (CABG) and stenting outcomes to determine the optimal revascularization option for the treatment of complex coronary artery disease.

Methods.—Patients (n = 1,800) with left main or three-vessel disease or both were randomly allocated to treatment with a TAXUS Express[2] paclitaxel-eluting stent (PES) or CABG, and were included in predefined nondiabetic (n = 1,348) or diabetic subgroups (n = 452); 258 patients with diabetes also had metabolic syndrome.

Results.—Among diabetic patients, the 3-year major adverse cardiac and cerebrovascular event (MACCE) rate (22.9% CABG, 37.0% PES; $p = 0.002$) and revascularization rate (12.9% CABG, 28.0% PES; $p < 0.001$) were higher after PES treatment. Diabetes increased MACCE rates among PES-treated patients, but had little impact on results after CABG. Compared with CABG, PES treatment yielded comparable MACCE in diabetic patients (30.5% versus 29.8%, $p = 0.98$) and nondiabetic patients (20.2% versus 20.3%, $p = 0.99$) with low Synergy Between Percutaneous Coronary Intervention With Taxus and Cardiac Surgery (SYNTAX) study scores of 22 or less. For patients with SYNTAX Scores of 33 or greater, MACCE rates were lower with CABG (18.5% versus 45.9%, $p < 0.001$ diabetic; 19.8% versus 30.0%, $p = 0.01$ nondiabetic). Metabolic syndrome did not significantly predict MACCE or repeat revascularization.

Conclusions.—These exploratory analyses suggest that among diabetic patients with complex left main or three-vessel disease, or both, 3-year MACCE is higher after PES compared with CABG. Although PES is a potential treatment option in patients with less complex lesions, CABG should be the revascularization option of choice for patients with more complex anatomic disease, especially with concurrent diabetes. Metabolic syndrome had little impact on 3-year outcomes.

▶ The World Health Organization definition of metabolic syndrome is the presence of diabetes and any 2 of the following: hypertension, central obesity (body mass index > 30 kg/m^2), dyslipidemia, or microalbuminuria. The impact of diabetes mellitus as a significant risk factor for cardiovascular disease and its deleterious effects following both coronary artery bypass grafting (CABG) and percutaneous coronary interventions (PCI) have been well documented and studied. However, the effects of metabolic syndrome in relation to coronary artery disease are still not fully understood. This interval analysis (3 years) of subgroups of the SYNTAX trial patients evaluates the outcomes of CABG versus paclitaxel drug-eluting stent (PES) in patients with or without diabetes and patients with metabolic syndrome. The goal of this study and the SYNTAX trial is to guide in the optimal strategy, CABG versus PES, for patients with cardiovascular disease in a prospective, randomized fashion. According to the results, diabetic patients had worse major adverse cardiac and cerebrovascular events (MACCE) and repeat revascularization rates following PES. In patients with less complex coronary artery disease, both with or without diabetes, PCI is a potential treatment option. However, CABG was shown to be the treatment of choice for patients with complex coronary disease and in patients with diabetes. This analysis failed to show a significant effect of metabolic syndrome in this set of patients in relation to MACCE or repeat revascularization. A limitation of this study was that it was a post-hoc analysis of patients with metabolic syndrome in the SYNTAX trial. Future studies need to be focused on the evaluation of metabolic syndrome and cardiovascular disease, specifically. The 5-year results and eventual completion of the SYNTAX trial will greatly help in the guidance of the best treatment options of patients with cardiovascular disease.

A. R. Khan, MD

V. H. Thourani, MD

Changing outcomes in patients bridged to heart transplantation with continuous- versus pulsatile-flow ventricular assist devices: An analysis of the registry of the International Society for Heart and Lung Transplantation
Nativi JN, Drakos SG, Kucheryavaya AY, et al (Univ of Utah, Salt Lake City; International Society for Heart and Lung Transplantation, Addison, TX; et al)
J Heart Lung Transplant 30:854-861, 2011

Background.—Patients bridged to heart transplantation with left ventricular assist devices (LVADs) have been reported to have higher post-transplant mortality compared with those without LVADs. Our aim was to determine the impact of the type of LVAD and implant era on post-transplant survival.

Methods.—In this study we included 8,557 patients from the registry of the International Society for Heart and Lung Transplantation. We examined post-transplant outcomes in 1,100 patients bridged to transplant with pulsatile-flow LVADs between January 2000 and June 2004 (first era), 880 patients bridged with pulsatile-flow LVADs between July 2004 and May 2008 (second era), and 417 patients bridged with continuous-flow LVADs in the second era. Patients who required intravenous inotropes but not LVAD support ($n = 2,728$) and patients who did not require either LVAD or inotropes ($n = 3,432$) served as controls.

Results.—Post-transplant survival of patients bridged with pulsatile LVADs improved significantly between the first and the second era ($p = 0.03$). In the second era, there was no significant difference in post-transplant survival of patients bridged with pulsatile- vs continuous-flow LVADs ($p = 0.26$), and survival rates in the 2 groups were not statistically different from that of the non-LVAD group. Graft rejection was similar in patients bridged with LVADs compared to those without LVADs.

Conclusions.—In the most recent era, the use of either pulsatile- or continuous-flow LVADs did not result in increased post-transplant mortality. This finding is important as the proportion of patients with LVADs at the time of transplant has been rising.

▶ The advent of continuous flow, left ventricular assist devices (LVADs) has led to a paradigm shift in the management of end-stage heart failure. The efficacy of newer, more efficient nonpulsatile LVADs as a bridge to transplant (BTT) is assessed in this article by analyzing the outcome data from registry of the International Society for Heart and Lung Transplant (ISHLT). This article addresses the concern for negative outcomes from the current trend toward using LVADs. In the ISHLT database, 880 patients received pulsatile-flow LVADs at the same time period that 417 patients received LVADs as a bridge to transplant.

A number of different devices were used at multiple transplant centers around the world, although Heartmate II was used most commonly. The demographic data, preoperative status, and overall posttransplant outcomes were also compared with patients who did not receive any LVAD before transplant. It is encouraging to find that the overall outcomes for all heart transplant patients who were bridged with LVADs have significantly improved. In the recent group of patients with the pulsatile LVADs, about 68%were not hospitalized before being placed on LVAD compared with only 37% before 2004. This likely reflects better understanding and management of patients before and after heart transplant. Of note, this data analysis shows the use of pulsatile or nonpulsatile LVADs as a bridge to heart transplant had equally good outcomes across multiple institutions worldwide. This is in contrast to prior data from 2000 to 2004, which showed an increased risk of mortality after transplant following BTT. BTT patients did have a higher rate of renal failure compared with non-LVAD transplant patients. One interesting finding was an increased level in allosensitization in pulsatile-versus continuous-flow LVAD patients, although this was not associated with increase in rejection. Although allosensitization is thought to impact long-term survival, it is unclear based on this study if this is a clinically significant difference. This large registry review shows promising results for BTT, which would encourage more widespread use of LVADs, especially the newer-generation continuous-flow LVADs.

S. R. Neravetla, MD
V. H. Thourani, MD

36 Coronary Heart Disease

Acute coronary syndrome and cocaine use: 8-year prevalence and inhospital outcomes
Carrillo X, Curós A, Muga R, et al (Hospital Universitari Germans Trias i Pujol, Badalona, Spain)
Eur Heart J 32:1244-1250, 2011

Aims.—The use of cocaine as a recreational drug has increased in recent years. The aims of this study were to analyse the prevalence and inhospital evolution of acute coronary syndrome (ACS) associated with cocaine consumption (ACS-ACC).

Methods and Results.—Prospective analysis of ACS patients admitted to a coronary care unit from January 2001 to December 2008. During the study period, 2752 patients were admitted for ACS, and among these 479 were ≤50 years of age. Fifty-six (11.7%) patients had a medical history of cocaine use with an increase in prevalence from 6.8% in 2001 to 21.7% in 2008 ($P = 0.035$). Among patients younger than 30 years of age, 25% admitted to being users compared with 5.5% of those aged 45−50 years ($P = 0.007$). Similarly, the prevalence of positive urine tests for cocaine was four times higher in the younger patients (18.2 vs. 4.1%, $P = 0.035$). Acute coronary syndrome associated with cocaine consumption patients ($n = 24$; those who had a positive urine test for cocaine or who admitted to being users upon admission) had larger myocardial infarcts as indicated by troponin I levels (52.9 vs. 23.4 ng/mL, $P < 0.001$), lower left ventricular ejection fraction (44.5 vs. 52.2%, $P = 0.049$), and increased inhospital mortality (8.3 vs. 0.8%, $P = 0.030$).

Conclusions.—The association between cocaine use and ACS has increased significantly over the past few years. Young adults with ACS-ACC that require admission to the coronary care unit have greater myocardial damage and more frequent complications (Figs 1 and 2).

▶ This is an unusual study confined to patients younger than 50 years with acute coronary syndromes from the University Hospital in Barcelona. The authors analyze the prevalence of cocaine use in patients admitted with acute coronary syndromes and the impact of this on the natural history. Cocaine is said to cause more cardiovascular complications than any other illegal drug, including arterial hypertension, aortic dissection, arrhythmias, acute pulmonary

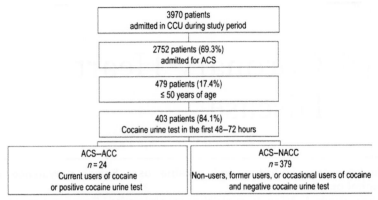

FIGURE 1.—Patients admitted to the coronary care unit between 1 January 2001 and 31 December 2008. ACS-ACC, acute coronary syndrome associated with cocaine consumption; ACS-NACC, acute coronary syndrome not associated with cocaine consumption. (Reprinted from Carrillo X, Curós A, Muga R, et al, Acute coronary syndrome and cocaine use: 8-year prevalence and inhospital outcomes. *Eur Heart J.* 2011;32:1244-1250, by permission of The European Society of Cardiology.)

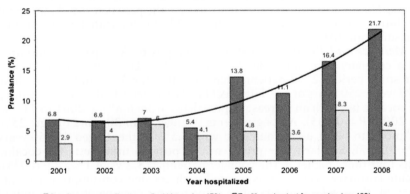

FIGURE 2.—Annual prevalence of cocaine use according to patient history and urine test for cocaine. (Reprinted from Carrillo X, Curós A, Muga R, et al, Acute coronary syndrome and cocaine use: 8-year prevalence and inhospital outcomes. *Eur Heart J.* 2011;32:1244-1250, by permission of The European Society of Cardiology.)

edema, coronary vasospasm, cardiomyopathy, and sudden cardiac death.[1] An association between cocaine and acute coronary syndromes was first documented in the early 1980s and then in a large series in the 1990s.[2]

Among patients younger than 50 years 11.7% had a medical history of cocaine use. As expected, the prevalence of a history of cocaine use increased steadily between 2001 and 2008 from 6.8% to an alarming 21.7%. What is also notable but not surprising is the young age of the patients, and in patients under the age of 45 years, cocaine use ranged from 17.3% (age 40–44 years) to 25% in those younger than 30 years. Mortality and infarct size were greater in cocaine users, and left ventricular ejection fraction was lower. Moreover, the impact on mortality was huge (8.3% in cocaine users vs 0.8% among nonusers). The marked adverse prognosis is particularly disturbing given the young age of the patients. Interestingly, acute coronary syndromes occurred among both acute and chronic cocaine users, and the prevalence of 2- and 3-vessel disease was significantly higher among cocaine users.

The explanation for these adverse outcomes is multifactorial and might reflect a lack of prior beta-blocker use, adrenergic hyperactivity secondary to cocaine leading to increased myocardial oxygen demands, and perhaps concomitant vasospasm or vasoconstriction. In addition, cocaine users had more Q-wave myocardial infarctions and a greater proportion of multivessel disease. These data certainly reinforce the need for a physician to take a specific medical history with regard to cocaine use and to use urine testing, particularly in younger patients with acute coronary syndromes. I suspect that these data also reinforce the need for beta-blockers, and although there is no evidence to support this, there are data to suggest a hyperadrenergic state in cocaine users, which might interfere with them.

B. J. Gersh, MB, ChB, DPhil, FRCP

References

1. Lange RA, Hillis LD. Cardiovascular complications of cocaine use. *New Engl J Med*. 2001;345:351-358.
2. Mittleman MA, Mintzer D, Maclure M, Tofler GH, Sherwood JB, Muller JE. Triggering of myocardial infarction by cocaine. *Circulation*. 1999;99:2737-2741.

Association Between Adoption of Evidence-Based Treatment and Survival for Patients With ST-Elevation Myocardial Infarction
Jernberg T, for SWEDEHEART/RIKS-HIA (Karolinska Univ Hosp, Stockholm, Sweden; et al)
JAMA 305:1677-1684, 2011

Context.—Only limited information is available on the speed of implementation of new evidence-based and guideline-recommended treatments and its association with survival in real life health care of patients with ST-elevation myocardial infarction (STEMI).

Objective.—To describe the adoption of new treatments and the related chances of short- and long-term survival in consecutive patients with STEMI in a single country over a 12-year period.

Design, Setting, and Participants.—The Register of Information and Knowledge about Swedish Heart Intensive Care Admission (RIKS-HIA) records baseline characteristics, treatments, and outcome of consecutive patients with acute coronary syndrome admitted to almost all hospitals in Sweden. This study includes 61 238 patients with a first-time diagnosis of STEMI between 1996 and 2007.

Main Outcome Measures.—Estimated and crude proportions of patients treated with different medications and invasive procedures and mortality over time.

Results.—Of evidence based-treatments, reperfusion increased from 66% (95%, confidence interval [CI], 52%-79%) to 79% (95% CI, 69%-89%; $P < .001$), primary percutaneous coronary intervention from 12% (95% CI, 11%-14%) to 61% (95% CI, 45%-77%; $P < .001$), and revascularization from 10% (96% CI, 6%-14%) to 84% (95% CI, 73%-95%; $P < .001$). The use of aspirin, clopidogrel, β-blockers, statins, and angiotensin-converting enzyme (ACE) inhibitors all increased: clopidogrel from 0% to 82% (95% CI, 69%-95%; $P < .001$), statins from 23% (95% CI, 12%-33%) to 83% (95% CI, 75%-91%; $P < .001$), and ACE inhibitor or angiotensin II receptor blockers from 39% (95% CI, 26%-52%) to 69% (95% CI, 58%-70%; $P < .001$). The estimated in-hospital, 30-day and 1-year mortality decreased from 12.5% (95% CI, 4.3%-20.6%) to 7.2% (95% CI, 1.7%-12.6%; $P < .001$); from 15.0% (95% CI, 6.2%-23.7%) to 8.6% (95% CI, 2.7%-14.5%; $P < .001$); and from 21.0% (95% CI, 11.0%-30.9%) to 13.3% (95% CI, 6.0%-20.4%; $P < .001$), respectively. After adjustment, there was still a consistent trend with lower standardized mortality over the years. The 12-year survival analyses showed that the decrease of mortality was sustained over time.

Conclusion.—In a Swedish registry of patients with STEMI, between 1996 and 2007, there was an increase in the prevalence of evidence-based treatments. During this same time, there was a decrease in 30-day and 1-year mortality that was sustained during long-term follow-up.

▶ The results of this national registry from Sweden, which includes all 72 hospitals that provide care for patients with acute cardiac diseases, are indeed gratifying. This analysis was confined to the 61 238 patients with ST-elevation myocardial infarction (STEMI), and the strength of the study is the inclusion of every STEMI patient in the whole of Sweden for 10 years and the fact that most patients were included for an additional 2 years. This virtually eliminates selection bias; follow-up was also complete.

Over the last 12 years there has been a steady increase in the use of evidence-based pharmacologic therapies, an increase in the proportion of patients receiving reperfusion therapy, and a marked switch from fibrinolysis to primary percutaneous coronary intervention. At the same time, there has been a marked reduction in both early and late mortality, and it would appear that this trend is continuing. This appears to be a great example of translating the results of clinical trials into evidence-based clinical practice.

Notably, however, there was a wide variation between hospitals as to how quickly new therapies based on guidelines and evidence were implemented into the clinical protocols, and in many centers the adoption of these treatments was slow and gradual. This is one area amenable to a quality improvement initiative that apparently is already an ongoing process in Sweden.

An accompanying editorial does point out that data do not definitively confirm a cause-and-effect relationship between new therapies and the decline in mortality.[1] Nonetheless, the results certainly suggest a strong association and at a minimum confirm that guideline-based treatment works. What is also encouraging is to see the efficacy outcomes of clinical trials reflected in clinical practice.

B. J. Gersh, MB, ChB, DPhil, FRCP

Reference

1. Mukherjee D. Implementation of evidence-based therapies for myocardial infarction and survival. *JAMA*. 2011;305:1710-1711.

Association of Door-In to Door-Out Time With Reperfusion Delays and Outcomes Among Patients Transferred for Primary Percutaneous Coronary Intervention

Wang TY, Nallamothu BK, Krumholz HM, et al (Duke Univ Med Ctr, Durham, NC; Univ of Michigan Med School, Ann Arbor; Yale Univ School of Medicine and Yale—New Haven Hosp Ctr for Outcomes Res and Evaluation, CT; et al)
JAMA 305:2540-2547, 2011

Context.—Patients with ST-elevation myocardial infarction (STEMI) requiring interhospital transfer for primary percutaneous coronary intervention (PCI) often have prolonged overall door-to-balloon (DTB) times from first hospital presentation to second hospital PCI. Door-in to door-out (DIDO) time, defined as the duration of time from arrival to discharge at the first or STEMI referral hospital, is a new clinical performance measure, and a DIDO time of 30 minutes or less is recommended to expedite reperfusion care.

Objective.—To characterize time to reperfusion and patient outcomes associated with a DIDO time of 30 minutes or less.

Design, Setting, and Patients.—Retrospective cohort of 14 821 patients with STEMI transferred to 298 STEMI receiving centers for primary PCI in the ACTION Registry—Get With the Guidelines between January 2007 and March 2010.

Main Outcome Measures.—Factors associated with a DIDO time greater than 30 minutes, overall DTB times, and risk-adjusted in-hospital mortality.

Results.—Median DIDO time was 68 minutes (interquartile range, 43-120 minutes), and only 1627 patients (11%) had DIDO times of 30 minutes or less. Significant factors associated with a DIDO time greater than 30 minutes included older age, female sex, off-hours presentation, and non—emergency medical services transport to the first hospital. Patients with a DIDO time of 30 minutes or less were significantly more likely to have an overall DTB time of 90 minutes or less compared with patients with DIDO times greater than 30 minutes (60% [95% confidence interval {CI}, 57%-62%] vs 13% [95% CI, 12%-13%]; *P* < .001). Among patients with DIDO times greater than 30 minutes, only 0.6% (95% CI, 0.5%-0.8%) had an absolute contraindication to fibrinolysis. Observed in-hospital mortality was significantly higher among patients with DIDO times greater than 30 minutes vs patients with DIDO times of 30 minutes or less (5.9% [95% CI, 5.5%-6.3%] vs 2.7% [95% CI, 1.9%-3.5%]; $P < .001$; adjusted odds ratio for in-hospital mortality, 1.56 [95% CI, 1.15-2.12]).

Conclusion.—A DIDO time of 30 minutes or less was observed in only a small proportion of patients transferred for primary PCI but was associated with shorter reperfusion delays and lower in-hospital mortality.

▶ It is generally accepted that primary percutaneous coronary intervention (PPCI) is the optimal method of reperfusion therapy, but 75% of US hospitals do not have acute PCI capability and, as such, need to transfer patients to a PCI center when logistically feasible. The processes involved in transfer are a potential Achilles heel, and several studies have documented substantial delays both in patients receiving lytics and in those transferred directly for PPCI.[1] Moreover, these delays have been associated with worse outcomes, although it is unclear whether this is directly a time-related phenomenon or a reflection of the overall standard of care.

The door-in to door-out (DIDO) measure is increasingly being recognized as an important metric that places the burden of responsibility on both the transferring and receiving hospitals. This large study makes several important points. First, only 11% of patients had DIDO times of 30 minutes or less, and factors associated with longer times were older age, female sex, off-hours presentation, and nonemergency medical services transportation to the first hospital. Moreover, a DIDO time of less than 30 minutes was associated with an overall door-to-balloon time of 90 minutes or less (the guideline recommendation for PPCI without preceding lytics). In addition, there was a statistically significant reduction in risk-adjusted in-hospital mortality in patients with a DIDO of 30 minutes or less versus greater than 30 minutes (2.7% vs 5.9% $P > .001$).

These data suggest that DIDO is important as a metric for assessing the quality of reperfusion therapy, and the data really do also show that there is ample room for improvement. We have done well in shortening door-to-balloon times, but the major advances in the delivery of reperfusion therapy will come from steps taken outside the PCI-capable hospital.

B. J. Gersh, MB, ChB, DPhil, FRCP

Reference

1. McMullan JT, Hinckley W, Bentley J, et al. Reperfusion is delayed beyond guideline recommendations in patients requiring interhospital helicopter transfer for treatment of ST-segment elevation myocardial infarction. *Ann Emerg Med.* 2011;57: 213-220.

Causes of Delay and Associated Mortality in Patients Transferred With ST-Segment—Elevation Myocardial Infarction

Miedema MD, Newell MC, Duval S, et al (Minneapolis Heart Inst Foundation at Abbott Northwestern Hosp, MN)
Circulation 124:1636-1644, 2011

Background.—Regional ST-segment—elevation myocardial infarction systems are being developed to improve timely access to primary percutaneous coronary intervention (PCI). System delays may diminish the mortality benefit achieved with primary PCI in ST-segment—elevation myocardial infarction patients, but the specific reasons for and clinical impact of delays in patients transferred for PCI are unknown.

Methods and Results.—This was a prospective, observational study of 2034 patients transferred for primary PCI at a single center as part of a regional ST-segment—elevation myocardial infarction system from March 2003 to December 2009. Despite long-distance transfers, 30.4% of patients (n = 613) were treated in ≤ 90 minutes and 65.7% (n = 1324) were treated in ≤ 120 minutes. Delays occurred most frequently at the referral hospital (64.0%, n = 1298), followed by the PCI center (15.7%, n = 317) and transport (12.6%, n = 255). For the referral hospital, the most common reasons for delay were awaiting transport (26.4%, n = 535) and emergency department delays (14.3%, n = 289). Diagnostic dilemmas (median, 95.5 minutes; 25th and 75th percentiles, 72—127 minutes) and nondiagnostic initial ECGs (81 minutes; 64—110.5 minutes) led to delays of the greatest magnitude. Delays caused by cardiac arrest and/or cardiogenic shock had the highest in-hospital mortality (30.6%), in contrast with nondiagnostic initial ECGs, which, despite long treatment delays, did not affect mortality (0%). Significant variation in both the magnitude and clinical impact of delays also occurred during the transport and PCI center segments.

Conclusions.—Treatment delays occur even in efficient systems for ST-segment—elevation myocardial infarction care. The clinical impact of specific delays in interhospital transfer for PCI varies according to the cause of the delay.

▶ The major advances in reperfusion therapy are going to be made outside the referral hospital setting. The emphasis has swung away from the specific nature of reperfusion therapy to the efficacy of its delivery, and the key to this is the establishment of regional systems or networks.[1] In this respect, one size does not fit all, and networks need to be adaptable and flexible in regard to local factors, including resources, ambulance systems, distances, climate, and the numbers and characteristics of hospitals in the area.

This prospective observational study from the state of Minnesota draws attention to the causes of delay and their effects on mortality. Approximately two-thirds of the delays occurred at the referral hospital and not the percutaneous coronary intervention (PCI) center. The most common reasons for delays at the referral hospital were awaiting transport and delays in the emergency department and other areas, and what is important is that these are all areas that are amenable to improvement. There were also significant variations in the magnitude and clinical impact of delays occurring during transport and at the PCI center. At the latter, the greatest delay was due to a diagnostic dilemma with little impact on mortality, whereas delays incurred by cardiogenic shock had the highest mortality.

This very nicely done study demonstrates opportunities for improvement in an already efficient system. Ongoing auditing and continuous quality improvement are essential components of a successful network.

B. J. Gersh, MB, ChB, DPhil, FRCP

Reference

1. Jollis JG, Roettig ML, Aluko AO, et al; Reperfusion of Acute Myocardial Infarction in North Carolina Emergency Departments (RACE) Investigators. Implementation of a statewide system for coronary reperfusion for ST-segment elevation myocardial infarction. *JAMA.* 2007;298:2371-2380.

Heparin plus a glycoprotein IIb/IIIa inhibitor versus bivalirudin monotherapy and paclitaxel-eluting stents versus bare-metal stents in acute myocardial infarction (HORIZONS-AMI): final 3-year results from a multicentre, randomised controlled trial
Stone GW, on behalf of the HORIZONS-AMI Trial Investigators (Columbia Univ Med Ctr and The Cardiovascular Res Foundation, NY; et al)
Lancet 377:2193-2204, 2011

Background.—Primary results of the HORIZONS-AMI trial have been previously reported. In this final report, we aimed to assess 3-year outcomes.

Method.—HORIZONS-AMI was a prospective, open-label, randomised trial undertaken at 123 institutions in 11 countries. Patients aged 18 years or older were eligible for enrolment if they had ST-segment elevation myocardial infarction (STEMI), presented within 12 h after onset of symptoms, and were undergoing primary percutaneous coronary intervention. By use of a computerised interactive voice response system, we randomly allocated patients 1:1 to receive bivalirudin or heparin plus a glycoprotein IIb/IIIa inhibitor (GPI; pharmacological randomisation; stratified by previous and expected drug use and study site) and, if eligible, randomly allocated 3:1 to receive a paclitaxel-eluting stent or a bare metal stent (stent randomisation; stratified by pharmacological group assignment, diabetes mellitus status, lesion length, and study site). We produced Kaplan-Meier estimates of major adverse cardiovascular events at 3 years by intention to treat. This study is registered with ClinicalTrials. gov, number NCT00433966.

Findings.—Compared with 1802 patients allocated to receive heparin plus a GPI, 1800 patients allocated to bivalirudin monotherapy had lower rates of all-cause mortality ($5 \cdot 9\%$ vs $7 \cdot 7\%$, difference $-1 \cdot 9\%$ [$-3 \cdot 5$ to $-0 \cdot 2$], HR $0 \cdot 75$ [$0 \cdot 58-0 \cdot 97$]; $p = 0 \cdot 03$), cardiac mortality ($2 \cdot 9\%$ vs $5 \cdot 1\%$, $-2 \cdot 2\%$ [$-3 \cdot 5$ to $-0 \cdot 9$], $0 \cdot 56$ [$0 \cdot 40-0 \cdot 80$]; $p = 0 \cdot 001$), reinfarction ($6 \cdot 2\%$ *vs* $8 \cdot 2\%$, $-1 \cdot 9\%$ [$-3 \cdot 7$ to $-0 \cdot 2$], $0 \cdot 76$ [$0 \cdot 59-0 \cdot 99$];

$p = 0.04$), and major bleeding not related to bypass graft surgery (6.9% *vs* 10.5%, -3.6% [-5.5 to -1.7], 0.64 [$0.51-0.80$]; $p = 0.0001$) at 3 years, with no significant differences in ischaemia-driven target vessel revascularisation, stent thrombosis, or composite adverse events. Compared with 749 patients who received a bare-metal stent, 2257 patients who received a paclitaxel-eluting stent had lower rates of ischaemia-driven target lesion revascularisation (9.4% *vs* 15.1%, -5.7% [-8.6 to -2.7], 0.60 [$0.48-0.76$]; $p < 0.0001$) after 3 years, with no significant differences in the rates of death, reinfarction, stroke or stent thrombosis. Stent thrombosis was high ($\geq4.5\%$) in both groups.

Interpretation.—The effectiveness and safety of bivalirudin monotherapy and paclitaxel-eluting stenting are sustained at 3 years for patients with STEMI undergoing primary percutaneous coronary intervention.

▶ This is the 3-year follow-up of a large multicenter trial of patients with ST-segment elevation myocardial infarction (STEMI) randomly assigned to bare-metal versus drug-eluting stents and also to bivalirudin or the combination of heparin plus a glycoprotein IIb/IIIa inhibitor.

There are 2 interesting aspects of this trial. First, the trial essentially puts to rest previously expressed concerns about late outcomes with drug-eluting stents versus bare-metal stents.[1] Late stent thrombosis did not differ between the 2 groups but was quite high at 4% to 5%. The reduction in the need for ischemia-driven target revascularization was 5.7% less with paclitaxel-eluting stents, a finding that one would expect. Nonetheless, among patients not undergoing routine angiographic follow-up, the rates of revascularization were quite low in both groups, and this is perhaps a manifestation of the fact that stenotic lesions are supplying infracted myocardium and as such not causing symptoms. From a clinical perspective, however, these data are reassuring and support the use of bare-metal stents in patients undergoing primary percutaneous coronary intervention (PCI) in the presence of discrete, short lesions, and good distal vessels, particularly when one does not have the crucial information about compliance, ability to take long-term antiplatelet agents, and knowledge about the presence of comorbidities that might require noncardiac surgery. On the other hand, the relatively high rate of late stent thrombosis in both groups opens the window for additional improved antiplatelet medications.

Bivalirudin has in other studies been associated with less bleeding, and bleeding has been identified as a powerful independent predictor of subsequent mortality in patients with acute coronary syndromes and after PCI.[2] The mechanisms underlying this association are multifactorial and certainly complex.[3] To what extent the lower early and late mortality with bivalirudin in this trial is due to a reduction in major bleeding is uncertain. Moreover, the reduction in late mortality and reinfarction after the 30-day period is also difficult to explain since the half-life of the drug and duration of its administration is short lived. The limitations of the HORIZONS trial[4] have been previously discussed, but this is a landmark study that establishes the safety of drug-eluting stents in acute STEMI and raises intriguing questions in regard to the association between bivalirudin and a reduction in mortality.

B. J. Gersh, MB, ChB, DPhil, FRCP

References

1. Kaltoft A, Kelbaek H, Thuesen L, et al. Long-term outcome after drug-eluting versus bare-metal stent implantation in patients with ST-segment elevation myocardial infarction: 3-year follow-up of the randomized DEDICATION (Drug Elution and Distal Protection in Acute Myocardial Infarction) Trial. *J Am Coll Cardiol.* 2010;56:641-645.
2. Rao SV, Jollis JG, Harrington RA, et al. Relationship of blood transfusion in clinical outcomes in patients with acute coronary syndromes. *JAMA.* 2004;292: 1555-1562.
3. Pocock SJ, Mehran R, Clayton TC, et al. Prognostic modeling of individual patient risk and mortality impact of ischemic and hemorrhagic complications: assessment from the Acute Catheterization and Urgent Intervention Triage Strategy trial. *Circulation.* 2010;121:43-51.
4. Stone GW, Witzenbichler B, Guagliumi G, et al. Bivalirudin during primary PCI in acute myocardial infarction. *N Engl J Med.* 2008;358:2218-2230.

Intramyocardial, Autologous CD34+ Cell Therapy for Refractory Angina
Losordo DW, the ACT34-CMI Investigators (Northwestern Univ, Chicago, IL; et al)
Circ Res 109:428-436, 2011

Rationale.—A growing number of patients with coronary disease have refractory angina. Preclinical and early-phase clinical data suggest that intramyocardial injection of autologous CD34+ cells can improve myocardial perfusion and function.

Objective.—Evaluate the safety and bioactivity of intramyocardial injections of autologous CD34+ cells in patients with refractory angina who have exhausted all other treatment options.

Methods and Results.—In this prospective, double-blind, randomized, phase II study (ClinicalTrials.gov identifier: NCT00300053), 167 patients with refractory angina received 1 of 2 doses (1×10^5 or 5×10^5 cells/kg) of mobilized autologous CD34+ cells or an equal volume of diluent (placebo). Treatment was distributed into 10 sites of ischemic, viable myocardium with a NOGA mapping injection catheter. The primary outcome measure was weekly angina frequency 6 months after treatment. Weekly angina frequency was significantly lower in the low-dose group than in placebo-treated patients at both 6 months (6.8 ± 1.1 versus 10.9 ± 1.2, $P = 0.020$) and 12 months (6.3 ± 1.2 versus 11.0 ± 1.2, $P = 0.035$); measurements in the high-dose group were also lower, but not significantly. Similarly, improvement in exercise tolerance was significantly greater in low-dose patients than in placebo-treated patients (6 months: 139 ± 151 versus 69 ± 122 seconds, $P = 0.014$; 12 months: 140 ± 171 versus 58 ± 146 seconds, $P = 0.017$) and greater, but not significantly, in the high-dose group. During cell mobilization and collection, 4.6% of patients had cardiac enzyme elevations consistent with non-ST segment elevation myocardial infarction. Mortality at 12 months was 5.4% in the placebo-treatment group with no deaths among cell-treated patients.

Conclusions.—Patients with refractory angina who received intramyocardial injections of autologous CD34+ cells (10^5 cells/kg) experienced significant improvements in angina frequency and exercise tolerance. The cell-mobilization and -collection procedures were associated with cardiac enzyme elevations, which will be addressed in future studies (Figs 2 and 3).

▶ This double-blind, randomized trial of autologous CD34+ cells mobilized with granulocyte colony-stimulating factor in patients with refractory angina is extremely encouraging in that there appears to be a significant improvement in symptom status and exercise duration. Moreover, the trial was double blinded. In the current era, in which late mortality from symptomatic coronary disease has declined because of revascularization, improved medical therapy, and aggressive secondary prevention, we are now faced with an expanding population of "revascularization survivors" who are severely limited by refractory angina. Current estimates are that more than 850 000 people in the United States fall into this category.[1] The therapeutic options are limited but include enhanced external counterpulsation, spinal cord stimulation, transcutaneous nerve stimulation, and, until randomized trials demonstrated that it was ineffective, transcutaneous laser myocardial revascularization. New antianginal drugs have been slow to reach the market.

This trial is based on the fact that human CD34+ hematopoietic stem cells have also been shown to have endothelial lineage potential in vitro and in vivo. Furthermore, preclinical studies have suggested that the administration of these cells may improve perfusion and ischemia, perhaps by the stimulation of neovascularization in ischemic tissue and, in particular, the microvasculature.[2] This trial not only provides data on safety and efficacy but also demonstrates that the techniques of mobilizing, collecting, purifying, and delivering the cells via an intramyocardial approach is feasible at a large number of centers and is exemplified by those who took part in the trial.

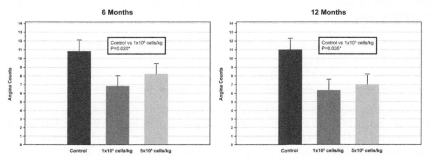

FIGURE 2.—Weekly angina incidence at 6 and 12 months. Least squares means and standard errors. *Probability values from pairwise comparisons of ratios from Poisson regression (log of baseline used as covariate). (Reprinted from Losordo DW, the ACT34-CMI Investigators. Intramyocardial, autologous CD34+ cell therapy for refractory angina. *Circ Res.* 2011;109:428-436. © American Heart Association, Inc.)

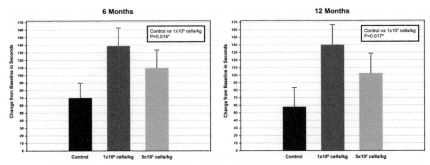

FIGURE 3.—Change in exercise time at 6 months and 12 months. Means and standard errors. *Probability values from analysis of covariance with repeated measures (baseline value used as covariate). (Reprinted from Losordo DW, the ACT34-CMI Investigators. Intramyocardial, autologous CD34+ cell therapy for refractory angina. *Circ Res.* 2011;109:428-436. © American Heart Association, Inc.)

What is a little puzzling about the data is the apparent decline in efficacy in the higher dose subgroup, but as pointed out by the authors, there is an extensive body of literature suggesting that the response to biological manipulation of angiogenesis may be biphasic.[3] The next step is a larger phase 3 clinical trial, but the data from this trial are certainly very encouraging.

B. J. Gersh, MB, ChB, DPhil, FRCP

References

1. Mannheimer C, Camici P, Chester MR, et al. The problem of chronic refractory angina: report from the esc joint study group on the treatment of refractory angina. *Eur Heart J.* 2002;23:355-370.
2. Kawamoto A, Iwasaki H, Kusano K, et al. CD34-positive cells exhibit increased potency and safety for therapeutic neovascularization after myocardial infarction compared with total mononuclear cells. *Circulation.* 2006;114:2163-2169.
3. Folkman J. Angiogenesis. *Annu Rev Med.* 2006;57:1-18.

Comparison of coronary bypass surgery with drug-eluting stenting for the treatment of left main and/or three-vessel disease: 3-year follow-up of the SYNTAX trial

Kappetein AP, Feldman TE, MacK MJ, et al (Erasmus Med Centre, Rotterdam, The Netherlands; NorthShore Univ Health System, Evanston, IL; Baylor Healthcare System, Dallas, TX; et al)
Eur Heart J 32:2125-2134, 2011

Aims.—Long-term randomized comparisons of percutaneous coronary intervention (PCI) to coronary artery bypass grafting (CABG) in left main coronary (LM) disease and/or three-vessel disease (3VD) patients have been limited. This analysis compares 3-year outcomes in LM and/or 3VD patients treated with CABG or PCI with TAXUS Express stents.

Methods and Results.—SYNTAX is an 85-centre randomized clinical trial ($n = 1800$). Prospectively screened, consecutive LM and/or 3VD patients were randomized if amenable to equivalent revascularization using either technique; if not, they were entered into a registry. Patients in the randomized cohort will continue to be followed for 5 years. At 3 years, major adverse cardiac and cerebrovascular events [MACCE: death, stroke, myocardial infarction (MI), and repeat revascularization; CABG 20.2% vs. PCI 28.0%, $P < 0.001$], repeat revascularization (10.7 vs. 19.7%, $P < 0.001$), and MI (3.6 vs. 7.1%, $P = 0.002$) were elevated in the PCI arm. Rates of the composite safety endpoint (death/stroke/MI 12.0 vs. 14.1%, $P = 0.21$) and stroke alone (3.4 vs. 2.0%, $P = 0.07$) were not significantly different between treatment groups. Major adverse cardiac and cerebrovascular event rates were not significantly different between arms in the LM subgroup (22.3 vs. 26.8%, $P = 0.20$) but were higher with PCI in the 3VD subgroup (18.8 vs. 28.8%, $P < 0.001$).

Conclusions.—At 3 years, MACCE was significantly higher in PCI-compared with CABG-treated patients. In patients with less complex disease (low SYNTAX scores for 3VD or low/intermediate terciles for LM patients), PCI is an acceptable revascularization, although longer follow-up is needed to evaluate these two revascularization strategies (Figs 2 and 5).

► The SYNTAX trial is the most contemporary and largest randomized trial comparing coronary bypass surgery with drug-eluting stenting. It is confined

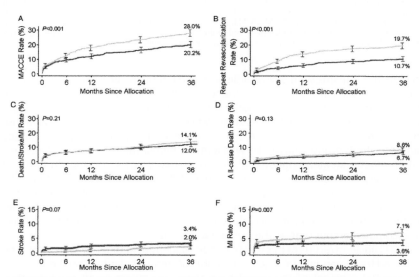

FIGURE 2.—Rates of clinical outcomes among randomized treatment groups. Time-to-event curves in patients treated with coronary artery bypass grafting (blue line) or percutaneous coronary intervention (yellow line) for the composite of major adverse cardiac and cerebrovascular events (A), repeat revascularization (B), death/stroke/myocardial infarction (C), all-cause death (D), stroke (E), and myocardial infarction (F) to 3 years. P-values from log-rank test. For interpretation of the references to color in this figure legend, the reader is referred to web version of this article. (Reprinted from Kappetein AP, Feldman TE, MacK MJ, et al. Comparison of coronary bypass surgery with drug-eluting stenting for the treatment of left main and/or three-vessel disease: 3-year follow-up of the SYNTAX trial. *Eur Heart J.* 2011;32:2125-2134, by permission of The European Society of Cardiology.)

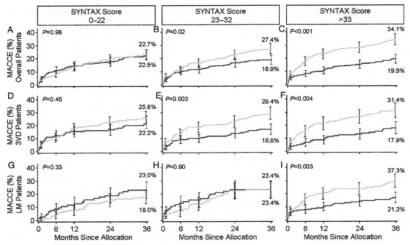

FIGURE 5.—Major adverse cardiac and cerebrovascular event rates according to the subset, treatment group, and SYNTAX score category. Time-to-event curves in the coronary artery bypass grafting (blue line) or percutaneous coronary intervention (yellow line) overall cohorts to 3 years according to the low (0–22, A), intermediate (23–32, B), or high (≥33, C) SYNTAX scores. (D–F) Major adverse cardiac and cerebrovascular events in three-vessel disease patients with low, intermediate, or high SYNTAX scores, respectively. (G–I) Major adverse cardiac and cerebrovascular events in patients with left main disease with low, intermediate, or high SYNTAX scores. P-value from log-rank test. For interpretation of the references to color in this figure legend, the reader is referred to web version of this article. (Reprinted from Kappetein AP, Feldman TE, MacK MJ, et al. Comparison of coronary bypass surgery with drug-eluting stenting for the treatment of left main and/or three-vessel disease: 3-year follow-up of the SYNTAX trial. *Eur Heart J.* 2011;32:2125-2134, by permission of The European Society of Cardiology.)

to high-risk patients with 3-vessel disease and left main coronary artery disease. The initial results at 1 year demonstrated no difference in mortality between the 2 procedures, but the risk of stroke was higher in patients undergoing coronary artery bypass grafting (CABG), and the rate of myocardial infarction was higher in the percutaneous coronary intervention (PCI) group. The major difference between the 2 groups, however, was a much higher rate of repeat revascularization among stented patients—a finding that was not surprising. In terms of the primary composite endpoint of the trial, PCI failed to show a noninferiority, but this was driven by the higher rate of repeat revascularization.[1] Not surprisingly, perceptions of the trial results vary substantially between surgeons and interventional cardiologists, which is a problem often introduced by the use of a composite endpoint as the primary endpoint.

The long-term results of this trial have been eagerly awaited, and patients will be followed for 5 years in total. The high number of stents implanted and the length of the stented segment of the vessel have raised questions about the long-term outcome in stented patients, and as such these 3-year data are important.

In regard to death, there remains no difference at 3 years, but the stroke rate remains slightly higher after CABG, although not quite statistically significant, but the difference in nonfatal myocardial infarction has increased and is significantly higher after stenting. The higher rate of repeat revascularization after PCI persists, and the gap is widening. However, among the triple-vessel disease patients, mortality and the combined endpoint of death, stroke, and myocardial infarction were increased in the PCI group.

Some of the most interesting data relate to the SYNTAX score, which is an index of lesion complexity and the severity and extent of disease. What we see is that in patients in the lowest tercile of the SYNTAX score, PCI is an acceptable form of revascularization, bearing in mind that these are patients with 3-vessel and left main coronary artery disease. On the other hand, among the highest tercile, CABG is clearly superior, and in the intermediate tercile of SYNTAX score, therapy with CABG is superior to stenting in those with triple-vessel disease, but the 2 therapies were equivalent for left main coronary disease. In regard to left main disease, we need to await the results of larger ongoing trials of drug-eluting stents and coronary bypass surgery. In regard to SYNTAX, the 5-year data will be equally interesting.

B. J. Gersh, MB, ChB, DPhil, FRCP

Reference

1. Serruys PW, Morice MC, Kappetein AP, et al. Percutaneous coronary intervention versus coronary-artery bypass grafting for severe coronary artery disease. *N Engl J Med.* 2009;360:961-972.

Optimal timing of coronary angiography and potential intervention in non-ST-elevation acute coronary syndromes
Katritsis DG, Siontis GCM, Kastrati A, et al (Athens Euroclinic, Greece; Univ of Ioannina School of Medicine, Greece; Technische Universität München, Munich, Germany; et al)
Eur Heart J 32:32-40, 2011

Aims.—An invasive approach is superior to medical management for the treatment of patients with acute coronary syndromes without ST-segment elevation (NSTE-ACS), but the optimal timing of coronary angiography and subsequent intervention, if indicated, has not been settled.

Methods and Results.—We conducted a meta-analysis of randomized trials addressing the optimal timing (early vs. delayed) of coronary angiography in NSTE-ACS. Four trials with 4013 patients were eligible (ABOARD, ELISA, ISAR-COOL, TIMACS), and data for longer follow-up periods than those published became available for this meta-analysis by the ELISA and ISAR-COOL investigators. The median time from admission or randomization to coronary angiography ranged from 1.16 to 14 h in the early and 20.8—86 h in the delayed strategy group. No statistically significant difference of risk of death [random effects risk ratio (RR) 0.85, 95% confidence interval (CI) 0.64—1.11] or myocardial infarction (MI) (RR 0.94, 95% CI 0.61—1.45) was detected between the two strategies. Early intervention significantly reduced the risk for recurrent ischaemia (RR 0.59, 95% CI 0.38—0.92, $P = 0.02$) and the duration of hospital stay (by 28%, 95% CI 22—35%, $P < 0.001$). Furthermore, decreased major bleeding events (RR 0.78, 95% CI 0.57—1.07, $P = 0.13$), and less major events (death, MI, or stroke) (RR 0.91, 95% CI 0.82−1.01, $P = 0.09$) were observed with the early strategy but these differences were not nominally significant.

Conclusion.—Early coronary angiography and potential intervention reduces the risk of recurrent ischaemia, and shortens hospital stay in patients with NSTE-ACS (Fig 1).

▶ Non-ST-segment elevation acute coronary syndromes (NSTE-ACS) represent a major burden of cardiovascular care, and the literature to some extent has been dominated by trials of antiplatelet and anticoagulant therapies in this patient subset. In addition, the role of an aggressive strategy of early intervention as opposed to a more conservative ischemia-driven strategy has been the focus of several randomized controlled trials in what appears to be a barrage of meta-analyses.[1] A prevailing consensus, however, is that the superior strategy for NSTE-ACS in centers with the requisite facilities and expertise is an invasive approach. The evidence is particularly strong in high-risk patients on the basis of elevated troponin, prior angina, diabetes, older age, ST-segment depression, and transient heart failure, among other variables, and a variety of risk scores are being developed for this purpose.[2]

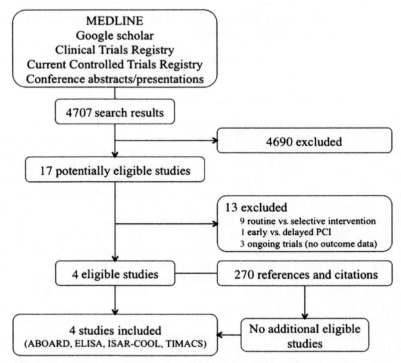

FIGURE 1.—Selection of studies. (Reprinted from Katritsis DG, Siontis GCM, Kastrati A, et al. Optimal timing of coronary angiography and potential intervention in non-ST-elevation acute coronary syndromes. *Eur Heart J.* 2011;32:32-40, by permission of The European Society of Cardiology.)

A different issue is the optimal timing of angiography, which is addressed by this meta-analysis of 4 trials that enrolled 4300 patients. The conclusion is that early angiography reduces the risk of recurrent ischemia and shortens the duration of hospital stay.

Personally, I am not sure that a meta-analysis is needed because the trials all addressed slightly different questions. ABOARD demonstrated no benefit from emergency primary percutaneous coronary intervention (PCI) versus waiting for up to 24 hours, and in the "delayed" group, the time to angiography was 20.8 hours (median range 17.5—24.6 hours). This conclusion probably created a sense of relief among many interventionists given the exigencies of emergency primary PCI 24 hours around the clock. The TIMACS supported a policy of angiography within 24 hours but not as an emergency, and the ISAR-COOL trial showed no advantage in waiting for several days for "plaque passivation."

In summary, early catheterization with a view to coronary revascularization within the first 24 hours is superior to a conservative strategy, but emergency primary PCI is not necessary in patients with NSTE-ACS.

B. J. Gersh, MB, ChB, DPhil, FRCP

References

1. Bavry AA, Kumbhani DJ, Rassi AN, Bhatt DL, Askari AT. Benefit of early invasive therapy in acute coronary syndromes: a meta-analysis of contemporary randomized clinical trials. *J Am Coll Cardiol.* 2006;48:1319-1325.
2. Eagle KA, Lim MJ, Dabbous OH, et al; GRACE Investigators. A validated prediction model for all forms of acute coronary syndrome: estimating the risk of 6-month postdischarge death in an international registry. *JAMA.* 2004;291:2727-2733.

37 Hypertension

ACCF/AHA 2011 Expert Consensus Document on Hypertension in the Elderly: A Report of the American College of Cardiology Foundation Task Force on Clinical Expert Consensus Documents Developed in Collaboration With the American Academy of Neurology, American Geriatrics Society, American Society for Preventive Cardiology, American Society of Hypertension, American Society of Nephrology, Association of Black Cardiologists, and European Society of Hypertension
Aronow WS, Fleg JL, Pepine CJ, et al (National Heart, Lung, and Blood Institute, USA)
J Am Coll Cardiol 57:2037-2114, 2011

Background.—Hypertension is common in persons age 65 years or older, so these individuals are more likely to suffer organ damage or clinical cardiovascular disease (CVD). Because the Hypertension in the Very Elderly Trial (HYVET) has documented the benefits of antihypertensive treatment for persons even age 80 years or older, it is important to understand the issues relevant to hypertension management in older patients.

Physical Findings and Diagnosis.—Age-associated increases in the prevalence of hypertension result from changes in arterial structure and function. With age, vessel distensibility diminishes, pulse wave velocity increases, late systolic blood pressure (SBP) is augmented, myocardial oxygen demand rises, and organ perfusion is limited. Adding coronary stenosis or a drug-induced excessive reduction in diastolic blood pressure (DBP) enhances these adverse conditions. Other causes of hypertension include renal artery stenosis, obstructive sleep apnea, primary aldosteronism, and thyroid disorders. Contributing factors are lifestyle, substance use, and medication effects. Elderly persons with poor BP control can suffer cerebrovascular disease, coronary artery disease, disorders of left ventricular (LV) structure and function, cardiac rhythm disorders, aortic and peripheral arterial disease, chronic kidney disease, ophthalmologic disorders, and quality of life deterioration.

The diagnosis of hypertension is based on at least three BP measurements done on at least two separate office visits. Patients should be seated comfortably for at least 5 minutes with the feet on the floor, the back supported, the arm supported horizontally, and the BP cuff at heart level. Findings should consider possible pseudohypertension (falsely increased SBP caused by sclerotic arteries) and white-coat hypertension, which must be ruled out. Besides accurately determining that the patient's BP is elevated, the clinician must identify reversible and/or treatable causes, evaluate for organ damage, assess for other CVD risk factors and/or comorbid conditions, and identify barriers to treatment compliance. Clinicians conduct a thorough history, physical examination, and laboratory testing, which should focus on urinalysis to detect renal damage, blood chemistries, cholesterol and triglyceride status, fasting blood sugar levels, and electrocardiographic results. Certain patients may benefit from two-dimensional electrocardiography to detect LV hypertrophy and LV dysfunction. Quality of life and cognitive function should also be determined.

Management.—Evidence-based guidelines are currently unavailable, so the management of hypertension relies on expert opinion. Lifestyle modification can be sufficient for milder forms of hypertension. Drug therapy is begun at the lowest dose and gradually increased based on BP responses until one reaches the maximum tolerated dose. If BP response is insufficient with a single agent, a second drug from another class is added, with adjustments to ensure tolerance and effectiveness. If BP response is insufficient with two agents at full dose levels, a third drug from another class is added. Treatment must be individualized in elderly patients, with evaluation of possible reasons for inadequate BP response conducted before adding new antihypertensive drugs. Elderly patients take an average of at least six prescription drugs so the clinician must be concerned about polypharmacy, nonadherence, and potential drug interactions.

The principal drug classes used to manage hypertension are thiazide diuretics, often the initial agent given; non-thiazide diuretics such as indapamide, furosemide, mineralocorticoid antagonists, epithelial sodium transport channel antagonists, beta blockers, calcium antagonists, and angiotensin-converting enzyme inhibitors (ACEIs); direct renin inhibitors such as aliskiren; and nonspecific vasodilators, which have unfavorable side effects and should be used only in combination therapy. Combination therapy is efficacious, avoids adverse effects, is convenient, and facilitates compliance. Some combinations of ACEIs, angiotensin receptor blockers, and calcium antagonists provide even greater protection for the cardiovascular system. Most elderly patients will need at least two drugs. If the initial BP is over 20/10 mm Hg above the goal, initiation of therapy may be best accomplished with two drugs. Patients with complicated hypertension are given multiple agents based on their comorbid conditions. Special recommendations are also applicable to elderly black individuals, octogenarians, and persons with resistant hypertension.

Conclusions.—Current recommendations recognize that elderly patients with hypertension can benefit from nonpharmacologic interventions but should receive drug therapy if they remain hypertensive. SBP values of < 140 mm Hg are an appropriate goal for most patients 79 years of age or younger. The goal for patients 80 years or older is 140 to 145 mm Hg, if tolerated. Further research is needed to define the pathogenesis of increased vascular and LV stiffness, set appropriate treatment thresholds and goals, compare the effectiveness of various treatment strategies, and assess the relative safety and efficacy of various approaches in preventing mortality and morbidity.

▶ These guidelines were assembled using old-fashioned methods, rather than by the new paradigm, which involves gathering all the available evidence, ranking it by study design, performing rigorous meta-analyses of trials that addressed a similar question, and deciding that there is no significant benefit to any more intensive or more expensive intervention.[1,2] It is anticipated, for example, that the Eighth Report of the Joint National Committee on Prevention, Detection, Evaluation, and Treatment of High Blood Pressure is using this new paradigm. Instead, these authors gathered expert opinion about many important questions and synthesized these opinions to form recommendations that many would argue are not very evidence-based.

Perhaps not surprisingly, these guidelines differ only in small ways from the Seventh Report of the Joint National Committee on Prevention, Detection, Evaluation, and Treatment of High Blood Pressure.[3] Many of these authors served on that committee, and their opinions have generally changed very little. One surprising omission from this set of guidelines is the recommendation to achieve a blood pressure of less than 130/80 mm Hg for patients with established heart disease, and less than 125/75 mm Hg in those with heart failure.[4] There was little overlap between these authors and the authors of that Scientific Statement from the American Heart Association in 2007, which may be part of the reason why these specific recommendations were not accepted for older patients. It does appear, however, from the long discussion (and the 740 references) in this document that there is more concern about lowering blood pressure too far by this expert panel than in many others, which may be perfectly appropriate for a guideline written about elderly patients.

Although these guidelines are interesting, they differ little from national guidelines about hypertension in general published more than 8 years ago,[3] they do not use the evidence-based approach, and they do not break much new ground.[5,6] These features make it less likely that these will be widely discussed or implemented, particularly because the Joint National Committee will likely update these guidelines soon.

W. J. Elliott, MD, PhD

References

1. NICE clinical guideline 127: Hypertension: Clinical management of primary hypertension in adults. http://www.nice.org.uk/CG127. Accessed August 24, 2011.
2. Smith SC Jr, Benjamin EJ, Bonow RO, et al. AHA/ACCF secondary prevention and risk reduction therapy for patients with coronary and other atherosclerotic vascular disease: 2011 update: a guideline from the American Heart Association and American College of Cardiology Foundation. *Circulation.* 2011;124:2458-2473.
3. Chobanian AV, Bakris GL, Black HR, et al; Joint National Committee on Prevention, Detection, Evaluation, and Treatment of High Blood Pressure, National High Blood Pressure Education Program Coordinating Committee. Seventh Report of the Joint National Committee on Prevention, Detection, Evaluation, and Treatment of High Blood Pressure. *Hypertension.* 2003;42:1206-1252.
4. Rosendorff C, Black HR, Cannon CP, et al; American Heart Association Council for High Blood Pressure Research, American Heart Association Council on

Clinical Cardiology, American Heart Association Council on Epidemiology and Prevention. Treatment of hypertension in the prevention and management of ischemic heart disease: a Scientific Statement from the American Heart Association Council for High Blood Pressure Research and the Councils on Clinical Cardiology and Epidemiology and Prevention. *Circulation.* 2007;115:2761-2788.

5. Elliott WJ. What should be the blood pressure target for diabetic patients? *Curr Opin Cardiol.* 2011;26:308-313.

6. Upadhyay A, Earley A, Haynes SM, Uhlig K. Systematic review: blood pressure target in chronic kidney disease and proteinuria as an effect modifier. *Ann Intern Med.* 2011;154:541-548.

NICE clinical guideline 127: Hypertension: Clinical management of primary hypertension in adults

Williams B, for The Guideline Development Groups, National Collaborating Centres, and NICE Project Team. United Kingdom National Health Service: National Institute for Health and Clinical Excellence (Univ of Leicester and Univ Hosps of Leicester NHS Trust, London, UK)

United Kingdom Natl Health Serv 1-36, 2011

Objectives and Targets.—This guidance updates and replaces the United Kingdom's National Institute for Health and Clinical Excellence (NICE) hypertension guidelines issued in 2004 and 2006. It is intended to provide advice about patient-centered care for persons with elevated blood pressure, but no other conditions for which NICE guidance has already been offered.

Major New Points.—Diagnosis: 24-hour ambulatory blood pressure monitoring (with at least 14 measurements/day) should be offered for every newly-diagnosed person with hypertension. Home blood pressure monitoring can be used to confirm a diagnosis of hypertension if two consecutive measurements are taken at least 1 minute apart, morning and evening, for at least 4, but preferably 7 days. Drug therapy: Drug treatment should be offered to all people with stage 2 hypertension, and all people with stage 1 hypertension younger than 80 years of age with target organ damage, established cardiovascular disease, renal disease, diabetes, or a 10-year risk of cardiovascular disease > 20%. Seek specialist advice for people with stage 1 hypertension younger than 40 years for assessment of target organ damage and secondary causes of hypertension. Monitoring and target blood pressures: For people who display the "white-coat effect," consider using home or ambulatory blood pressures as an adjunct to office measurements. Step 1 antihypertensive treatment for people over age 55 or blacks should be a calcium antagonist, with either chlorthalidone or indapamide as an alternative. Otherwise an ACE-inhibitor (or an angiotensin receptor blocker, if cough or angioedema) should be offered. For people with resistant hypertension (already taking a calcium antagonist, ACE-inhibitor, and thiazide-like diuretic), consider low-dose spironolactone or higher-dose chlorthalidone or indapamide, depending on the serum potassium. Target blood pressures should be <140/90 mm Hg for people less than 80 years of age, and <150/90 mm Hg otherwise.

Rationale.—The NICE Economics Team has performed incremental cost-utility analyses, typically based on meta-analyses of clinical trial data, to formulate each of these recommendations, using national data and recent costs of interventions (including drug therapy) to the National Health Service. Most of these are (or soon will be) available either on the NICE website, or published in the medical literature.

Conclusions.—These recommendations are for primary care of people with raised blood pressure. Other NICE guidances provide advice about appropriate treatments for complicated hypertension, including type 2 diabetes (CG 87), heart failure (CG 108), pregnancy (CG 107), chronic kidney disease (CG 73), stroke (CG 68), secondary prevention of myocardial infarction (CG 48), etc.

▶ There is new pervasive emphasis among guideline writers to require that all recommendations be very evidence based, using clinical trials or meta-analyses of clinical trials as the highest-ranking evidence.[1] The United Kingdom National Institute for Health and Clinical Excellence (NICE) guidelines have taken these new paradigms 1 step further, however, because their Economics Group performed cost-utility analyses, informed by the clinical trial results, and populated by nationwide costs to the National Health Service (NHS) of all procedures and drugs. It is remarkable, for example, that the cost of amlodipine to the UK NHS is about 10- to 50-fold lower than the average wholesale price of the very same medication in the United States. This makes translation of the NICE guidelines across the Atlantic Ocean very challenging.

The NICE hypertension guidelines are also clearly meant to apply ONLY to people with raised blood pressure—no further complications or other diseases that might reasonably influence treatment. On first reading, therefore, there appears to be no lower blood pressure target for diabetics or people with chronic kidney disease, which is consistent with several recent meta-analyses. However, the NICE Clinical Guideline 127 makes specific reference to earlier NICE guidelines about each of these conditions. Only after accessing other guidelines, for example, does one learn that a blood pressure target of less than 130/80 mm Hg is recommended for diabetics with chronic kidney disease, nondiabetics with chronic kidney disease, and greater than 1 gm/d of proteinuria[2] or diabetics with kidney, eye, or cerebrovascular damage.[3]

The new NICE recommendations to routinely use 24-hour ambulatory blood pressure monitoring for the initial diagnosis of hypertension are a departure from previous NICE guidelines,[4,5] but the economic and clinical advantages of using it to rule out "white-coat hypertension" have been published nearly 15 years ago and have recently been published in detail.[6] Because of its huge purchasing power, the UK NHS has obtained a very low price for the technology, approximately 25% to 33% of current US prices. The NICE recommendations about antihypertensive drug therapy are little changed from the 2006 recommendations, relegating β-blockers to step 4 therapy and recommending amlodipine as initial therapy for all but white people less than 55 years of age. This is presumably based on the results of the Anglo-Scandinavian Cardiac Outcomes Trial, in which the amlodipine-based regimen was superior in some secondary endpoints over an atenolol-based regimen.[7] The new NICE guidelines recommend spirono-lactone as fourth-line therapy (again as used in ASCOT[8]), which is now becoming more common in many centers across the world.

Many of these NICE recommendations are implementable in health care systems other than the UK NHS, but one wonders if the unique acquisition costs for many of the recommended procedures and agents will make them cost prohibitive elsewhere. This is especially likely to be true in low-income countries.[9]

W. J. Elliott, MD, PhD

References

1. Sackett DL, Rosenberg WM, Gray JA, Haynes RB, Richardson WS. Evidence based medicine: what it is and what it isn't. *BMJ.* 1996;312:71-72.
2. National Institute for Health and Clinical Excellence. CG 73 Chronic kidney disease: Early identification and management of chronic kidney disease in adults in primary and secondary care: NICE guideline. http://www.nice.org.uk/nicemedia/live/12069/42117/42117.pdf. Accessed October 31, 2011.
3. National Institute for Health and Clinical Excellence. CG 87 Type 2 diabetes—Newer agents (a partial update of CG 66): NICE guideline. http://guidance.nice.org.uk/CG87/NICEGuidance/pdf/English. Accessed October 31, 2011.
4. National Institute for Health and Clinical Excellence. CG 34 Hypertension: Management of hypertension in adults in primary care: NICE guideline. http://www.nice.org.uk/CG034. Accessed October 31, 2011.
5. Essential Hypertension: Managing Adult Patients in Primary Care. 2004. NICE Clinical Guideline 18. http://www.nice.org.uk/nicemedia/live/10986/30118/30118.pdf. Accessed June 03, 2011.
6. Lovibond K, Jowett S, Barton P, et al. Cost-effectiveness of options for the diagnosis of high blood pressure in primary care: a modelling study. *Lancet.* 2011; 378:1219-1230.
7. Dahlöf B, Sever PS, Poulter NR, et al. Prevention of cardiovascular events with an antihypertensive regimen of amlodipine adding perindopril as required versus atenolol adding bendroflumethiazide as required, in the Anglo-Scandinavian Cardiac Outcomes Trial-Blood Pressure Lowering Arm (ASCOT-BPLA): a multicentre randomised controlled trial. *Lancet.* 2005;366:895-906.
8. Chapman N, Dobson J, Wilson S, et al; Anglo-Scandinavian Cardiac Outcomes Trial Investigators. Effect of spironolactone on blood pressure in subjects with resistant hypertension. *Hypertension.* 2007;49:839-845.
9. Danaei G, Finucane MM, Lin JK, et al; Global Burden of Metabolic Risk Factors of Chronic Diseases Collaborating Group (Blood Pressure). National, regional, and global trends in systolic blood pressure since 1980: systematic analysis of health examination surveys and epidemiological studies with 786 country-years and 5·4 million participants. *Lancet.* 2011;377:568-577.

Relative effectiveness of clinic and home blood pressure monitoring compared with ambulatory blood pressure monitoring in diagnosis of hypertension: systematic review

Hodgkinson J, Mant J, Martin U, et al (Univ of Birmingham, Edgbaston; Univ of Cambridge, UK; et al)
BMJ 342:d3621, 2011

Objective.—To determine the relative accuracy of clinic measurements and home blood pressure monitoring compared with ambulatory blood pressure monitoring as a reference standard for the diagnosis of hypertension.

Design.—Systematic review with meta-analysis with hierarchical summary receiver operating characteristic models. Methodological quality was appraised, including evidence of validation of blood pressure measurement equipment.

Data Sources.—Medline (from 1966), Embase (from 1980), Cochrane Database of Systematic Reviews, DARE, Medion, ARIF, and TRIP up to May 2010.

Eligibility Criteria for Selecting Studies.—Eligible studies examined diagnosis of hypertension in adults of all ages using home and/or clinic blood pressure measurement compared with those made using ambulatory monitoring that clearly defined thresholds to diagnose hypertension.

Results.—The 20 eligible studies used various thresholds for the diagnosis of hypertension, and only seven studies (clinic) and three studies (home) could be directly compared with ambulatory monitoring. Compared with ambulatory monitoring thresholds of 135/85 mm Hg, clinic measurements over 140/90 mm Hg had mean sensitivity and specificity of 74.6% (95% confidence interval 60.7% to 84.8%) and 74.6% (47.9% to 90.4%), respectively, whereas home measurements over 135/85 mm Hg had mean sensitivity and specificity of 85.7% (78.0% to 91.0%) and 62.4% (48.0% to 75.0%).

Conclusions.—Neither clinic nor home measurement had sufficient sensitivity or specificity to be recommended as a single diagnostic test. If ambulatory monitoring is taken as the reference standard, then treatment decisions based on clinic or home blood pressure alone might result in substantial overdiagnosis. Ambulatory monitoring before the start of life-long drug treatment might lead to more appropriate targeting of treatment, particularly around the diagnostic threshold.

► Many different methods of obtaining blood pressure measurements have been developed, which have advantages and disadvantages for many patients. Office blood pressure readings have been the gold standard for research for more than a century, but few medical offices routinely take the standardized approach that takes time, effort, and testing and retraining of observers.[1] Automated office blood pressures have recently been advanced as a reasonably accurate alternative for busy primary care settings.[2] Home readings reduce the risk of the "white-coat response," and correlate better with target-organ damage, but can have their own disadvantages for some patients.[3] Twenty-four—hour ambulatory blood pressure monitoring has recently been recommended by the recently issued British hypertension guidelines for people suspected of having hypertension,[4] because the procedure is cost-effective in their National Health Service.[5]

These authors therefore performed a systematic review and meta-analysis of the diagnostic characteristics of office versus home blood pressure measurements, using the 24-hour ambulatory blood pressure monitoring results as the gold standard. Perhaps because this is a very hot topic and has been addressed by well-done, widely cited studies in many countries, the authors' main conclusions are not surprising, as they reflect the conclusions of the summarized studies. The contentious and rather subjective issue is whether office or home reading is sufficiently insensitive and nonspecific for diagnosing hypertension to recommend the more technically challenging 24-hour blood pressure monitoring, especially if it must be performed more than annually. The economics of 24-hour blood pressure monitoring differ in the United Kingdom and the United States, which is likely why their respective governmental health care authorities have nearly diametrically opposite policies regarding implementation and reimbursement for the procedure.

The authors believe that their analysis has several limitations, including the lack of a quality score for the included studies, lack of direct comparisons across the methods, variability of diagnostic thresholds for hypertension, variability in the number of measurements used for each technique, and major differences in the demographic characteristics of the studied populations. It is nonetheless likely that when 24-hour ambulatory blood pressure monitoring is not available, home readings would be wise in selected patients to supplement information from traditional office readings. Unfortunately, in the United States, interpretation of home readings is not currently reimbursed, although it has been recommended.[6]

W. J. Elliott, MD, PhD

References

1. Pickering TG, Hall JE, Appel LJ, et al; Subcommittee of Professional and Public Education of the American Heart Association Council on High Blood Pressure Research. Recommendations for blood pressure measurement in humans and experimental animals: Part 1: blood pressure measurement in humans: a statement for professionals from the Subcommittee of Professional and Public Education of the American Heart Association Council on High Blood Pressure Research. *Hypertension*. 2005;45:142-161.
2. Myers MG, Godwin M, Dawes M, et al. Conventional versus automated measurement of blood pressure in primary care patients with systolic hypertension: randomised parallel design controlled trial. *BMJ*. 2011;342:d286.
3. Bray EP, Holder R, Mant J, McManus RJ. Does self-monitoring reduce blood pressure? Meta-analysis with meta-regression of randomized controlled trials. *Ann Med*. 2010;42:371-386.
4. Williams B, Williams H, Northedge J, et al; for The Guideline Development Groups, National Collaborating Centres, and NICE Project Team. NICE Clinical Guideline 127: Hypertension: Clinical Management of Primary Hypertension in Adults. United Kingdom National Health Service: National Institute for Health and Clinical Excellence. http://www.nice.org.uk/CG127. Accessed August 24, 2011.
5. Lovibond K, Jowett S, Barton P, et al. Cost-effectiveness of options for the diagnosis of high blood pressure in primary care: a modelling study. *Lancet*. 2011; 378:1219-1230.
6. Pickering TG, Miller NH, Ogedegbe G, Krakoff LR, Artinian NT, Goff D; American Heart Association, American Society of Hypertension, Preventive Cardiovascular Nurses Association. Call to action on use and reimbursement for home blood pressure monitoring: executive summary. A joint scientific statement from the American Heart Association, American Society of Hypertension, and Preventive Cardiovascular Nurses Association. *Hypertension*. 2008;52:1-9.

Association of blood pressure in late adolescence with subsequent mortality: cohort study of Swedish male conscripts

Sundström J, Neovius M, Tynelius P, et al (Uppsala Univ, Sweden; Karolinska Institutet, Stockholm, Sweden)

BMJ 342:d643, 2011

Objective.—To investigate the nature and magnitude of relations of systolic and diastolic blood pressures in late adolescence to mortality.

Design.—Nationwide cohort study.

Setting.—General community in Sweden.

Participants.—Swedish men (n = 1 207 141) who had military conscription examinations between 1969 and 1995 at a mean age of 18.4 years, followed up for a median of 24 (range 0-37) years.

Main Outcome Measures.—Total mortality, cardiovascular mortality, and non-cardiovascular mortality.

Results.—During follow-up, 28 934 (2.4%) men died. The relation of systolic blood pressure to total mortality was U shaped, with the lowest risk at a systolic blood pressure of about 130 mm Hg. This pattern was driven by the relation to non-cardiovascular mortality, whereas the relation to cardiovascular mortality was monotonically increasing (higher risk with higher blood pressure). The relation of diastolic blood pressure to mortality risk was monotonically increasing and stronger than that of systolic blood pressure, in terms of both relative risk and population attributable fraction (deaths that could be avoided if blood pressure was in the optimal range). Relations to cardiovascular and non-cardiovascular mortality were similar, with an apparent risk threshold at a diastolic blood pressure of about 90 mm Hg, below which diastolic blood pressure and mortality were unrelated, and above which risk increased steeply with higher diastolic blood pressures.

Conclusions.—In adolescent men, the relation of diastolic blood pressure to mortality was more consistent than that of systolic blood pressure. Considering current efforts for earlier detection and prevention of risk, these observations emphasise the risk associated with high diastolic blood pressure in young adulthood.

▶ Blood pressure is a potent risk factor for cardiovascular morbidity and mortality,[1] but the focus changes from diastolic blood pressure in younger people to systolic blood pressure past 50 years of age.[2] Some have suggested that because the absolute risk of cardiovascular events is small in younger people, a more focused approach solely on systolic blood pressure is warranted.[3] This study was therefore undertaken to compare the predictive value of systolic and diastolic blood pressures in a large cohort of male Swedes who were examined before joining the armed services at around age 18 and were then followed prospectively for more than 24 years.

The methods used to measure blood pressure in the Swedish military conscription service differ from current US guidelines and practice.[4] A single blood pressure reading was taken after 5 to 10 minutes of quiet rest in the supine position and was repeated (and replaced) if it was either high or low. The authors used standard techniques for the remainder of their methodologies and, amazingly, lost no subjects to follow-up; they even knew which men emigrated and when. The finding that is most difficult to explain was the J- or U-shaped curve for diastolic blood pressure, because the military conscription service routinely excluded young men with disabilities and chronic diseases, so the likelihood of "reverse causality" is remote. The authors discuss a number of other possibilities, including chronic cerebral hypoperfusion and ischemia (perhaps related to accidental death), suicide, and other options, but none seems a clear favorite.

These data are consistent with many other data sets in even larger cohorts of older people,[1] but these are perhaps the most useful population-based data from a white, northern European cohort. The obvious limitations of including no women, minorities, or non-Swedes do not lessen their impact. They remind us of the importance of measuring blood pressure in adolescent men, despite the fact that most of them have many decades before cardiovascular events occur.

W. J. Elliott, MD, PhD

References

1. Lewington S, Clarke R, Qizilbash N, Peto R, Collins R; Prospective Studies Collaboration. Age-specific relevance of usual blood pressure to vascular mortality: a meta-analysis of individual data for one million adults in 61 prospective studies. *Lancet.* 2002;360:1903-1913.
2. Burt VL, Cutler JA, Higgins M, et al. Trends in the prevalence, awareness, treatment, and control of hypertension in the adult US population. Data from the health examination surveys, 1960 to 1991. *Hypertension.* 1995;26:60-69.
3. Izzo JL Jr, Levy D, Black HR. Clinical advisory statement. Importance of systolic blood pressure in older Americans. *Hypertension.* 2000;35:1021-1024.
4. Pickering TG, Hall JE, Appel LJ, et al; Subcommittee of Professional and Public Education of the American Heart Association Council on High Blood Pressure Research. Recommendations for blood pressure measurement in humans and experimental animals: Part 1: blood pressure measurement in humans: a statement for professionals from the Subcommittee of Professional and Public Education of the American Heart Association Council on High Blood Pressure Research. *Hypertension.* 2005;45:142-161.

Reliability of palpation of the radial artery compared with auscultation of the brachial artery in measuring SBP

van der Hoeven NV, van den Born B-JH, van Montfrans GA (Academic Med Ctr, Amsterdam, The Netherlands)
J Hypertens 29:51-55, 2011

Background.—Systolic blood pressure contributes more to cardiovascular disease than DBP, especially in elderly persons. Palpation of the radial artery to assess SBP — Riva-Rocci's technique — may be an attractive alternative for auscultatory SBP in these patients. Therefore, we investigated the difference between SBP determined by palpation of the radial artery (pSBP) and SBP assessed by auscultation of the brachial artery (aSBP).

Methods.—Patients were included from the waiting room of a hypertension outpatient clinic. In each patient eight simultaneous pSBP and aSBP measurements were assessed by two observers in the same arm. After every two readings the observers switched between pSBP and aSBP.

Results.—Forty patients were included, 25 men (62.5%), mean age 55.3 years (range 24—78). From a total of 320 measurements, mean difference between pSBP and aSBP was −5.2 mm Hg (range −12—26 mm Hg) ($P < 0.01$). This difference correlated significantly with BMI ($r = 0.51$, $P < 0.01$), but not with age ($r = 0.15$, $P = 0.35$), pulse rate ($r = 0.29$, $P = 0.09$) or mean SBP ($r = 0.03$, $P = 0.85$). After averaging the first three comparisons, reproducibility did not improve when increasing the number of comparisons. When correcting for the underestimation of 6 mm Hg over the first three comparisons, Riva-Rocci's technique estimates SBP with an acceptable accuracy.

Conclusion.—In clinical practice, Riva-Rocci's palpatory technique offers an acceptable alternative for auscultatory SBP measurement. It is recommended to take three measurements and then correct for the average underestimation of 6 mm Hg (Fig 2).

▶ Sometimes, what's old is what's new, and sometimes what's old becomes classic. Perhaps that is the message of this article, which compared 2 century-old methods of estimating systolic blood pressure in a convenience sample of 40 consecutive subjects attending a hypertension center in Holland. The rationale for this comparison is reasonably compelling: A Clinical Advisory Statement from the American Heart Association more than 10 years ago suggested that systolic is the most important, single blood pressure compared with diastolic or pulse pressure[1]; this conclusion was subsequently corroborated by an analysis from the Prospective Studies Collaboration.[2] The authors of this article assert that a proper comparison of the palpatory method of Riva-Rocci and the ausculatory method of Korotkoff has never been published, but it seems likely that such comparisons were done sometime during the last millennium and simply not deemed worthy of completing the manuscript. Modern statistical methods and Bland-Altman plots make it more likely that the finding of no significant difference between the 2 methods would be more likely to be publishable today.

The most important point of this article is that the 2 methods provide very similar information that is highly correlated. The unfortunate aspect is that there seems to be a systematic underestimation of the systolic pressure by 6 mm Hg using the Riva-Rocci method, which might be very difficult to explain from first principles. There is a hint in the pseudo Bland-Altman plot (Fig 2, which uses the mean of the palpated and auscultated systolic blood pressures on the x-axis) of the article, which indicates that systolic blood pressure was underestimated by about 22 mm Hg in 2 subjects and by more than 20 mm Hg in 5 (of 40!) subjects, using the palpatory method. The authors discuss the history and possible reasons for this discrepancy, noting that Korotkoff observed a systolic blood pressure higher than 10 to 12 mm Hg using his auscultatory method compared with the palpatory method.[3-6] The rationale is that the palpatory

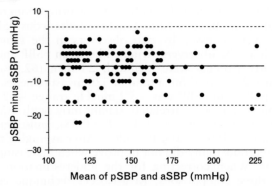

FIGURE 2.—Comparison of the first three SBP measurements assessed by palpation and the first three SBP measurements assessed by auscultation for all patients ($n = 120$). On the horizontal axis of the Bland–Altman plot the mean palpatory SBP (pSBP) and auscultatory SBP (aSBP) measurement is shown. The vertical axis shows the difference between pSBP and aSBP. The solid line represents the mean at −5.7 mmHg. The dashed lines represent 1.96 times the SD above and below the mean at 5.6mmHg and −17.0 mmHg, respectively. pSBP, SBP assessed by palpation; aSBP, SBP assessed by auscultation. (Reprinted from van der Hoeven NV, van den Born BJ, van Montfrans GA. Reliability of palpation of the radial artery compared with auscultation of the brachial artery in measuring SBP. *J Hypertens.* 2011;29:51-55. © Lippincott Williams & Wilkins.)

method takes about 3 heartbeats before the pulse is detected, compared with the auscultatory method, which would average about a 6-mm Hg difference with a heart rate of 60 per minute.

The authors admit to some limitations of their study, including the fact that a small number of subjects were studied, and all were recruited from a waiting room of a hypertension center. This provided a wide range of measured systolic blood pressures (about 105–230 mm Hg, according to Fig 2) but may not be representative of the broader population. They recommend that the Riva-Rocci method not be forgotten but used in addition to, and possibly instead of, the Korotkoff method, at least for determining the peak inflation level before applying the stethoscope.[7]

W. J. Elliott, MD, PhD

References

1. Izzo JL Jr, Levy D, Black HR. Clinical advisory statement. Importance of systolic blood pressure in older Americans. *Hypertension.* 2000;35:1021-1024.
2. Lewington S, Clarke R, Qizilbash N, Peto R, Collins R; Prospective Studies Collaboration. Age-specific relevance of usual blood pressure to vascular mortality: a meta-analysis of individual data for one million adults in 61 prospective studies. *Lancet.* 2002;360:1903-1913.
3. Korotkoff NC. To the question of methods of determining the blood pressure (from the clinic of Professor CP Federoff). *Rep Imperial Mil Acad [in Russian].* 1905;11:365-367.
4. Dock W. Korotkoff's sounds. *N Engl J Med.* 1980;302:1264-1267.
5. Korotkov NS. Concerning the problem of the methods of blood pressure measurement. *J Hypertens.* 2005;23:5.
6. Paskalev D, Kircheva A, Krivoshiev S. A centenary of auscultatory blood pressure measurement: a tribute to Nikolai Korotkoff. *Kidney Blood Press Res.* 2005;28:259-263.

7. Pickering TG, Hall JE, Appel LJ, et al; Subcommittee of Professional and Public Education of the American Heart Association Council on High Blood Pressure Research. Recommendations for blood pressure measurement in humans and experimental animals: Part 1: blood pressure measurement in humans: a statement for professionals from the Subcommittee of Professional and Public Education of the American Heart Association Council on High Blood Pressure Research. *Hypertension.* 2005;45:142-161.

38 Non-Coronary Heart Disease in Adults

Mortality Reduction of Cardiac Resynchronization and Implantable Cardioverter-Defibrillator Therapy in Heart Failure: An Updated Meta-Analysis. Does Recent Evidence Change the Standard of Care?
Bertoldi EG, Polanczyk CA, Cunha V, et al (Federal Univ of Rio Grande do Sul, Porto Alegre, Brazil; et al)
J Card Fail 17:860-866, 2011

Background.—The recent publication of the MADIT-CRT and RAFT trials has more than doubled the number of patients in which a direct comparison of the combination of cardiac resynchronization therapy (CRT) and implantable cardioverter-defibrillator (ICD) versus ICD alone was carried out. The present meta-analysis aims to assess the impact of combined CRT and ICD therapy on survival of heart failure (HF) patients.

Methods and Results.—Medline, Embase, and the Cochrane Library databases were searched, and all randomized controlled trials of CRT alone or combined with ICDs in HF resulting from left ventricular systolic dysfunction were included. Main outcome was all-cause mortality. Summary relative risk (RR) and 95% confidence interval (CI) were calculated employing random-effects models. Twelve studies were included, with a total of 8,284 randomized patients. For the comparison of CRT alone versus medical therapy, pooled analysis of 5 available trials demonstrated a significant reduction in all-cause mortality with CRT (RR 0.76, 95% CI: 0.64–0.9). Pooled analysis of 6 trials that compared the combination of CRT and ICD therapy to ICD alone also showed a statistically significant reduction in all-cause mortality (RR 0.83, 95% CI: 0.72–0.96). Stratified analysis showed significant mortality reductions in all New York Heart Association class subgroups, with greater effect in classes III–IV (RR 0.70; 95% CI: 0.57–0.88). Pooled estimates of implant-related risks were 0.6% for death and 8% for implant failure.

Conclusion.—Combined CRT and ICD therapy reduces overall mortality in HF patients when compared with ICD alone (Figs 2B, 3, and 4).

▶ The introduction of implantable cardioverter-defibrillators (ICD) and cardiac resynchronization therapy (CRT) has been a major advance in the treatment of patients with advanced heart failure (HF).[1] There is good evidence that both of these devices in appropriate patients with HF prolong life and, in the case of

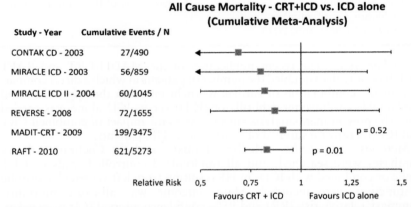

Study or Subgroup	CRT+ICD Events	Total	ICD Events	Total	Weight	Risk Ratio IV, Random, 95% CI	Year
CONTAK CD	11	245	16	245	3.7%	0.69 [0.33, 1.45]	2003
MIRACLE ICD	14	187	15	182	4.2%	0.91 [0.45, 1.83]	2003
MIRACLE ICD II	2	85	2	101	0.5%	1.19 [0.17, 8.26]	2004
REVERSE	9	419	3	191	1.2%	1.37 [0.37, 4.99]	2008
MADIT-CRT	74	1089	53	731	17.8%	0.94 [0.67, 1.32]	2009
RAFT	186	894	236	904	72.5%	0.80 [0.67, 0.94]	2010
Total (95% CI)		**2919**		**2354**	**100.0%**	**0.83 [0.72, 0.96]**	
Total events	296		325				

Heterogeneity: Tau² = 0.00; Chi² = 1.72, df = 5 (P = 0.89); I² = 0%
Test for overall effect: Z = 2.58 (P = 0.010)

FIGURE 2.—All-cause mortality—CRT + ICD versus ICD alone. CRT, cardiac resynchronization therapy; ICD, implantable cardioverter defibrillator therapy; IV, inverse variance method. (Reprinted from the Journal of Cardiac Failure, Bertoldi EG, Polanczyk CA, Cunha V, et al. Mortality reduction of cardiac resynchronization and implantable cardioverter-defibrillator therapy in heart failure: an updated meta-analysis. Does recent evidence change the standard of care? *J Card Fail.* 2011;17:860-866. Copyright 2011 with permission from Elsevier.)

All Cause Mortality - CRT+ICD vs. ICD alone (Cumulative Meta-Analysis)

Study - Year	Cumulative Events / N
CONTAK CD - 2003	27/490
MIRACLE ICD - 2003	56/859
MIRACLE ICD II - 2004	60/1045
REVERSE - 2008	72/1655
MADIT-CRT - 2009	199/3475
RAFT - 2010	621/5273

FIGURE 3.—Cumulative meta-analysis of all-cause mortality with CRT+ICD versus ICD alone. CRT, cardiac resynchronization therapy; ICD, implantable cardioverter defibrillator therapy; IV, inverse variance method. Note that the point estimate suggests a reduction in mortality since the earlier trials, but statistical significance only appears after addition of the RAFT trial. (Reprinted from the Journal of Cardiac Failure, Bertoldi EG, Polanczyk CA, Cunha V, et al. Mortality reduction of cardiac resynchronization and implantable cardioverter-defibrillator therapy in heart failure: an updated meta-analysis. Does recent evidence change the standard of care? *J Card Fail.* 2011;17:860-866. Copyright 2011 with permission from Elsevier.)

CRT when added to optimal medical therapy, reduce symptoms.[2,3] Most previous trials compared the use of either ICD or CRT with optimal medical therapy.[4-6] Earlier studies are not convincing that the combination added significant improvement in all-cause mortality. Recently, the MADIT-CRT and the RAFT trials compared the combination of CRT and ICD with ICD alone.[7,8] Because these studies more than doubled the number of patients involved in this comparison, this study does a combined analysis of all trials, allowing greater reliability to whether the combination of the 2 devices brings incremental benefit over either treatment alone. To be included, the studies had to be randomized controlled trials of more than 2 weeks duration that included HF patients with left ventricular (LV) systolic dysfunction and evaluated CRT, either alone or

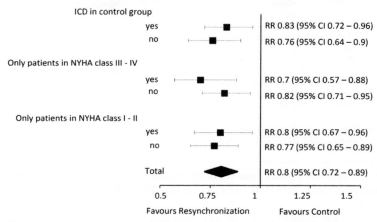

All-Cause Mortality - Resynchronization vs. Control

ICD in control group
yes — RR 0.83 (95% CI 0.72 – 0.96)
no — RR 0.76 (95% CI 0.64 – 0.9)

Only patients in NYHA class III - IV
yes — RR 0.7 (95% CI 0.57 – 0.88)
no — RR 0.82 (95% CI 0.71 – 0.95)

Only patients in NYHA class I - II
yes — RR 0.8 (95% CI 0.67 – 0.96)
no — RR 0.77 (95% CI 0.65 – 0.89)

Total — RR 0.8 (95% CI 0.72 – 0.89)

0.5   0.75   1   1.25   1.5
Favours Resynchronization   Favours Control

FIGURE 4.—Stratified analysis of all-cause mortality according to NYHA class and inclusion of ICD therapy. CI, confidence interval; ICD, implantable cardioverter-defibrillator; NYHA, New York Heart Association; RR, relative risk. (Reprinted from the Journal of Cardiac Failure, Bertoldi EG, Polanczyk CA, Cunha V, et al. Mortality reduction of cardiac resynchronization and implantable cardioverter-defibrillator therapy in heart failure: an updated meta-analysis. Does recent evidence change the standard of care? *J Card Fail.* 2011;17:860-866. Copyright 2011 with permission from Elsevier.)

with an ICD, versus ICD therapy alone. The primary outcome was all-cause mortality. Twelve trials met the criteria, all with prolonged QRS interval and, most commonly, ischemic etiology of the HF, and follow-up time in various series was from 6 to 40 months. The pooled analysis of trials found that when comparing CRT with medical therapy, CRT reduced all-cause mortality by 24% and with CRT + ICD versus ICD alone, CRT + ICD reduced all-cause mortality 17%, both highly significant reductions. Implant failure rate of CRT in the pooled studies was 8%, and risk of major peri-implant complication was 13.2%. These complication rates declined progressively from earlier to more recent studies. Earlier trials that found no difference in mortality were either too small in number or with too short a follow-up time.

M. D. Cheitlin, MD

References

1. Jessup M, Abraham WT, Casey DE, et al. 2009 focused update: ACCF/AHA Guidelines for the Diagnosis and Management of Heart Failure in Adults: a report of the American College of Cardiology Foundation/American Heart Association Task Force on Practice Guidelines: developed in collaboration with the International Society for Heart and Lung Transplantation. *Circulation.* 2009;119:1977-2016.
2. Ezekowitz JA, Armstrong PW, McAlister FA. Implantable cardioverter defibrillators in primary and secondary prevention: a systematic review of randomized, controlled trials. *Ann Intern Med.* 2003;138:445-452.
3. Bradley DJ, Bradley EA, Baughman KL, et al. Cardiac resynchronization and death from progressive heart failure: a meta-analysis of randomized controlled trials. *JAMA.* 2003;289:730-740.

4. Freemantle N, Tharmanathan P, Calvert MJ, Abraham WT, Ghosh J, Cleland JG. Cardiac resynchronisation for patients with heart failure due to left ventricular systolic dysfunction—a systematic review and meta-analysis. *Eur J Heart Fail.* 2006;8:433-440.
5. McAlister FA, Ezekowitz JA, Wiebe N, et al. Systematic review: cardiac resynchronization in patients with symptomatic heart failure. *Ann Intern Med.* 2004;141: 381-390.
6. Lam SK, Owen A. Combined resynchronisation and implantable defibrillator therapy in left ventricular dysfunction: Bayesian network meta-analysis of randomised controlled trials. *BMJ.* 2007;335:925.
7. Moss AJ, Hall WJ, Cannom DS, et al. Cardiac-resynchronization therapy for the prevention of heart-failure events. *N Engl J Med.* 2009;361:1329-1338.
8. Tang AS, Wells GA, Talajic M, et al. Cardiac-resynchronization therapy for mild-to-moderate heart failure. *N Engl J Med.* 2010;363:2385-2395.

Effects of selective heart rate reduction with ivabradine on left ventricular remodelling and function: results from the SHIFT echocardiography substudy

Tardif J-C, on behalf of the SHIFT Investigators (Université de Montréal, Quebec, Canada; et al)

Eur Heart J 32:2507-2515, 2011

Aims.—The SHIFT echocardiographic substudy evaluated the effects of ivabradine on left ventricular (LV) remodelling in heart failure (HF).

Methods and Results.—Eligible patients had chronic HF and systolic dysfunction [LV ejection fraction (LVEF) ≤35%], were in sinus rhythm, and had resting heart rate ≥70 bpm. Patients were randomly allocated to ivabradine or placebo, superimposed on background therapy for HF. Complete echocardiographic data at baseline and 8 months were available for 411 patients (ivabradine 208, placebo 203). Treatment with ivabradine reduced LVESVI (primary substudy endpoint) vs. placebo [−7.0 ± 16.3 vs. −0.9 ± 17.1 mL/m²; difference (SE), −5.8 (1.6), 95% CI −8.8 to −2.7, $P < 0.001$]. The reduction in LVESVI was independent of beta-blocker use, HF aetiology, and baseline LVEF. Ivabradine also improved LV end-diastolic volume index (−7.9 ± 18.9 vs. −1.8 ± 9.0 mL/m², $P = 0.002$) and LVEF (+2.4 ± 7.7 vs. −0.1 ± 8.0%, $P < 0.001$). The incidence of the SHIFT primary composite outcome (cardiovascular mortality or hospitalization for worsening HF) was higher in patients with LVESVI above the median (59 mL/m²) at baseline (HR 1.62, 95% CI 1.03−2.56, $P = 0.04$). Patients with the largest relative reductions in LVESVI had the lowest event rates.

Conclusion.—Ivabradine reverses cardiac remodelling in patients with HF and LV systolic dysfunction (Figs 2 and 3).

▶ In 2010, the Systolic Heart Failure Treatment with the I(f) Inhibitor Ivabradine Trial (SHIFT) investigators reported that provoking slowing of sinus rhythm in heart failure (HF) patients with a heart rate ≥70 beats per minute, and with an ejection fraction ≤35% by ivabradine, a specific inhibitor of the I(f) current in the sinoatrial node, there was an 18% reduction in the primary composite endpoint

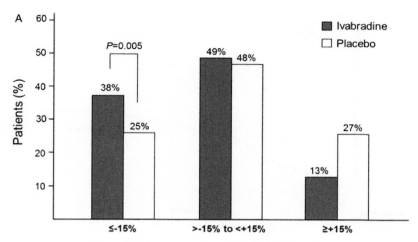

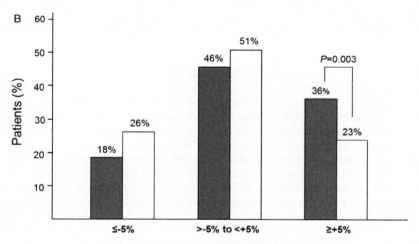

FIGURE 2.—(*A*) Relative change in left ventricular end-systolic volume index (LVESVI) and (*B*) absolute change in left ventricular ejection fraction (LVEF) from baseline to 8 months. The grey and white bars represent percentages of patients reaching echocardiographic criteria for the ivabradine and placebo groups, respectively. (Reprinted from Tardif J-C, on behalf of the SHIFT Investigators. Effects of selective heart rate reduction with ivabradine on left ventricular remodelling and function: results from the SHIFT echocardiography substudy. *Eur Heart J.* 2011;32:2507-2515, by permission of The European Society of Cardiology.)

of cardiovascular death or hospitalization for worsening HF.[1] Left ventricular (LV) enlargement predicts adverse cardiovascular events,[2] and reduced LV ejection fraction is a powerful predictor of cardiovascular outcomes and all-cause mortality.[3] This substudy of the SHIFT study using echocardiography evaluates

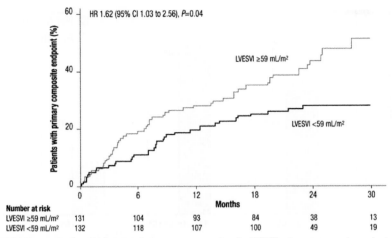

FIGURE 3.—Kaplan–Meier cumulative event curves for the SHIFT primary composite endpoint of cardiovascular death or hospitalization for worsening heart failure in the placebo group split by median left ventricular end-systolic volume index (LVESVI) ≥59 vs. <59 mL/m². (Reprinted from Tardif J-C, on behalf of the SHIFT Investigators. Effects of selective heart rate reduction with ivabradine on left ventricular remodelling and function: results from the SHIFT echocardiography substudy. *Eur Heart J*. 2011;32:2507-2515, by permission of The European Society of Cardiology.)

the effects of ivabradine versus placebo on left ventricular remodeling (LVR). Because ivabradine affects only the heart rate and has no effect on myocardial contractility and intracardiac conduction, ivabradine's effect is related to isolated heart rate reduction. After 8 months from the baseline echocardiogram, the finding of a significantly greater reduction in LV end-systolic and end-diastolic volumes and increase in LV ejection fraction with ivabradine compared with placebo shows a positive effect of ivabradine on LVR. Larger decreases in heart rate were associated with greater increases in LV ejection fraction. In contrast, there was no significant relationship between changes in heart rate and changes in LV volumes for all patients. However, when split by baseline median heart rate of 77 beats per minute, those patients with higher heart rates had larger LV end volumes and lower ejection fractions at baseline. In evaluating the impact of the baseline values of the echocardiographic parameters of LV function, the authors divided the LV end-systolic volume index in the placebo group by the median baseline of 59 mL/m² and found the incidence of the combined endpoint of hospitalization for worsening HF or CV mortality was greater in those with the higher values. There were too few composite endpoints in the echocardiographic SHIFT substudy to evaluate the effect of treatment on outcomes according to the effect of ivabradine on LV volumes. However, when dividing the ivabradine and placebo groups into tertiles of change in LV end-systolic volume indices and determining the incidence of composite endpoints after 8 months of therapy for each third, those with the greatest relative reductions in LV end-systolic volume index had lower event rates than those with smaller reductions or increases. This study shows reversal of LVR with ivabradine over 8 months of therapy in patients, 90% of whom were on beta-blockers and renin-angiotensin-aldosterone system

(RAAS) antagonists. These findings are supported by studies in animal models of HF showing effects of ivabradine on reduction of fibrosis, RAAS, and sympathetic stimulation, and improvement in endothelial function.[4-6] How important these findings of the effect of ivabradine in patients with heart failure will be is questionable. First, it is possible that the same effects can be accomplished by pushing beta-blockers to the same level of heart rate reduction. Second, Cullington and colleagues[7] evaluated more than 2200 patients with systolic dysfunction (LV ejection fraction < 50%) attending an HF clinic and reported that if a high resting heart rate greater than 70 beats per minute in patients on optimum HF therapy is necessary for ivabradine's use, then only about 5% would be suitable candidates.

M. D. Cheitlin, MD

References

1. Swedberg K, Komajda M, Böhm M, et al; SHIFT Investigators. Ivabradine and outcomes in chronic heart failure (SHIFT): a randomised placebo-controlled study. *Lancet.* 2010;376:875-885.
2. St John Sutton M, Pfeffer MA, Plappert T, et al. Quantitative two-dimensional echocardiographic measurements are major predictors of adverse cardiovascular events after acute myocardial infarction. The protective effects of captopril. *Circulation.* 1994;89:68-75.
3. Solomon SD, Anavekar N, Skali H, et al; Candesartan in Heart Failure Reduction in Mortality (CHARM) Investigators. Influence of ejection fraction on cardiovascular outcomes in a broad spectrum of heart failure patients. *Circulation.* 2005; 112:3738-3744.
4. Dedkov EI, Zheng W, Christensen LP, Weiss RM, Mahlberg-Gaudin F, Tomanek RJ. Preservation of coronary reserve by ivabradine-induced reduction in heart rate in infarcted rats is associated with decrease in perivascular collagen. *Am J Physiol Heart Circ Physiol.* 2007;293:H590-H598.
5. Milliez P, Messaoudi S, Nehme J, Rodriguez C, Samuel JL, Delcayre C. Beneficial effects of delayed ivabradine treatment on cardiac anatomical and electrical remodeling in rat severe chronic heart failure. *Am J Physiol Heart Circ Physiol.* 2009;296:H435-H441.
6. Vercauteren M, Favre J, Mulder P, Mahlberg-Gaudin F, Thuillez C, Richard V. Protection of endothelial function by long-term heart rate reduction induced by ivabradine in a rat model of chronic heart failure. *Eur Heart J.* 2007;28:48. P468.
7. Cullington D, Goode KM, Cleland JG, Clark AL. Limited role for ivabradine in the treatment of chronic heart failure. *Heart.* 2011;97:1961-1966.

Eplerenone Survival Benefits in Heart Failure Patients Post-Myocardial Infarction Are Independent From its Diuretic and Potassium-Sparing Effects: Insights From an EPHESUS (Eplerenone Post-Acute Myocardial Infarction Heart Failure Efficacy and Survival Study) Substudy

Rossignol P, Ménard J, Fay R, et al (INSERM, Nancy, France; INSERM, Paris, France; et al)
J Am Coll Cardiol 58:1958-1966, 2011

Objectives.—The purpose of this study was to determine whether a diuretic effect may be detectable in patients treated with eplerenone, a mineralocorticoid receptor antagonist, as compared with placebo during the first month of EPHESUS (Eplerenone Post-Acute Myocardial

Infarction Heart Failure Efficacy and Survival study) (n = 6,080) and whether this was associated with eplerenone's beneficial effects on cardiovascular outcomes.

Background.—The mechanism of the survival benefit of eplerenone in patients with heart failure post-myocardial infarction remains uncertain.

Methods.—A diuretic effect was indirectly estimated by changes at 1 month that was superior to the median changes in the placebo group in body weight (−0.05 kg) and in the estimated plasma volume reduction (+1.4%). A potassium-sparing effect was defined as a serum potassium increase greater than the median change in the placebo group: +0.11 mmol/l.

Results.—In the eplerenone group, body weight ($p < 0.0001$) and plasma volume ($p = 0.047$) decreased, whereas blood protein and serum potassium increased (both, $p < 0.0001$), as compared with the placebo group, suggesting a diuretic effect induced by eplerenone, associated with a potassium-sparing effect. A diuretic effect, as defined by an estimated plasma volume reduction, was independently associated with 11% to 19% better outcomes (lower all-cause death, cardiovascular death or cardiovascular hospitalization, all-cause death or hospitalization, hospitalization for heart failure). Potassium sparing was also independently associated with 12% to 34% better outcomes. There was no statistically significant interaction between the observed beneficial effects of eplerenone (9% to 17%) on cardiovascular outcomes and potassium-sparing or diuretic effects.

Conclusions.—Eplerenone's beneficial effects on long-term survival and cardiovascular outcomes are independent from early potassium-sparing or diuretic effects, suggesting that mineralocorticoid receptor antagonism provides cardiovascular protection beyond its diuretic and potassium-sparing properties (Figs 2 and 3).

▶ Congestion in patients with heart failure (HF) is associated with a poor outcome.[1,2] Diuretics in patients with HF are valuable in that they reduce symptoms and improve the quality of life. However, diuretic use is associated with a worse prognosis and is not supported by large clinical, randomized, placebo-controlled studies. Furthermore, diuretics stimulate the renin-angiotensin and sympathetic nervous systems and are associated with a decrease in glomerular filtration rate. The EPHESUS (Eplerenone Post-Acute Myocardial Infarction Heart Failure Efficacy and Survival) study showed that eplerenone, a mineralocorticoid receptor blocker, added to standard optimal therapy that included diuretic use, in more than 6000 patients with an acute myocardial infarction and HF with systolic dysfunction, improved survival by 15% and significantly reduced cardiovascular deaths, sudden deaths, and hospitalization for HF.[3] Because eplerenone is a diuretic, spares potassium loss, and has other pleiotropic effects, this study was done to examine which of these effects could be detected and whether these effects related to cardiovascular outcomes. This substudy of the EHESUS trial showed an early diuretic and potassium-sparing effect of eplerenone compared with the control group and, independent of eplerenone use, that plasma volume depletion was significantly associated with a 11% to 19%

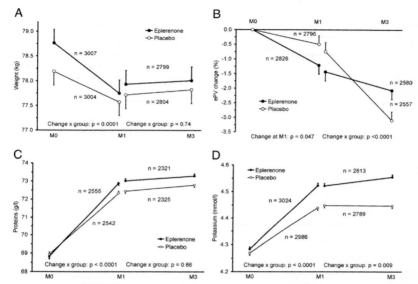

FIGURE 2.—Eplerenone Exerts Early (1-Month) Diuretic-Like and K-Sparing Effects. Diuretic-like (**A to C**) and K-sparing (**D**) effects are shown. As a result of missing data, frequencies did not sum to 6,080 (M1) nor 5,692 (M3). M0-M1 and M1-M3 mean values are those for patients with available data at both ends of the period. Change at M1: single comparison of plasma volume change (Mann-Whitney test). Baseline values were set to zero for the graphical presentation. Change × group: interaction between change from M1 to M3 and study group (repeated measures analysis of variance). ePV = estimated plasma volume; M0 = inclusion; M1 = month 1; M3 = month 3. (Reprinted from the Journal of the American College of Cardiology, Rossignol P, Ménard J, Fay R, et al. Eplerenone survival benefits in heart failure patients post-myocardial infarction are independent from its diuretic and potassium-sparing effects: insights from an EPHESUS (Eplerenone Post-Acute Myocardial Infarction Heart Failure Efficacy and Survival Study) substudy. *J Am Coll Cardiol.* 2011;58:1958-1966. Copyright 2011, with permission from the American College of Cardiology.)

improvement in all-cause death, cardiovascular death or cardiovascular hospitalization, and hospitalization for HF, but not for sudden death. Furthermore, plasma volume depletion, across the spectrum of cardiovascular outcomes except for sudden death, showed a significant linear trend in the crude event rates in the whole study population. This was not true with the weight-based definition of diuretic effect, representing intracellular and extracellular volume depletion that was not associated with any of the assessed outcomes. Multivariate analysis of the main cardiovascular outcomes confirmed that the effect of eplerenone on outcomes was independent from early diuretic and potassium-sparing effects. This is the first time in patients with systolic dysfunction and HF after an acute myocardial infarction that an initial and short-term diuretic-like effect as defined by plasma volume depletion after 1 month is associated with better cardiovascular outcomes, independent of potassium-sparing effect. Also, the benefit of eplerenone on outcomes was independent of the diuretic and potassium-sparing effects. Another important finding of this study is the independent early potassium-sparing effect, consistent with eplerenone's mineralocorticoid receptor antagonism, which was associated with improved

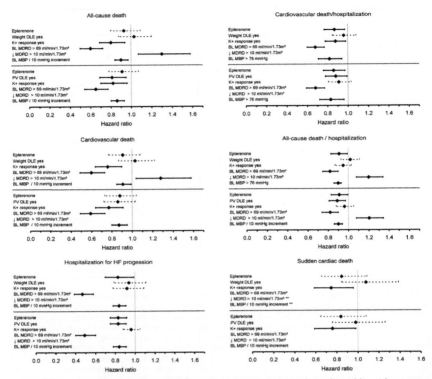

FIGURE 3.—Determinants of the Cardiovascular Outcomes. Relationships of variables with outcomes are shown with the assessment of a diuretic effect either by body weight changes (**upper half of each plot**) or by estimated plasma volume changes (**lower half of each plot**) added into the model. Weight DLE indicates weight-based diuretic-like effect (included in the **upper panels**); ePV DLE indicates estimated plasma volume–based diuretic-like effect (included in the **lower panels**). Potassium response indicates the potassium-sparing effect; ↓MDRD (Modification of Diet in Renal Disease) >10 ml/min/1.73 m² indicates a decrease between inclusion and month 1 in estimated glomerular filtration rate using the MDRD formula >10 ml/min/1.73 m². Covariables were removed from the models when they did not reach significance or have to be used as stratification factors in order to meet the models validity assumptions. BL = baseline; MBP = mean blood pressure. (Reprinted from the Journal of the American College of Cardiology, Rossignol P, Ménard J, Fay R, et al. Eplerenone survival benefits in heart failure patients post-myocardial infarction are independent from its diuretic and potassium-sparing effects: insights from an EPHESUS (Eplerenone Post-Acute Myocardial Infarction Heart Failure Efficacy and Survival Study) substudy. *J Am Coll Cardiol*. 2011;58:1958-1966. Copyright 2011, with permission from the American College of Cardiology.)

long-term cardiovascular outcomes. The conclusions of the authors is that this study supports the hypothesis that pleiotropic effects of the eplerenone may involve left ventricular and vascular remodeling, including effects on collagen synthesis and endothelial and immune function. It remains to be seen whether the same effects are seen in patients with HF not caused by acute myocardial infarction.

M. D. Cheitlin, MD

References

1. Drazner MH, Rame JE, Stevenson LW, Dries DL. Prognostic importance of elevated jugular venous pressure and a third heart sound in patients with heart failure. *N Engl J Med.* 2001;345:574-581.
2. Lucas C, Johnson W, Hamilton MA, et al. Freedom from congestion predicts good survival despite previous class iv symptoms of heart failure. *Am Heart J.* 2000;140: 840-847.
3. Pitt B, Remme W, Zannad F, et al. Eplerenone, a selective aldosterone blocker, in patients with left ventricular dysfunction after myocardial infarction. *N Engl J Med.* 2003;348:1309-1321.

Anticoagulant therapy in pregnant women with mechanical prosthetic heart valves: no easy option

McLintock C (Auckland City Hosp, New Zealand)
Thromb Res 127:S56-S60, 2011

The choice of anticoagulant agent for pregnant women with mechanical prosthetic heart valves introduces a clinical dilemma for women and the clinicians caring for them. Options include continuing oral anticoagulants (OAC) such as warfarin throughout pregnancy, switching from warfarin to unfractionated heparin or low molecular weight heparin (LMWH) in the first trimester then back to warfarin until close to delivery or taking unfractionated heparin or LMWH throughout pregnancy. The dilemma is that warfarin is the most effective at preventing maternal thromboembolic complications but causes significant fetal morbidity and mortality; unfractionated heparin and in particular LMWH have good fetal outcomes but the risk of thromboembolic complications is high. What is considered to be an "acceptable level" of risk to mother and infant may differ from one clinician to another and of equal importance, it may also differ from one woman to the next. An unbiased discussion of the pros and cons of each option is required to allow women to make and informed and confident choice in this very difficult clinical situation (Fig 1).

▶ The first Starr-Edwards mechanical valve was inserted in 1960.[1] Since then, there has been a difficult dilemma when a patient with a mechanical prosthetic heart valve (MPHV) becomes pregnant. These valves have such a high incidence of thromboembolism without anticoagulation (over 70% in 10 years) that anticoagulation, almost always with warfarin, is mandatory. Even with anticoagulation, the annual risk of thromboembolic events is about 1%.[2] Pregnancy is associated with changes that produce a prothrombotic environment, so anticoagulation is even more essential in patients with MPHV. Oral anticoagulants like warfarin have small molecules that cross the placenta and are teratogenic. Unfractionated heparin and low-molecular-weight heparin don't cross the placenta and avoid the danger of teratogenicity but may be less effective than warfarin in preventing thromboembolism in patients with MPHV. Thus, the dilemma. This article discusses the problems associated with pregnancy in patients with MPHV, the various alternative approaches to keeping the patient

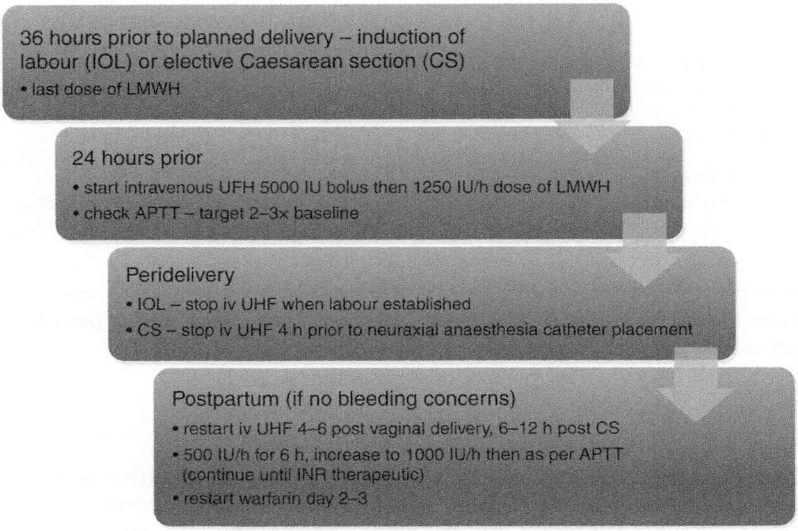

36 hours prior to planned delivery – induction of labour (IOL) or elective Caesarean section (CS)
- last dose of LMWH

24 hours prior
- start intravenous UFH 5000 IU bolus then 1250 IU/h dose of LMWH
- check APTT – target 2–3x baseline

Peridelivery
- IOL – stop iv UHF when labour established
- CS – stop iv UHF 4 h prior to neuraxial anaesthesia catheter placement

Postpartum (if no bleeding concerns)
- restart iv UHF 4–6 post vaginal delivery, 6–12 h post CS
- 500 IU/h for 6 h, increase to 1000 IU/h then as per APTT (continue until INR therapeutic)
- restart warfarin day 2–3

FIGURE 1.—Suggested regimen for peripartum anticoagulation in women with mechanical prosthetic heart valves. APTT: activated partial thromboplastin time; LMWH: low molecular weight heparin; UFH: unfractionated heparin. (Reprinted from Thrombosis Research, McLintock C. Anticoagulant therapy in pregnant women with mechanical prosthetic heart valves: no easy option. *Thromb Res.* 2011;127:S56-S60. Copyright 2011, with permission from Elsevier.)

on warfarin after the first trimester as long as possible, and the possible bridges for maintaining a reasonable state of anticoagulation during the time of the pregnancy that warfarin should not be used. There are discussions of the arguments for and against unfractionated and low-molecular-weight heparin, the peridelivery management of anticoagulation, and the emergency reversal of anticoagulation in the event of overanticoagulation or frank hemorrhage. Pregnant women with an MPHV are at great risk. The only greater risk is to go through the pregnancy unanticoagulated. The physician must inform the patient with the MPHV of the risks of anticoagulation with warfarin and heparin and recommend a program of anticoagulation throughout the pregnancy.

Ultimately, the decision of which drug to take must be made by the informed woman and her family.

M. D. Cheitlin, MD

References

1. Starr A, Edwards ML. Mitral replacement: clinical experience with a ball-valve prosthesis. *Ann Surg.* 1961;154:726-740.
2. McLintock C. Prosthetic heart valves. In: Pavord S, Hunt B, eds. *The Obstetric Haematology Manual.* Cambridge University Press; 2010:109-119.

39 Pediatric Cardiovascular Disease

Comparison of Risk of Hypertensive Complications of Pregnancy Among Women With Versus Without Coarctation of the Aorta

Krieger EV, Landzberg MJ, Economy KE, et al (Children's Hosp Boston, MA; Brigham and Women's Hosp, Boston, MA; et al)
Am J Cardiol 107:1529-1534, 2011

Hypertension is a common consequence of coarctation of the aorta. The frequency of hypertensive complications of pregnancy in women with coarctation in the general population is undefined. In this study, we used the 1998 to 2007 Nationwide Inpatient Sample, a nationally representative data set, to identify patients admitted to an acute care hospital for delivery. The frequency of hypertensive complications of pregnancy was compared between women with and without coarctation. Secondary outcomes, including length of stay, hospital charges, Caesarean delivery, and adverse maternal outcomes, were also assessed. There were an estimated 697 deliveries among women with coarctation, compared to 42,601,409 deliveries by women without coarctation. The frequency of hypertensive complications of pregnancy was 24.1 ± 3.3% for women with coarctation compared to 8.0 ± 0.1% for women without coarctation (multivariate odds ratio [OR] 3.6, 95% confidence interval [CI] 2.5 to 5.2). Preexisting hypertension complicating pregnancy (10.2 ± 2.5% vs 1.0% ± 0.02%, multivariate OR 10.8, 95% CI 5.9 to 19.8) and pregnancy-induced hypertension (13.9 ± 3.0% vs 7.0% ± 0.1%, multivariate OR 2.1, 95% CI 1.3 to 3.3) were more common in women with coarctation. Women with coarctation were more likely to deliver by Caesarean section (41.6 ± 3.3% vs 26.4% ± 0.2%, multivariate OR 2.0, 95% CI 1.4 to 2.8), have adverse cardiovascular outcomes (4.8 ± 2.2% vs 0.3 ± 0.01%, multivariate OR 16.7, 95% CI 6.7 to 41.5), have longer hospital stays, and incur higher hospital charges (both p values <0.0001) than women without coarctation. In conclusion, women with coarctation are more likely to have hypertensive complications of pregnancy, deliver by Caesarean section, have adverse cardiovascular outcomes, have longer hospitalizations, and incur higher hospital charges than women without coarctation.

▶ This article documents the presence of an increased risk of hypertensive problems and cesarean delivery in women with coarctation. Many women have had coarctation surgical repair or percutaneous treatment; these all need follow-up in a center for adults with congenital heart disease and planned obstetric care in collaboration with such a center.

T. P. Graham, Jr, MD

Best Practices in Managing Transition to Adulthood for Adolescents With Congenital Heart Disease: The Transition Process and Medical and Psychosocial Issues: A Scientific Statement From the American Heart Association
Sable C, on behalf of the American Heart Association Congenital Heart Defects Committee of the Council on Cardiovascular Disease in the Young, Council on Cardiovascular Nursing, Council on Clinical Cardiology, and Council on Peripheral Vascular Disease
Circulation 123:1454-1485, 2011

Background.—Children with complex childhood diseases are more likely to survive into adulthood than previously and can expect to live meaningful, productive lives. Ultimately it is necessary to transition them from their pediatric care providers to adult care practitioners. Often there are no structured programs to guide this transition, causing patients and their families as well as the healthcare delivery system emotional and financial stress. Many patients are simply lost to follow-up at this point. At least half of the adults with congenital heart disease (CHD) have complex disease and require specialized providers. Looking ahead, adolescent patients with CHD will require a well-planned, well-executed transition process to be able to successfully transfer to adult care providers. A formal transition program should prepare young adults for the transfer of care while providing uninterrupted care that is patient centered, age and developmentally appropriate, flexible, and comprehensive. The ultimate goal is to optimize the patient's quality of life (QOL), life expectancy, and future productivity. The American Heart Association (AHA) has offered recommendations for this transition process, which were presented in the context of topics pertaining to the care of adolescents and young adults with CHD.

Topics.—The topics explored included underlying concepts specific to transition care; timing for transitions; social and/or family dynamics; health supervision issues; anticipatory guidance with respect to genetic counseling, sexuality, pregnancy, and reproductive issues, exercise, education and career choices, end-of-life, mortality, and advance directives; and issues relevant to patients with developmental delay or disabilities. These were approached from the standpoint of the patient, the family, and the health care practitioner. Also offered was a description of the transition clinic and how it would facilitate the process of transferring care from pediatric to adult providers. The key elements relate to the pretransition phase, which involves preparation for transitioning and focuses on educating the patient and family about what is to come; the transition itself, which is only undertaken when the patient is developmentally mature and includes a standard core educational curriculum; and the transfer phase, which is ideally accomplished after the successful completion of a thoughtful transition process. It is recommended that there be a policy on timing, but that this policy be flexible to meet individual patient needs.

Recommendations.—AHA recommendations and levels of evidence for practice guidelines were provided as appropriate. These were also directed toward the adolescent, parents, or health care provider and offered specific actions to be taken.

Conclusions.—There is an urgent need for programs designed to facilitate the smooth transition of adolescent CHD patients to adult CHD care situations. It is hoped that transition programs will soon become the standard of care so that these patients can achieve their full potential under excellent medical supervision and live meaningful and productive lives.

▶ This very comprehensive statement regarding transition from pediatric cardiac centers to adult congenital heart disease centers contains information for all who are involved with these patients. I have not seen any center that has seamlessly, completely solved the multiple issues involved with this process. This treatise gives the optimal management all can strive for.

T. P. Graham, Jr, MD

Cardiovascular Screening with Electrocardiography and Echocardiography in Collegiate Athletes

Magalski A, McCoy M, Zabel M, et al (Saint Luke's Mid America Heart and Vascular Inst, Kansas City, MO; Lawrence Memorial Hosp, KS; et al)
Am J Med 124:511-518, 2011

Background.—Current guidelines for preparticipation screening of competitive athletes in the US include a comprehensive history and physical examination. The objective of this study was to determine the incremental value of electrocardiography and echocardiography added to a screening program consisting of history and physical examination in college athletes.

Methods.—Competitive collegiate athletes at a single university underwent prospective collection of medical history, physical examination, 12-lead electrocardiography, and 2-dimensional echocardiography. Electrocardiograms (ECGs) were classified as normal, mildly abnormal, or distinctly abnormal according to previously published criteria. Eligibility for competition was determined using criteria from the 36th Bethesda Conference on Eligibility Recommendations for Competitive Athletes with Cardiovascular Abnormalities.

Results.—In 964 consecutive athletes, ECGs were classified as abnormal in 334 (35%), of which 95 (10%) were distinctly abnormal. Distinct ECG abnormalities were more common in men than women (15% vs 6%, $P < .001$) as well as black compared with white athletes (18% vs 8%, $P < .001$). Echocardiographic and electrocardiographic findings initially resulted in exclusion of 9 athletes from competition, including 1 for long QT syndrome and 1 for aortic root dilatation; 7 athletes with Wolff-Parkinson-White patterns were ultimately cleared for participation. (Four received further evaluation and treatment, and 3 were determined to not need treatment.) After multivariable adjustment, black race was a statistically significant predictor of distinctly abnormal ECGs (relative risk 1.82, 95% confidence interval, 1.22-2.73; $P = .01$).

Conclusions.—Distinctly abnormal ECGs were found in 10% of athletes and were most common in black men. Noninvasive screening using both electrocardiography and echocardiography resulted in identification of 9 athletes with important cardiovascular conditions, 2 of whom were excluded from competition. These findings offer a framework for performing preparticipation screening for competitive collegiate athletes.

▶ This study indicates that the addition of an electrocardiogram (ECG) to history and physical exam is useful to identify athletes with cardiovascular abnormalities that require further evaluation and possible treatment before participation in competitive sports. Interestingly, there were no athletes found with hypertrophic cardiomyopathy. The majority of abnormalities were Wolff-Parkinson-White, which resulted in 4 of 7 receiving further evaluation and treatment, and 3 of 7 were determined not to require treatment. Ultimately, 2 athletes were excluded from competition. These data suggest that ECG screening can be useful in this screening process.

T. P. Graham, Jr, MD

PART SEVEN

THE DIGESTIVE SYSTEM

NICHOLAS J. TALLEY, MD, PHD

Introduction

Welcome to this year's selection of the top articles in Gastroenterology. In this year's set, the focus has been on key advances in the luminal gut.

You will read about how to improve outcomes in Crohn disease and the latest on biologic therapy. New insights into eradication therapy options for *Helicobacter pylori* are presented, as standard triple therapy (proton pump inhibitor, clarithromycin, and amoxicillin) is increasingly unsuccessful in curing infection. Furthermore, the controversy surrounding offering *H pylori* therapy to patients with nonulcer dyspepsia is put to bed (yes, eradication therapy does work and is superior to placebo in this setting).

Management of difficult esophageal strictures remains highly challenging and this is included because internists in such cases are often asked by their patients about the plan and prognosis. Complications arising from proton pump inhibitor (PPI) therapy are topical and more on these is included. The possible role of esophagitis in the genesis of Barrett esophagus, a premalignant condition, is newsworthy.

Gastroparesis presents with recurrent vomiting, pain, and weight loss and remains a very challenging condition to manage, so it is worth it to pay attention to nutritional deficiencies. A very rare condition, chronic idiopathic intestinal pseudo-obstruction (CIIP), is encountered by internists, and the benefit of a potent prokinetic available in Europe and Asia (prucalopride) provides some hope that management will improve. Can feeding tube placement complications be eliminated? Maybe so. New information on celiac disease and T-cell lymphoma is presented, and a similar entity after solid organ transplant has been recognized. The natural history of a rare but important and treatable entity, eosinophilic gastroenteritis, is presented.

One of the commonest gastrointestinal disorders encountered day to day by internists is irritable bowel syndrome (IBS) so advances here are welcome. While psychological therapies can definitely help IBS sufferers, the sparse availability of expert practitioners has hindered therapy as an option; now the internet provides a viable alternative based on new trial evidence.

There are other fascinating insights. For example, constipation is now recognized as an early symptom of Parkinson disease that presents before the classic central neurological manifestations. The long-term outcome of surgery for Hirschprung disease is new and fascinating. You will learn whether a vegetarian diet affects diverticular disease. The diagnostic yield of *Clostridium difficile* testing is discussed. The complex topic of when radiofrequency ablation should be offered over surgery in hepatocellular carcinoma (HCC) is included, and new weight loss data are presented.

Summarized in this year's volume is all this and more. We hope you find the offerings interesting and clinically applicable.

Nicholas J. Talley, MD, PhD

40 Esophagus

Systematic review: the use of proton pump inhibitors and increased susceptibility to enteric infection
Bavishi C, DuPont HL (Univ of Texas Health Science Ctr at Houston School of Public Health)
Aliment Pharmacol Ther 34:1269-1281, 2011

Background.—The use of proton pump inhibitors (PPIs) is increasing worldwide. Suppression of gastric acid alters the susceptibility to enteric bacterial pathogens.

Aim.—This systematic review was undertaken to examine the relationship between PPI use and susceptibility to enteric infections by a specific pathogen based on published literature and to discuss the potential mechanisms of PPI enhanced pathogenesis of enteric infections.

Methods.—PubMed, OVID Medline Databases were searched. Search terms included proton pump inhibitors and mechanisms of, actions of, gastric acid, enteric infections, diarrhoea, *Clostridium difficile*, *Salmonella*, *Shigella* and *Campylobacter*.

Results.—The use of PPIs increases gastric pH, encourages growth of the gut microflora, increases bacterial translocation and alters various immunomodulatory and anti-inflammatory effects. Enteric pathogens show variable gastric acid pH susceptibility and acid tolerance levels. By multiple mechanisms, PPIs appear to increase susceptibility to the following bacterial enteropathogens: *Salmonella*, *Campylobacter jejuni*, invasive strains of *Escherichia coli*, vegetative cells of *Clostridium difficile*, *Vibrio cholerae* and *Listeria*. We describe the available evidence for enhanced susceptibility to enteric infection caused by *Salmonella*, *Campylobacter* and *C. difficile* by PPI use, with adjusted relative risk ranges of 4.2–8.3 (two studies); 3.5–11.7 (four studies); and 1.2–5.0 (17 of 27 studies) for the three respective organisms.

Conclusions.—Severe hypochlorhydria generated by PPI use leads to bacterial colonisation and increased susceptibility to enteric bacterial infection. The clinical implication of chronic PPI use among hospitalized patients placed on antibiotics and travellers departing for areas with high incidence of diarrhoea should be considered by their physicians.

▶ Proton pump inhibitors (PPIs) are widely prescribed and until recently felt to be very safe. Over the past few years, several concerns have arisen for patients treated with long-term, particularly high-dose PPIs, including increased risks of hip fracture, pneumonia (both hospital- and community-acquired),

Clostridium difficile infection, and others. This article is a systematic review of increased risk of enteric infections in PPI-treated patients.

Gastric acid has two major functions: it aids in the digestion of food and kills bacteria that may enter the gastrointestinal tract with our food. It has been long known that patients with a total lack of gastric acid (achlorhydria) have changes in both upper and lower gut flora and an increased risk of certain infections. It is important to remember that PPI therapy (even high-dose, twice-daily) does not completely eliminate gastric acid, which has led to a sense of security (perhaps false security) in the use of these agents. These authors were able to make a case for a small, but statistically significant increase in *Salmonella, Campylobacter jejuni,* and *C difficile* infections in PPI-treated patients. There were not enough studies to confirm increased risks of *Escherichia coli*, shigella, cholera, or listeria infections, although they provide some data to suggest an association with these infections as well.

The authors suggest that patients on PPIs should take extra care and avoid high-risk foods and activities, particularly when traveling to areas with an increased risk of the above infections. These seem to be reasonable suggestions. In addition, many patients on high-dose PPIs can be weaned down to lower doses with continued symptom control, and a proportion of patients can even stop their acid blockers all together. These concerns and others have reinvigorated the concept of stepping patients with acid-related symptoms down to the lowest effective dose that provides acceptable control of those symptoms, which should minimize, but perhaps not eliminate, these adverse effects.

K. R. DeVault, MD

Erosive Esophagitis Is a Risk Factor for Barrett's Esophagus: A Community-Based Endoscopic Follow-Up Study
Ronkainen J, Talley NJ, Storskrubb T, et al (Univ of Oulu, Finland; Univ of Newcastle, Australia; Kalix Hosp, Sweden; et al)
Am J Gastroenterol 106:1946-1952, 2011

Objectives.—Symptomatic gastroesophageal reflux disease (GERD) is associated with a significantly increased risk of esophageal adenocarcinoma, but its natural history in the general population is poorly understood. Whether nonerosive reflux disease (NERD) is a risk factor for Barrett's esophagus (BE), the precursor of esophageal adenocarcinoma, is unknown. Furthermore, quantifying the risk of incident BE in those with untreated reflux esophagitis has not been possible. We aimed, in a prospective follow-up study with endoscopy, to evaluate the risk of BE in a cohort from the Swedish general population (the Kalixanda Study).

Methods.—Those with endoscopic or histological findings suggestive of GERD and randomly half of those with NERD ($n = 481$) were invited for follow-up investigation including endoscopy and a validated symptom questionnaire 5 years after the initial study. Multinomial logistic regression was used to estimate relative risk ratios (RRRs) and 95% confidence intervals (CIs) for change in presentation of GERD.

Results.—Of the 405 subjects available for inclusion, endoscopy was performed in 284 (response rate 70.1%). The incidence of BE was 9.9/ 1,000 person-years. Of those with NERD at baseline ($n = 113$), progression to erosive esophagitis was found in 11; 2 developed BE. Erosive esophagitis ($n = 90$) progressed to a more severe grade in 12 and to BE in 8 cases. Erosive esophagitis at baseline was independently associated with BE at follow-up (RRR 5.2; 95% CI 1.2—22.9).

Conclusions.—Compared with being free of GERD at follow-up, erosive esophagitis is a major risk factor for BE (with a fivefold increased risk) after 5 years in the general population.

▶ Current guidelines suggest screening patients with appropriate risk factors for Barrett esophagus (BE), and many experts have advocated that additional screening is not needed unless BE is diagnosed on that original endoscopy. This is unsettling since we believe BE is an acquired condition and it has to start sometime! This group followed patients with erosive esophagitis (EE) or nonerosive reflux disease (NERD) for 5 years. In the 113 with NERD, 11 progressed to EE (9.7%) and 2 progressed to BE (1.8%). Among the 90 with EE, 12 developed a more severe grade of EE (13.3%) and 8 progressed to BE (11.3%). EE was therefore an independent risk factor for the development of BE.

On the surface it appears that this study disproves the concept of a once in a lifetime endoscopy to exclude BE, since it did develop over time. On the other hand, it could be that Barrett was present at the initial endoscopy and actually was prevalent not incident. This could be because of EE masking the appearance of the BE, but could also be because of changes in endoscopic practices (more aggressive approach to biopsy for BE and improved optics) over the 5-year span of the study. Pathology was obtained in a systematic fashion at both endoscopies, and the same endoscopists did both sets of endoscopies, making missed BE less likely. These data also suggest that even in the NERD patients, a normal endoscopy does not get you off the hook for BE, since 1.8% developed BE, but more importantly, 11.3% developed EE, which if you believe these data, puts an additional 1% or 2% at risk for BE. There is no financial analysis associated with this article, but other studies have suggested that Barrett screening and surveillance are effective in a very limited patient profile (older, white men with long-term GERD symptoms). Adding future rescreening examinations would likely make the costs even less appealing.

Currently, reassuring patients with a negative endoscopy continues to seem appropriate. If a patient has continuous symptoms, an additional screening examination at some point (perhaps after 5 or 10 years) is supportable and perhaps may be somewhat cost-effective if combined with screening colonoscopy.

K. R. DeVault, MD

Efficacy of Large-Diameter Dilatation in Cricopharyngeal Dysfunction

Clary MS, Daniero JJ, Keith SW, et al (Thomas Jefferson Univ, Philadelphia, PA)
Laryngoscope 121:2521-2525, 2011

Objectives/Hypothesis.—To investigate patient outcomes with large-diameter bougienage in isolated cricopharyngeal dysfunction and understand how esophageal dilatation can be used as an effective diagnostic and therapeutic modality in treating dysphagia.

Study Design.—Retrospective review.

Methods.—A retrospective chart review was performed on 46 patients meeting the criteria for cricopharyngeal dysphagia from 2004 to 2008 presenting in the outpatient setting. Patients were treated with 60 French esophageal dilators. Outcomes were analyzed as a function of symptomatology, manometry, duration of benefit, and safety.

Results.—Over the period reviewed, 59 dilatations were performed on 46 patients with cricopharyngeal dysfunction. Eight patients were dilated more than once. Four patients were lost to follow-up. The average starting Functional Outcome Swallowing Score (FOSS) was 2.07. Of the patients reviewed, 64.29% experienced an improvement in their FOSS with a median duration of 741 days. There were five minor complications and no major complications.

Conclusions.—In the largest series of esophageal dilatation for cricopharyngeal dysfunction in the literature, we found large-bore bougienage to have significant utility due to its efficacy, ease of use, and safety when compared to other modalities such as botulinum injection, balloon dilatation, and cricopharyngeal myotomy.

▶ The appropriateness and utility of esophageal dilation in patients without a stenosis demonstrated by barium or endoscopic examination remains debatable. Among those who advocate for empiric dilation, the concept that dilating the cricopharyngeal (CP) region may improve dysphagia is often invoked. This study looked at the effect of dilation in patients diagnosed with CP dysfunction demonstrated by an abnormal appearance at barium or manometric examination.

Interestingly, in a previous study, manometric abnormalities were predictive of improvement after dilation.[1] On the other hand, an often quoted study compared balloon dilation (mostly of the distal esophagus) with an 18-mm balloon-to-sham dilation and found no difference.[2] It is possible that some of these patients had CP dysfunction that was not addressed by the dilation, although another small study compared a 56F with 40F dilator and also found no difference.[3] This article required evidence of CP dysfunction for inclusion. It is not clear that similar results would be expected from patients with proximal dysphagia symptoms in whom both studies were normal. The authors used good-sized dilators, starting at 45F and progressing to 60F, although it was not clear how many of the patients were able to be taken up to the maximal diameter. This study supports dilation of the CP area in patients with appropriate symptoms and abnormalities on functional testing. It also supports obtaining functional testing before endoscopy in these patients presenting with dysphagia to more rationally offer dilation.

K. R. DeVault, MD

References

1. Hatlebakk JG, Castell JA, Spiegel J, Paoletti V, Katz PO, Castell DO. Dilatation therapy for dysphagia in patients with upper esophageal sphincter dysfunction—manometric and symptomatic response. *Dis Esophagus*. 1988;11:254-259.
2. Scolapio JS, Gostout CJ, Schroeder KW, Mahoney DW, Lindor KD. Dysphagia without endoscopically evident disease: to dilate or not? *Am J Gastroenterol*. 2001;96:327-330.
3. Lavu K, Mathew TP, Minocha A. Effectiveness of esophageal dilation in relieving nonobstructive esophageal dysphagia and improving quality of life. *South Med J*. 2004;97:137-140.

Endoscopic Management of Difficult or Recurrent Esophageal Strictures
de Wijkerslooth LRH, Vleggaar FP, Siersema PD (Univ Med Ctr Utrecht, The Netherlands)
Am J Gastroenterol 106:2080-2091, 2011

Esophageal strictures are a common problem in gastroenterological practice. In general, the management of malignant or benign esophageal strictures is different and requires a different treatment approach. In daily clinical practice, stent placement is a commonly used modality for the palliation of incurable malignant strictures causing dysphagia, whereas, if available, intraluminal brachytherapy can be considered in patients with a good performance status. Recurrent dysphagia frequently occurs in malignant cases. In case of tissue in-or overgrowth, a second stent is placed. If stent migration occurs, the stent can be repositioned or a second (preferably partially covered) stent can be placed. Food obstruction of the stent lumen can be resolved by endoscopic cleansing. The cornerstone of the management of benign strictures is still dilation therapy (Savary-Gilliard bougie or balloon). There are a subgroup of strictures that are refractory or recur and an alternative approach is required. In order to prevent stricture recurrence, steroid injections into the stricture followed by dilation can be considered. In case of anastomotic strictures or Schatzki rings, incisional therapy is a safe method in experienced hands. Temporary stent placement is a third option before considering self-bougienage or surgery as a salvage treatment. In this review, the most frequently used endoscopic treatment modalities for malignant and benign stricture management will be discussed based on the available literature, and some practical information for the management in daily clinical practice will be provided.

▶ Patients presenting with difficult-to-control esophageal strictures represent a major challenge to endoscopic practice. If these lesions are not controlled, aspiration, weight loss, and the need for tube-based enteral nutrition may be

372 / The Digestive System

required. This systematic review addressed both benign and malignant strictures and offers a reasonable approach to each.

In the patient with malignant dysphagia who is not a candidate for curative resection, the initial approach should include radiation and chemotherapy if appropriate. The endoscopic approach surrounds the use of esophageal stents. The type of stent is dependent on the location with smaller, flexible stents preferred for proximal lesions and larger stents distally. The authors also outline an approach to recurrent obstruction, with poststenting with endoscopic clearance, and placement of additional stents as the options. Finally, some patients cannot maintain their nutrition despite our best efforts and will require enteral tube placement.

Common causes of benign stricture include severe reflux, strictures postsurgery, and radiation-induced strictures. Strictures caused by caustic ingestion and autoimmune diseases are less common but still may be seen. Progressive dilation with peroral dilators or balloons is suggested and may be repeated for up to 5 sessions with the goal of reaching a size of 16 to18 mm. The next step for refractory lesions can include steroid injection and, in the case of difficult rings and anastamotic strictures, incisional therapy. In those who still do not respond, a covered removable stent may be placed to attempt to remodel the stricture open. Finally, self-bougienage or surgery may rarely be needed.

This systematic review provides a very rational approach. Endoscopists who are not comfortable with some of these techniques should consider referral to a specialized esophageal center before giving up on a patient's swallowing function.

K. R. DeVault, MD

41 Gastrointestinal Motility Disorders/ Neurogastroenterology

A Randomized Study Comparing Levofloxacin, Omeprazole, Nitazoxanide, and Doxycycline versus Triple Therapy for the Eradication of *Helicobacter pylori*
Basu PP, Rayapudi K, Pacana T, et al (Columbia Univ, NY; Forest Hills Hosp, NY; et al)
Am J Gastroenterol 106:1970-1975, 2011

Objectives.—Resistance to standard *Helicobacter pylori* (HP) treatment regimens has led to unsatisfactory cure rates in HP-infected patients. This study was designed to evaluate a novel four-drug regimen (three antibiotics and a proton pump inhibitor (PPI)) for eradication of HP infection in treatment-naive patients.

Methods.—Patients with a diagnosis of HP gastritis or peptic ulcer disease confirmed using endoscopy and stool antigen testing were eligible for inclusion in this study. All patients underwent a washout period of 6 weeks from any prior antibiotic or PPI usage. Patients were then randomized to either levofloxacin, omeprazole, nitazoxanide, and doxycycline (LOAD) therapy for 7 days (LOAD-7) or 10 days (LOAD-10), including levofloxacin 250 mg with breakfast, omeprazole 40 mg before breakfast, nitazoxanide (Alina) 500 mg twice daily with meals and doxycycline 100 mg at dinner, or lansoprozole, amoxicillin, and clarithromycin (LAC) therapy for 10 days, which included lansoprozole 30 mg, amoxicillin 1 g with breakfast and dinner, and clarithromycin 500 mg with breakfast and dinner. HP eradication was confirmed by stool antigen testing at least 4 weeks after cessation of therapy.

Results.—Intention-to-treat analysis revealed significant differences ($P < 0.05$) in the respective eradication rates of the LOAD therapies (88.9% (80/90) LOAD-10, 90% (81/90) LOAD-7, 89.4% (161/180) for combined LOAD) compared with those receiving LAC, 73.3% (66/90). There were no differences in adverse effects between the groups.

Conclusions.—This open-label, prospective trial demonstrates that LOAD is a highly active regimen for the treatment of HP in treatment-naive patients.

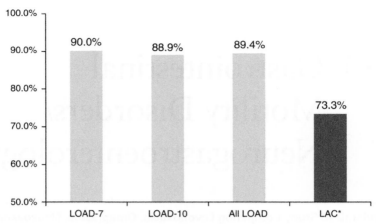

FIGURE 1.—Comparative efficacy, intent-to-treat analysis. *LAC vs. all LOAD, $P = 0.0001$; LAC vs. LOAD-7, $P = 0.006$; LAC vs. LOAD-10, $P = 0.013$. There was no difference between the LOAD regimens as compared with each other. LAC, lansoprozole 30 mg, amoxicillin 1 g with breakfast and dinner, and clarithromycin 500 mg with breakfast and dinner; LOAD, levofloxacin 250 mg with breakfast, omeprazole 40 mg before breakfast, nitazoxanide (Alina®) 500 mg twice daily with meals and doxycycline 100 mg at dinner. (Reprinted from Basu PP, Rayapudi K, Pacana T, et al. A randomized study comparing levofloxacin, omeprazole, nitazoxanide, and doxycycline versus triple therapy for the eradication of *Helicobacter pylori*. *Am J Gastroenterol*. 2011;106:1970-1975. Reprinted by permission from Macmillan Publishers Ltd: American Journal of Gastroenterology, copyright 2011.

A large randomized controlled trial is warranted to further evaluate the efficacy of this regimen (Fig 1).

▶ *Helicobacter pylori* infection may often be asymptomatic but clinically usually presents with dyspepsia. The infection is linked to functional dyspepsia (in a small minority of cases) but more importantly is a major cause of peptic ulcer disease (including bleeding ulcers) and gastric cancer (adenocarcinoma and the rare mucosa-associated lymphoid tissue lymphoma). Although current infection is usually easily diagnosed noninvasively (stool antigen or urea breath testing) or by endoscopy (gastric histology or rapid urease testing), treatment has become much more challenging. Currently approved triple therapy for *H pylori* (proton pump inhibitor, amoxicillin, and clarithromycin) fails in at least 30% of cases, even in compliant patients (and the failure rate is rising presumably secondary to increasing antibiotic resistance). Alternative regimens include bismuth quadruple therapy, but a meta-analysis of randomized controlled trials suggests that this approach is not superior to standard triple therapy. Clinically what is needed is a therapeutic approach that yields in practice at least a 90% cure rate (by intention to treat). This study suggests a levofloxacin-based quadruple regimen is superior to triple therapy (Fig 1). The therapy appeared well tolerated. However, this was an open-label trial, and the results need to be confirmed in blinded trials. Other limitations include questions about the study's generalizability; will the results apply to all ethnic groups (the majority in this study were of Asian descent), and will this work as well when applied as second-line therapy? Overall, these results suggest a 7-day regimen containing levofloxacin, omeprazole, nitazoxanide, and doxycycline may be a viable alternative to standard clarithromycin-based triple therapy in treatment-naïve patients, but more data are needed.

N. Talley, MD

Helicobacter pylori Eradication in Functional Dyspepsia: HEROES Trial
Mazzoleni LE, Sander GB, Francesconi CFDM, et al (Universidade Federal do Rio Grande do Sul, Porto Alegre, Brazil; et al)
Arch Intern Med 171:1929-1936, 2011

Background.—Eradication of *Helicobacter pylori* in patients with functional dyspepsia continues to be a matter of debate. We studied eradication effects on symptoms and quality of life of primary care patients.

Methods.—*Helicobacter pylori*—positive adult patients with functional dyspepsia meeting the Rome III International Consensus criteria were randomly assigned to receive omeprazole, amoxicillin trihydrate, and clarithromycin, or omeprazole plus placebo for 10 days. Endoscopy and *H pylori* tests were performed at screening and at 12 months. Outcome measures were at least 50% symptomatic improvement at 12 months using a validated disease-specific questionnaire (primary end point), patient global assessment of symptoms, and quality of life.

Results.—We randomly assigned 404 patients (78.7% were women; mean age, 46.1 years); 201 were assigned to be treated with antibiotics (antibiotics group) and 203 to a control group. A total of 389 patients (96.3%) completed the study. The proportion of patients who achieved the primary outcome was 49.0% (94 of 192) in the antibiotics group and 36.5% (72 of 197) in the control group ($P = .01$; number needed to treat, 8). In the patient global assessment of symptoms, 78.1% in the antibiotics group (157 of 201) answered that they were better symptomatically, and 67.5% in the control group (137 of 203) said that they were better ($P = .02$). The antibiotics group had a significantly larger increase in their mean (SD) Medical Outcomes Study 36-Item Short Form Health Survey physical component summary scores than the control group did (4.15 [8.5] vs 2.2 [8.1]; $P = .02$).

Conclusion.—*Helicobacter pylori* eradication provided significant benefits to primary care patients with functional dyspepsia.

Trial Registration.—clinicaltrials.gov Identifier: NCT00404534 (Fig 2).

▶ Functional dyspepsia (FD) affects 10% of Americans, although the syndrome is often misdiagnosed as gastroesophageal reflux disease (and accordingly mismanaged). The benefit of eradication of *Helicobacter pylori* in peptic ulcer disease is unequivocally in favor of testing and treating all documented cases (including those with a distant history of peptic ulcer disease). However, much more controversial has been the value of testing and treating patients with chronic dyspepsia (characterized by epigastric pain or epigastric burning or early satiety or postprandial fullness for at least 3 months) and a normal or near-normal endoscopy result (redness of the mucosa counts as normal). Meta-analyses, while mixed, have in

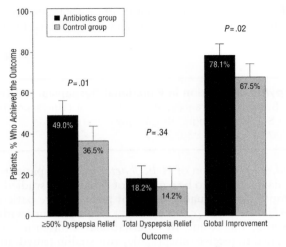

FIGURE 2.—Proportion of patients who achieved response in qualitative outcomes. (Initial: Archives of Internal Medicine, Mazzoleni LE, Sander GB, Francesconi CFDM, et al. *Helicobacter pylori* eradication in functional dyspepsia: HEROES trial. *Arch Intern Med.* 2011;171:1929-1936. American Medical Association. All rights reserved.)

general supported eradication of *H pylori* in improving FD symptoms, and benefits extended out at least a year after ceasing therapy (unlike any other therapies!). This well-conducted randomized, controlled trial from a single center should put any previous uncertainty to bed—all patients with current FD and documented *H pylori* infection deserve to be offered *H pylori* eradication, and a subset will definitely benefit over and above placebo (Fig 2). Concerns about *H pylori* eradication inducing gastroesophageal reflux disease appear overblown. The main limitation of the study is that, unfortunately, there was no control group included who were not infected with *H pylori* (so the apparent benefit of anti-*Helicobacter* therapy might possibly be related to effects elsewhere in the upper gut on the flora and not on elimination of *Helicobacter*). However, the adage "the only good *Helicobacter* is a dead one" seems to apply in FD based on all the available evidence.

N. Talley, MD

Risk of Gastroparesis in Subjects With Type 1 and 2 Diabetes in the General Population

Choung RS, Locke GR III, Schleck CD, et al (Mayo Clinic, Rochester, MN)
Am J Gastroenterol 107:82-88, 2012

Objectives.—In patients with diabetes mellitus (DM) and upper gastrointestinal symptoms, a diagnosis of diabetic gastroparesis is often considered, but population-based data on the epidemiology of diabetic gastroparesis are lacking. We aimed to estimate the frequency of and risk factors for gastroparesis among community subjects with DM.

Methods.—In this population-based, historical cohort study, the medical records linkage system of the Rochester Epidemiology Project was used to identify 227 Olmsted County, MN residents with type 1 DM in 1995, a random sample of 360 residents with type 2 DM, and an age- and sex-stratified random sample of 639 nondiabetic residents. Using defined diagnostic criteria, we estimated the subsequent risk of developing gastroparesis in each group through 2006. The risk in DM, compared with frequency-matched community controls, was assessed by Cox proportional hazards modeling.

Results.—The cumulative proportions developing gastroparesis over a 10-year time period were 5.2% in type 1 DM, 1.0% in type 2 DM, and 0.2% in controls. The age- and gender-adjusted hazard ratios (HRs) for gastroparesis (relative to controls) was 33 (95% confidence interval (CI): 4.0, 274) in type 1 DM and 7.5 (95% CI: 0.8, 68) in type 2 DM. The risk of gastroparesis in type 1 DM was significantly greater than in type 2 DM (HR: 4.4 (1.1, 17)). Heartburn (HR: 6.6 (1.7, 25)) at baseline was associated with diabetic gastroparesis in type 1 DM.

Conclusions.—Gastroparesis is relatively uncommon in patients with DM, although an increased risk for gastroparesis was observed in type 1 DM (Fig 2).

► Gastroparesis is usually diagnosed by a nuclear medicine gastric emptying study (preferably a 4-hour test using a standard meal) in the setting of otherwise unexplained upper gastrointestinal symptoms. However, this definition means some patients with functional dyspepsia (FD) will be mislabeled as

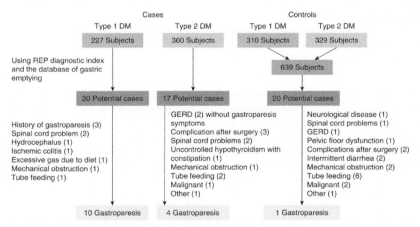

FIGURE 2.—Flow diagram for assessment of diabetic gastroparesis. In 227 cases with type 1 diabetes mellitus (DM), we identified 20 potential cases from the Rochester Epidemiology Project (REP) who may have had gastroparesis and 10 subjects were confirmed to have gastroparesis. In 360 cases with type 2 DM, 17 potential gastroparesis cases were identified and 4 cases were confirmed. Among 639 controls, 20 potential gastroparesis cases were identified, but only 1 subject had confirmed gastroparesis. GERD, gastroesophageal reflux disease. (Reprinted by permission from MacMillan Publishers Ltd. [Initial] American Journal of Gastroenterology, Choung RS, Locke GR III, Schleck CD, et al. Risk of gastroparesis in subjects with type 1 and 2 diabetes in the general population. *Am J Gastroenterol.* 2012;107:82-88. Copyright 2012.

suffering from gastroparesis, as about one-third of FD cases have slow gastric emptying (but treating the gastric emptying per se often fails to improve symptoms in FD). Some have even suggested that the gastric emptying cutoffs for gastroparesis should be tightened to avoid overcalling this disease. Regardless, recent population-based data suggest that idiopathic gastroparesis is really quite rare (and rarer than many expected); in tertiary referral centers even rare diseases can seem common because of referral bias, which seems to also be the case for gastroparesis (with the age-adjusted annual incidence in Olmsted County, Minnesota, being only 2.4 per 100 000 for men and 9.8 per 100 000 for women).[1] This study confirms that diabetes mellitus dramatically increases the risk of gastroparesis, particularly type 1 diabetes (by over 30-fold vs 8-fold in type 1 diabetes). Other evidence suggests poor glycemic control and neuropathy (particularly autonomic neuropathy) account for these dramatic differences between the rates of gastroparesis in types 1 and 2 diabetes. However, arguably the most important observation in this study is how rare gastroparesis is in diabetes (Fig 2). This is largely a disease of the tertiary referral center, and diabetics do not need to be overinvestigated if they present with upper gastrointestinal complaints (which are common).

N. Talley, MD

Reference

1. Jung HK, Choung RS, Locke GR III, et al. The incidence, prevalence, and outcomes of patients with gastroparesis in Olmsted County, Minnesota, from 1996 to 2006. *Gastroenterology.* 2009;136:1225-1233.

Dietary Intake and Nutritional Deficiencies in Patients With Diabetic or Idiopathic Gastroparesis
Parkman HP, for the NIDDK Gastroparesis Clinical Research Consortium (Temple Univ, Philadelphia, PA; et al)
Gastroenterology 141:486-498, 2011

Background & Aims.—Gastroparesis can lead to food aversion, poor oral intake, and subsequent malnutrition. We characterized dietary intake and nutritional deficiencies in patients with diabetic and idiopathic gastroparesis.

Methods.—Patients with gastroparesis on oral intake (N = 305) were enrolled in the National Institute of Diabetes and Digestive and Kidney Diseases Gastroparesis Registry and completed diet questionnaires at 7 centers. Medical history, gastroparesis symptoms, answers to the Block Food Frequency Questionnaire, and gastric emptying scintigraphy results were analyzed.

Results.—Caloric intake averaged 1168 ± 801 kcal/day, amounting to 58% ± 39% of daily total energy requirements (TER). A total of 194 patients (64%) reported caloric-deficient diets, defined as < 60% of estimated TER. Only 5 patients (2%) followed a diet suggested for patients with gastroparesis. Deficiencies were present in several vitamins and minerals; patients with idiopathic disorders were more likely to have diets with estimated deficiencies in vitamins A, B_6, C, K, iron, potassium, and zinc than diabetic patients. Only one-third of patients were taking multivitamin supplements. More severe symptoms (bloating and constipation) were characteristic of patients who reported an energy-deficient diet. Overall, 32% of patients had nutritional consultation after the onset of gastroparesis; consultation was more likely among patients with longer duration of symptoms and more hospitalizations and patients with diabetes. Multivariable logistic regression analysis indicated that nutritional consultation increased the chances that daily TER were met (odds ratio, 1.51; $P = .08$).

Conclusions.—Many patients with gastroparesis have diets deficient in calories, vitamins, and minerals. Nutritional consultation is obtained infrequently but is suggested for dietary therapy and to address nutritional deficiencies.

▶ Anecdotally, an antigastroparesis diet can be helpful in gastroparesis, although no randomized controlled trials of diet have been undertaken in this condition. This is an important study because it suggests that the vast majority of patients with gastroparesis fail to follow an appropriate diet for the disorder (and only one-third ever received any diet counseling); a poor diet may negatively affect outcome. Small frequent meals are better handled by the stomach, as is splitting of solids and liquids. High-fat diets delay gastric emptying, and high fiber may increase satiety and perhaps predispose to bezoar formation (thus a low-fat, low-fiber diet is worth prescribing). Vitamin supplements in this setting are important, as deficiencies are otherwise common. High-protein caloric drinks are useful if caloric intake is insufficient (although gastroparesis can be identified in the obese, and in this study more than 50% were overweight or obese). The results suggest that clinicians must be much more vigilant about dietary management once gastroparesis is diagnosed; referral to a dietician should probably now be standard of care at diagnosis with subsequently regular (eg, annual) dietary review.

N. Talley, MD

Internet-Delivered Exposure-Based Treatment vs. Stress Management for Irritable Bowel Syndrome: A Randomized Trial
Ljótsson B, Hedman E, Andersson E, et al (Karolinska Institutet, Stockholm, Sweden; et al)
Am J Gastroenterol 106:1481-1491, 2011

Objectives.—Our research group has developed an internet-delivered cognitive behavioral treatment (ICBT) for irritable bowel syndrome (IBS). We compared ICBT with internet-delivered stress management (ISM) for IBS to assess whether the effects of ICBT are specific.

Methods.—This was a randomized controlled trial, including 195 self-referred participants diagnosed with IBS. The treatment interventions lasted for 10 weeks and included an online therapist contact. The ICBT emphasized acceptance of symptoms through exposure to IBS symptoms and related negative feelings. The ICBT also included mindfulness training. The ISM emphasized symptom control through relaxation techniques, dietary adjustments, and problem-solving skills. Severity of IBS symptoms was measured with the gastrointestinal symptom rating scale—IBS version (GSRS-IBS). Credibility of the treatments and expectancy of improvement were assessed with the treatment credibility scale. The participants' perceived therapeutic alliance with their online therapist was measured with the working alliance inventory.

Results.—At post-treatment and 6-month follow-up, 192 (99%) and 169 (87%) participants returned data, respectively. At post-treatment and 6-month follow-up, we found significant differences on the GSRS-IBS, favoring ICBT. The difference on GSRS-IBS scores was 4.8 (95% confidence interval (CI): 1.2−8.4) at post-treatment and 5.9 (95% CI: 1.9−9.9) at 6-month follow-up. There were no significant differences on the treatment credibility scale or the working alliance inventory between the groups.

Conclusions.—Internet-delivered CBT has specific effects that cannot be attributed only to treatment credibility, expectancy of improvement, therapeutic alliance, or attention. Furthermore, a treatment based on exposure exercises specifically tailored for IBS may be a better treatment option than general stress and symptom management for IBS patients. ICBT is a promising treatment modality for IBS as it can be offered to IBS patients in much larger scale than conventional psychological treatments (Fig 2).

▶ The management of the irritable bowel syndrome (IBS) refractory to medical management incorporating diet and peripherally active medications (such as a bulking agent or an osmotic laxative for constipation or an antidiarrheal or

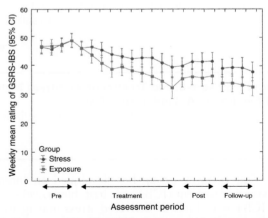

FIGURE 2.—Weekly scores on the GSRS-IBS for both groups during pretreatment, treatment, and post-treatment. Vertical bars denote 95 % confidence interval (CI). GSRS-IBS, gastrointestinal symptom rating scale—IBS version. (Reprinted by permission Ljótsson B, Hedman E, Andersson E, et al. Internet-delivered exposure-based treatment vs. stress management for irritable bowel syndrome: a randomized trial. *Am J Gastroenterol.* 2011;106:1481-1491. Copyright 2011. Reprinted by permission from Macmillan Publishers Ltd: *American Journal of Gastroenterology.*)

anticholinergic drug for loose stools) remains difficult; often antidepressant therapy is tried next, but many patients do not wish to consider centrally active drugs or fail such therapy. Psychological therapy is recognized to be a safe alternative but is unavailable in most practice settings. This article suggests that there is a new solution for some patients—delivery of efficacious psychological therapy over the Internet in the privacy of one's own home. There is reasonable evidence that psychological therapy delivered face-to-face by a therapist is superior to usual management or placebo in IBS; a meta-analysis reported the number needed to treat was 4, and although the best studied approach is cognitive-behavioral therapy (CBT), there is a lack of convincing evidence that one method of psychological therapy is superior to another in IBS.[1] The current trial used a novel type of CBT based on helping patients expose themselves to their IBS symptoms (eg, after eating) and the related negative feelings and reducing avoidance behaviors (eg, not going to the bathroom for relief), combined with specific mindfulness exercises, so that patients could learn to accept more readily their negative symptom experiences. Impressively, the CBT methodology applied was significantly better than standard stress reduction management (Fig 2). For example, at the end of therapy, 69% of those receiving Internet-delivered CBT over 10 weeks had adequate relief of IBS pain or discomfort compared with 58% receiving similarly Internet-delivered stress reduction (although this difference was not significant). However, at the 6-month follow-up off therapy, 65% who had undergone CBT versus 44% who had completed stress reduction therapy reported adequate relief (this was statistically significant). The results were not influenced by baseline symptom severity. Differences in patients' expectations regarding improvement or general support did not seem to explain the results. It therefore seems reasonable to conclude that Internet delivery of psychological therapy is feasible for patients with IBS, and a CBT approach, at least in this trial, was superior to standard stress reduction. Notably, psychological therapy was disappointing for at least one-third of patients applying this form of CBT, and these were largely well-educated, Internet-savvy and presumably motivated volunteers who may not be representative of IBS sufferers in general. Regardless, one suspects it will not be long before commercial companies begin to offer Internet-based psychological interventions for IBS sufferers, although sorting out genuine providers may then become problematic.

N. Talley, MD

Reference

1. Ford AC, Talley NJ, Schoenfeld PS, Quigley EM, Moayyedi P. Efficacy of antidepressants and psychological therapies in irritable bowel syndrome: systemic review and meta-analysis. *Gut.* 2009;58:367-378.

Double-Blind Randomized Controlled Trial of Rifaximin for Persistent Symptoms in Patients with Celiac Disease

Chang MS, Minaya MT, Cheng J, et al (Columbia Univ College of Physicians and Surgeons, NY; Virginia Commonwealth Univ, Richmond; et al)
Dig Dis Sci 56:2939-2946, 2011

Background.—Small intestinal bacterial overgrowth (SIBO) is one cause of a poor response to a gluten-free diet (GFD) and persistent symptoms in celiac disease. Rifaximin has been reported to improve symptoms in noncontrolled trials.

Aims.—To determine the effect of rifaximin on gastrointestinal symptoms and lactulose-hydrogen breath tests in patients with poorly responsive celiac disease.

Methods.—A single-center, double-blind, randomized, controlled trial of patients with biopsy-proven celiac disease and persistent gastrointestinal symptoms despite a GFD was conducted. Patients were randomized to placebo ($n = 25$) or rifaximin ($n = 25$) 1,200 mg daily for 10 days. They completed the Gastrointestinal Symptom Rating Scale (GSRS) and underwent lactulose-hydrogen breath tests at weeks 0, 2, and 12. An abnormal breath test was defined as: (1) a rise in hydrogen of ≥ 20 parts per million (ppm) within 100 min, or (2) two peaks ≥ 20 ppm over baseline.

Results.—GSRS scores were unaffected by treatment with rifaximin, regardless of baseline breath tests. In a multivariable regression model, the duration of patients' gastrointestinal symptoms significantly predicted their overall GSRS scores (estimate 0.029, $p < 0.006$). According to criteria 1 and 2, respectively, SIBO was present in 55 and 8% of patients at baseline, intermittently present in 28 and 20% given placebo, and 28 and 12% given rifaximin. There was no difference in the prevalence of SIBO between placebo and treatment groups at weeks 2 and 12.

Conclusions.—Rifaximin does not improve patients' reporting of gastrointestinal symptoms and hydrogen breath tests do not reliably identify who will respond to antibiotic therapy (Fig 2).

▶ A troubling problem in clinical practice is what to do with a patient who has biopsy-proven celiac disease who after several weeks or more of a gluten-free diet still complains about dyspepsia, gas, bloating, abdominal pain, and diarrhea or constipation. Checking into dietary compliance and confirming serological remission, followed by ensuring the diagnosis was correct in the first place, are reasonable first steps. But what next? Celiac disease, gluten intolerance without histological evidence for celiac disease, and irritable bowel syndrome (IBS) overlap more than expected by chance, so IBS may explain residual symptoms in some cases. In the textbooks and the literature, small intestinal bacterial overgrowth (SIBO) is listed as a reason why diet alone may fail in celiac disease,[1] and IBS has been associated with an increased rate of SIBO, although the association is controversial. One nonspecific method of identifying SIBO is by lactulose-hydrogen breath testing (although false-positive breath testing will occur if small bowel transit is fast and the sugar bolus reaches the cecum promptly). In

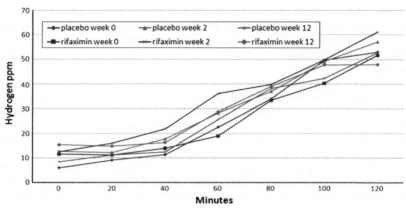

FIGURE 2.—Hydrogen breath test measurements for placebo and rifaximin at weeks 0, 2, and 12. (Reprinted from Chang MS, Minaya MT, Cheng J, et al. Double-blind randomized controlled trial of rifaximin for persistent symptoms in patients with celiac disease. *Dig Dis Sci.* 2011;56:2939-2946. Copyright 2011, with kind permission from Springer Science+Business Media, LLC.)

uncontrolled studies, rifaximin has been reported to induce symptom improvement in patients with celiac disease and residual gastrointestinal symptoms,[2] but these observations have not held up in the present randomized controlled trial. However, SIBO based on abnormal breath testing was uncommon in the population recruited and was not eliminated by rifaximin, which may reflect the poor utility of the test (Fig 2). Overall the results do suggest a nonabsorbable antibiotic is unlikely to help patients with celiac disease who have refractory gastrointestinal symptoms, and other management approaches need to be considered.

N. Talley, MD

References

1. Rubio-Tapia A, Barton SH, Rosenblatt JE, Murray JA. Prevalence of small intestine bacterial overgrowth diagnosed by quantitative culture of intestinal aspirate in celiac disease. *J Clin Gastroenterol.* 2009;43:157-161.
2. Tursi A, Brandimarte G, Giorgetti G. High prevalence of small intestinal bacterial overgrowth in celiac patients with persistence of gastrointestinal symptoms after gluten withdrawal. *Am J Gastroenterol.* 2003;98:839-843.

Randomised clinical trial: the efficacy of prucalopride in patients with chronic intestinal pseudo-obstruction - a double-blind, placebo-controlled, cross-over, multiple $n = 1$ study

Emmanuel AV, Kamm MA, Roy AJ, et al (Univ College, London, UK; St Vincent's Hosp & Univ of Melbourne, Australia; et al)
Aliment Pharmacol Ther 35:48-55, 2012

Background.—Chronic intestinal pseudo-obstruction is a disabling condition for which there are no established drug therapies. The condition is caused by a diverse range of intestinal myopathies and neuropathies.

Aim.—To assess the therapeutic efficacy of prucalopride, a selective high-affinity 5-HT$_4$ receptor agonist, we employed a multiple $n = 1$ study design. Each patient acted as his/her own control, each day counting as one treatment episode, allowing comparison of 168 days on each of active drug and placebo.

Methods.—Double-blind, randomised, placebo-controlled, cross-over trial of four 12-week treatment periods, with 2–4 mg prucalopride or placebo daily. In each of the first and second 6 months there was a prucalopride and a placebo treatment. Patients with proven chronic intestinal pseudo-obstruction, including dilated gut, were included. Evaluation was by patient diary and global evaluation.

Results.—Seven patients participated (mean 42 years, five female, median symptom duration 11 years). Three discontinued, two due to study length, and one on prucalopride due to unrelated malnutrition and bronchopneumonia. Four patients (three visceral myopathy and one visceral neuropathy) completed the study; prucalopride significantly improved pain in three of

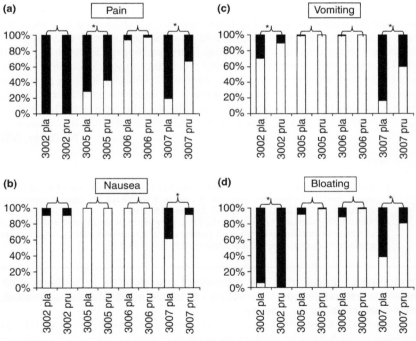

FIGURE 1.—Proportion of days with symptoms (dark) vs. no symptoms (light) for (a) pain, (b) nausea, (c) vomiting and (d) bloating for each of the four patients completing the study. Each number (pair of bars) represents a different patient, for whom all days on placebo and active drug have been summed. *Statistically significant reduction ($P < 0.05$) of symptoms with prucalopride vs. placebo. Pru, Prucalopride; Pla, Placebo. (Reprinted from Emmanuel AV, Kamm MA, Roy AJ, et al. Randomised clinical trial: the efficacy of prucalopride in patients with chronic intestinal pseudo-obstruction - a double-blind, placebo-controlled, cross-over, multiple $n = 1$ study. *Aliment Pharmacol Ther.* 2012;35:48-55, with permission from Blackwell Publishing Ltd. and John Wiley and Sons)

four patients, nausea in two, vomiting in one, bloating in four and analgesic intake. Bowel function was not changed substantially.

Conclusions.—$n = 1$ studies in rare conditions allow drug efficacy assessment. Prucalopride relieves symptoms in selected patients with chronic pseudo-obstruction (Fig 1).

▶ Chronic idiopathic intestinal pseudo-obstruction (CIIP) is a very rare but important condition, characterized by unexplained symptoms consistent with intestinal obstruction (pain, vomiting, distention, and constipation but sometimes diarrhea or both). It can overlap with gastroparesis and colonic inertia. Intestinal dilatation is characteristic but may be absent. The diagnosis is confirmed by excluding mechanical obstruction (don't miss a small hernia!) and either gastroduodenal manometry (to document a neuropathic or myopathic motility pattern) or more invasively by a full thickness intestinal biopsy at laparoscopy (to document neuropathy or myopathy). CIIP is usually idiopathic (we are the idiots—we don't know the cause), but sometimes may occur in the setting of degenerative neurological or autoimmune disease. Treatment is challenging—maintaining nutritional status, treating bacterial overgrowth if present, and managing symptoms (especially pain) are often necessary. Narcotics must be used very cautiously as they can worsen the problem. Prokinetics may help, but few are available aside from metoclopramide, which offers little in terms of effects on the small intestine. Cisapride has shown some very modest efficacy but is only available for compassionate use in some countries. Erythromycin and azithromycin (motilin agonists) are not of established efficacy, and domperidone probably is not of benefit. Prucalopride is a serotonin type 4 receptor agonist available in Europe and Australia that is established to be efficacious in chronic constipation. The current elegant multiple $n = 1$ randomized controlled study of prucalopride in CIIP suggests it is also of value for pain and bloating, and perhaps vomiting, in this difficult-to-manage syndrome (Fig 1). Referral to an expert center is recommended for patients with CIIP.

N. Talley, MD

Defecation Disorders in Children After Surgery for Hirschsprung Disease
Chumpitazi BP, Nurko S (Children's Hosp Boston, MA)
J Pediatr Gastroenterol Nutr 53:75-79, 2011

Background and Objective.—The majority of children with Hirschsprung disease (HD) after corrective surgery (CS) develop protracted defecation disorders (DDs) such as constipation, fecal incontinence, and/or enterocolitis. The aim of this investigation was to determine the diagnoses, therapies, and long-term clinical outcomes using a systematic algorithm to address protracted DD in children with HD after CS.

Methods.—Retrospective review of children with HD after CS cared for using a systematic algorithm at a tertiary care center. Potential anatomic etiologies were evaluated for first. Clinical outcome was categorized into 4 groups based on symptom severity, time interval from last enterocolitis episode, laxative usage, and/or rectal therapies at the time of last follow-up.

Results.—Fifty-seven children were identified, of whom 51 (89.5%) had obstructive symptoms and/or enterocolitis and 6 (10.5%) had nonretentive fecal incontinence. Nonintractable constipation responsive to laxatives was identified in 10 (17.5%), colonic dysmotility in 4 (7.0%), nonrelaxing anal sphincter as a primary etiology in 22 (38.6%), bacterial overgrowth in 2 (3.5%), food intolerance in 2 (3.5%), and rapid transit in 2 (3.5%). Further surgical intervention was undertaken in 22 (38.6%), including 9 (15.8%) for residual aganglionosis. Mean follow-up was 41.4 ± 4.5 months. Clinical outcomes were excellent in 16 (28.1%), good in 22 (38.6%), fair in 1 (1.8%), and poor in 18 (31.6%). Children with enterocolitis were more likely to have an excellent or good clinical outcome.

Conclusions.—The majority of children with HD and protracted DD after CS have a favorable long-term clinical outcome when following a systematic algorithm (Figs 1 and 2).

▶ Hirshsprung disease is a rare but important cause of chronic constipation; although usually diagnosed in children, it can also catch our adult gastroenterologists and surgeons treating patients with constipation. After a firm diagnosis has been made (anorectal manometry showing a failure of relaxation of the internal anal sphincter in response to distention, followed by deep rectal biopsies to confirm aganglionosis), corrective surgery is the treatment of choice. However, it is important to understand that a substantial number of patients (up to 60%) continue to be troubled by long-term constipation and other

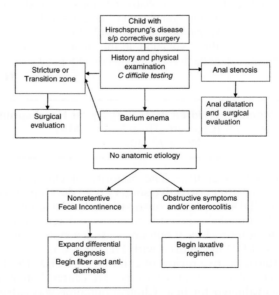

FIGURE 1.—Initial diagnostic and treatment algorithm for a child with Hirschsprung disease after corrective surgery presenting with a defecation disorder and/or enterocolitis. (Reprinted from Chumpitazi BP, Nurko S. Defecation disorders in children after surgery for Hirschsprung disease. *J Pediatr Gastroenterol Nutr.* 2011;53:75-79. © by the AAP

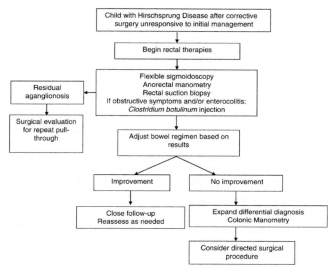

FIGURE 2.—Diagnostic and therapeutic algorithm for a child with Hirschsprung disease and defecation disorders and/or enterocolitis unresponsive to initial management. (Reprinted from Chumpitazi BP, Nurko S. Defecation disorders in children after surgery for Hirschsprung disease. *J Pediatr Gastroenterol Nutr.* 2011;53:75-79. © by the AAP.)

symptoms (including, less commonly, fecal incontinence). This article presents new data on long-term clinical outcomes and an approach to management in this difficult situation (Figs 1 and 2) and is worth a careful read by all who look after such cases. More than a quarter of cases required resurgery for residual aganglionosis or mechanical obstruction (eg, a stricture). Notably, making the correct diagnosis led to a good outcome in two-thirds of cases.

N. Talley, MD

A Prospective Study of Bowel Movement Frequency and Risk of Parkinson's Disease
Gao X, Chen H, Schwarzschild MA, et al (Brigham and Women's Hosp and Harvard Med School, Boston, MA; Natl Inst of Environmental Health Sciences, NC; Massachusetts General Hosp, Boston)
Am J Epidemiol 174:546-551, 2011

The authors prospectively examined bowel movement frequency at baseline in relation to future Parkinson's disease risk in the Health Professionals Follow-up Study (HPFS) during 2000–2006 (33,901 men) and the Nurses' Health Study (NHS) during 1982–2006 (93,767 women). During the follow-up (6 years for the HPFS and 24 years for the NHS), the authors identified 156 incident male Parkinson's disease cases (HPFS) and 402 female cases (NHS). In the HPFS, compared with men with daily bowel movements, men with a bowel movement every 3 days or less had a

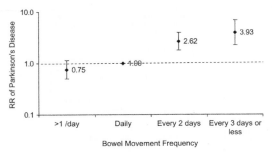

FIGURE 1.—Pooled relative risk (RR) of Parkinson's disease onset during the first 6 years of follow-up in the Health Professionals Follow-up Study (2000–2006) and the Nurses' Health Study (1982–1988). Adjusted for age (in months), smoking (never smoker, past smoker, or current smoker: cigarettes/day, 1–14 or ≥15), body mass index (<23, 23–24.9, 25–26.9, 27–29.9, or ≥30 kg/m^2), use of nonaspirin nonsteroidal antiinflammatory drugs (yes/no), laxatives (none, <1 time/month, 1–4 times/month, or ≥1 time/week), and intakes of alcohol (none, 1–4.9, 5–9.9, 10–14.9, or ≥15 g/day for women; none, 1–9.9, 10–19.9, 20–29.9, or ≥30 g/day for men), caffeine (quintiles), and lactose (quintiles). $P_{\text{trend}} < 0.0001$. Bars, confidence intervals. (Reprinted from Gao X, Chen H, Schwarzschild MA, et al. A prospective study of bowel movement frequency and risk of Parkinson's disease. *Am J Epidemiol.* 2011;174:546-551, with permission of Oxford University Press.)

multivariate-adjusted relative risk of 4.98 (95% confidence interval (CI): 2.59, 9.57) for developing Parkinson's disease in the next 6 years. In the NHS, the corresponding relative risk was 2.15 (95% CI: 0.76, 6.10), and the risk of Parkinson's disease was not elevated beyond 6 years of follow-up (relative risks = 1.25 for years 7–12, 0.54 for years 13–18, and 0.88 for years 19–24). When these 2 cohorts were combined, the pooled relative risks for Parkinson's disease in the next 6 years were 0.75, 1 (referent), 2.62, and 3.93 (95% CI: 2.26, 6.84) ($P_{\text{trend}} < 0.0001$) across 4 bowel movement categories. In conclusion, infrequent bowel movements may antedate the onset of cardinal motor symptoms of Parkinson's disease and may contribute to the identification of populations with higher than average Parkinson's disease risk (Fig 1).

▶ Constipation is common in Parkinson's disease, which may occur secondary to the disease process itself (from damage to the dorsal nucleus of the vagus or the myenteric plexus) or as a result of constipating medication use. However, accumulating data suggest that the new-onset constipation often precedes the onset of Parkinson's disease and represents a potential early marker of disease risk. In this large, well-conducted, prospective study of health professionals and nurses, the risk of Parkinson's disease increased with decreasing stool frequency (Fig 1). Presumably, this association reflects that constipation is an early marker of neurologic disease, but the remote possibility that constipation per se is causally linked to Parkinson's disease cannot be excluded, perhaps through changes in the intestinal microflora or via the accumulation of neurotoxins. In older patients in whom constipation newly develops, the possibility of the development of Parkinson's disease needs to be kept in mind by clinicians. Whether more aggressive treatment of constipation in this setting has any additional benefits is unknown.

N. Talley, MD

42 Inflammatory Bowel Disease

Is Obesity a Risk Factor for Crohn's Disease?

Mendall MA, Gunasekera AV, John BJ, et al (Mayday Univ Hosp, Croydon, UK)

Dig Dis Sci 56:837-844, 2011

Background.—Obesity is associated with a proinflammatory state.

Aim.—To determine whether obesity at diagnosis is a risk factor for Crohn's disease vs. ulcerative colitis and also vs. community controls and whether there is a U-shaped relationship between body mass index at diagnosis and risk of Crohn's disease versus ulcerative colitis.

Methods.—A total of 524 consecutive inflammatory bowel disease patients attending gastroenterology clinics were administered a questionnaire inquiring about weight at diagnosis and height as well as other risk factors for inflammatory bowel disease. An opportunistic control group of 480 community controls aged 50–70 were randomly selected from the registers of four local general practices as part of another study.

Results.—Obesity at diagnosis was more common in subjects with Crohn's disease versus ulcerative colitis odds ratio 2.02 (1.18–3.43) $p = 0.0096$ and also Crohn's disease versus community controls in the 50–70 year age group (odds ratio 3.22 (1.59–6.52) $p = 0.001$). There was evidence of a 'dose response' with increasing degrees of obesity associated with increased risk. Low BMI at diagnosis was also associated with risk of Crohn's disease versus ulcerative colitis. A U-shaped relationship between BMI and risk of Crohn's was supported by the strong inverse association of BMI at diagnosis ($p = 0.0001$) and positive association of BMI at diagnosis squared ($p = 0.0002$) when they were fitted together into the model.

Conclusions.—Obesity may play a role in the pathogenesis of Crohn's disease and it may be that obesity-related enteropathy is a distinct entity or a sub-type of Crohn's disease.

▶ Obesity has been linked to the onset of numerous diseases. In this article, the authors make a good case for biologic plausibility for obesity leading to older-age-onset inflammatory bowel disease. Their findings of higher risk of later-age-at-onset Crohn disease (CD) among those with obesity are interesting. Unfortunately, their ability to draw clear conclusions is hampered by limitations in their data. The main measurement of the study, body mass index (BMI), was left to patient recall and not verified in 25% of cases. They did find there was no difference overall in obesity rates between CD and ulcerative colitis (UC). However, in those diagnosed after age 45, over twice as many subjects with CD were obese compared with UC patients. They interpreted this finding as support against recall bias because there was no apparent reason that there should be differential recall between CD and UC. Numbers of subjects in the older age group were small. Unfortunately, we do not know what proportion of the reported BMI in each group was self-reported and not verified. They did, however, show that in a subset in which they compared reported BMI with verified BMI at diagnosis, the results were similar. Interestingly, site of CD did not matter, especially because in most series, the proportion with Crohn colitis is higher in those diagnosed at an older age. It was also surprising that a link to obesity was found at all, because many patients will have signs and symptoms of CD for years before diagnosis that would potentially lead to weight loss. Overall, they did a good job of adjusting for potential biases in their data and managed to demonstrate a consistent association of obesity with the development of CD. Although they do not claim to demonstrate causality, their results are provocative and suggest that obesity may be related to the development of older-age-onset CD.

M. F. Picco, MD

Does the severity of primary sclerosing cholangitis influence the clinical course of associated ulcerative colitis?

Marelli L, Xirouchakis E, Kalambokis G, et al (Royal Free Hosp, London, UK)
Gut 60:1224-1228, 2011

Background and Aims.—Ulcerative colitis (UC) associated with primary sclerosing cholangitis (PSC) is usually clinically mild. The aim of the study was to assess whether there is an association between severity of PSC and activity of UC, comparing the course of UC in patients with PSC not needing liver transplantation (LT) and those eventually transplanted.

Methods.—Between 1990 and 2009, 96 consecutive patients with PSC/UC were seen in the authors' institution. Data were evaluated from a database regarding UC activity (median follow-up 144 months). Follow-up was censored at time of LT or last clinical review.

Results.—Patients with PSC/UC were divided into two groups: 46 did not need LT (no-LT) and 50 were transplanted (LT). There were no significant differences concerning duration of UC or PSC and extent of UC. The LT group had significantly ($p = 0.002$) more clinically quiescent UC compared with the no-LT group. The LT group had fewer UC flare-ups ($p = 0.04$) and required fewer steroid courses ($p = 0.025$) with shorter duration ($p = 0.022$) and less use of azathioprine ($p = 0.003$). There was an increased need for surgery in the no-LT group ($p = 0.006$). Colon carcinoma and high grade dysplasia were more frequent in the no-LT group ($p = 0.004$). The no-LT group had increased inflammation in the colonic mucosa at histology ($p = 0.011$), but without visual difference at colonoscopy.

Conclusions.—Clinically progressive PSC requiring LT is associated with a milder course of UC (reduced disease activity and less use of steroids, azathioprine and surgery). This is paralleled by less histological activity and reduced incidence of dysplasia and colon carcinoma.

▶ The relationship between ulcerative colitis (UC) and primary sclerosing cholangitis (PSC) is complex and not clearly understood. UC tends to have a milder course when accompanied by PSC, but colon cancer risk is higher. Ursodiol, which is often prescribed for PSC, may result in a lower risk of colon cancer, but this remains controversial. The relationship of UC disease activity in the setting of PSC pre- and posttransplant is also not completely known. In this study, the authors found that PSC severity was inversely correlated with activity of UC and colorectal cancer (CRC) risk. Is this due to the severity of the PSC, or are there other potential explanations? The study was retrospective, and the liver transplant (LT) and nontransplant groups were reasonably matched, but the LT group was significantly younger. This could have resulted in a lower cancer risk compared with the non-LT group. Patients with more severe PSC in the LT group may have had different follow-up (ie, more clinic visits) compared with the non-LT group. LT patients may have had more colonoscopies, increasing the chance of dysplasia detection and lowering the risk of cancer. Despite this possibility, detection of low-grade dysplasia was higher in the non-LT group, suggesting a real effect, but high-grade dysplasia and CRC were higher in the non-LT group, which might suggest differences in the frequency of colonoscopies. More clinic visits could also lead fewer disease flares because of enhanced medication compliance and closer clinical attention. Data on number of follow-up visits and colonoscopies were not provided. We are also not provided information on mesalamine use, which could affect UC relapse rates, and ursodiol use, which might affect CRC rates. Azathioprine use was more common in the non-LT group, which supports the authors' conclusions on differences in severity. Unfortunately, a multivariate analysis was not performed to adjust for impact of important potential confounding variables such as age on disease course and CRC development. Overall, the study findings are interesting but do not definitively address the relationship of PSC to UC disease severity and CRC risk.

M. F. Picco, MD

Outcomes of Patients With Crohn's Disease Improved From 1988 to 2008 and Were Associated With Increased Specialist Care
Nguyen GC, Nugent Z, Shaw S, et al (Univ of Toronto, Ontario, Canada; Univ of Manitoba, Winnipeg, Canada)
Gastroenterology 141:90-97, 2011

Background & Aims.—We investigated factors that affect long-term outcomes in Crohn's disease (CD).

Methods.—We performed a retrospective study of 3403 patients with CD, diagnosed between 1988 and 2008 in Manitoba, Canada. Subjects were assigned to cohorts based on diagnosis year: cohort I (before 1996), cohort II (1996—2000), or cohort III (2001 and after). We compared risks for surgery and hospitalization among the cohorts and assessed use of immunomodulators and specialists.

Results.—The 5-year risks of first surgery were 30%, 22%, and 18% for cohorts I, II, and III, respectively. The adjusted hazard ratios for first surgery in cohorts II and III, compared with cohort I, were 0.72 (95% confidence interval [CI], 0.62—0.84) and 0.57 (95% CI, 0.48—0.68), respectively. The adjusted hazard ratio for cohort III, compared with cohort II, was 0.79 (95% CI, 0.65—0.97). There was a higher prevalence of visits to a gastroenterologist within the first year of diagnosis among cohorts II and III (cohort I, 53%; cohort II, 72%; and cohort III, 88%; $P < .0001$), which was associated with a reduced need for surgery (hazard ratio, 0.83; 95% CI, 0.71—0.98) and contributed to differences in surgery rates among the cohorts. The association between early gastroenterology care and lower risk for surgery was most evident 2 years after diagnosis (hazard ratio, 0.66; 95% CI, 0.53—0.82). Use of immunomodulators within the first year of diagnosis was higher in cohort III than in cohort II (20% vs 11%; $P < .0001$).

Conclusions.—Risk of surgery decreased among patients with CD diagnosed after, compared with before, 1996, and was associated with specialist care. Specialist care within 1 year of diagnosis might improve outcomes in CD.

▶ In this study, care of patients with Crohn disease (CD) by gastroenterologists was associated with a lower risk of surgery. This conclusion was supported by a carefully conducted analysis of data from Manitoba Health, which is the universal health care provider covering all of the 1.2 million residents of Manitoba, Canada. Surprisingly, overall rates of surgery were low (39% at 20 years) compared with reports as high as 70% at 15 years from other centers. Surgery rates did decrease with time and were lowest among those who had seen a gastroenterologist within 1 year of diagnosis. It took at least 2 years to see the difference, suggesting the effects may have been related to earlier use of immunomodulator or biologic therapy. Patients who did see a gastroenterologist were nearly 2 times more likely to receive an immunomodulator. Overall rates of immunomodulator use were low (32% within 5 years of diagnosis) but increased with time. Infliximab use was extremely low with only 5% of patients receiving this medication within 5 years of their diagnosis. These findings are important because, as the authors state, use of these agents was reserved for sicker patients and they were prescribed in a step-up manner. Earlier use of immunomodulators and biologics (top down) may lead to even more dramatic differences. More studies like this one are needed to justify early specialist care and intervention with aggressive therapy to alter the natural history of CD in select patients. Appropriate patient selection for aggressive top-down therapy and knowledge of the complexities of such therapy remain key to better outcomes. This intervention is best provided by specialists with expertise in this area.

M. F. Picco, MD

Adalimumab sustains steroid-free remission after 3 years of therapy for Crohn's disease

Kamm MA, Hanauer SB, Panaccione R, et al (St Vincent's Hosp and the Univ of Melbourne, Victoria, Australia; Univ of Chicago, IL; Univ of Calgary, Alberta, Canada; et al)

Aliment Pharmacol Ther 34:306-317, 2011

Background.—Treatments that achieve sustainable steroid-free clinical remission in Crohn's disease are needed; however, long-term steroid-sparing efficacy data are limited.

Aim.—To evaluate steroid-sparing efficacy and the impact of steroid discontinuation on adverse events during treatment of Crohn's disease with adalimumab in the phase III randomised, double-blind 1-year CHARM trial and for an additional 2 years in its open-label extension ADHERE.

Methods.—Steroid-free remission and response and steroid-sparing (≥50% steroid dose reduction) remission rates were evaluated over 3 years in patients who were taking corticosteroids at CHARM baseline.

Results.—Of 778 patients randomised in CHARM (including those who did not achieve clinical response to open-label induction therapy), 313 patients (40%) were on corticosteroids at baseline. In the 206 patients randomised to adalimumab, rates of steroid-free remission at 1 year and 3 years were 26% and 23% respectively; corresponding rates were 29% and 25% for steroid-sparing remission and 32% and 28% for steroid-free response. Although the incidence of serious infections with adalimumab treatment during CHARM was higher in patients taking steroids at baseline than those who were not, the rates of overall adverse events, serious infections and opportunistic infections were lower in patients who were able to discontinue corticosteroids than those who remained on steroids.

Conclusion.—Adalimumab therapy resulted in modest but clinically meaningful rates of steroid-free remission, sustained over 3 years of treatment, in a heavily pretreated population of patients with Crohn's disease receiving steroids at the start of therapy (http://www.clinicaltrials.gov number: NCT00077779).

▶ Adalimumab is a well-established biologic therapy in Crohn disease. It is generally considered equivalent to infliximab and certolizumab. Like these other agents, experience beyond 1 year of therapy is lacking. In this study, the authors followed patients over 3 years who had been previously enrolled in the CHARM study. CHARM enrolled patients after open-label adalimumab induction therapy with placebo, then weekly or every other week adalimumab for 1 year. Failures after week 12 could then move to open label every other week or weekly adalimumab. This study looked at patients who completed CHARM and were enrolled in an open-label extension study (ADHERE) for an additional 2 years. Patients were started on every-other-week adalimumab (40 mg) if they had received placebo or continued on every other week therapy if they received it during CHARM. The main objective was to measure steroid-sparing long term. Patients who were able to wean off steroids in CHARM managed to stay off steroids over the next 2 years. The study also showed that 50% of patients who received long-term adalimumab therapy eventually required weekly therapy. Patients who had received steroids for the shortest amount of time (< 3 months) before enrolling in CHARM were most likely to wean off steroids. This is not surprising because patients on steroids for longer periods may have more severe disease or have been more likely to experience complications and less likely to be treatment-responsive. These results are encouraging, demonstrate the benefit of long-term adalimumab therapy, and support accepted clinical practice.

M. F. Picco, MD

Crohn's Disease and Small Bowel Adenocarcinoma: A Population-Based Case–Control Study
Shaukat A, Virnig DJ, Howard D, et al (VA Med Ctr and Univ of Minnesota, Minneapolis; Emory Univ, Atlanta, GA; et al)
Cancer Epidemiol Biomarkers Prev 20:1120-1123, 2011

Background.—Although Crohn's disease (CD) is thought to predispose to adenocarcinomas of the small bowel, the association has not been well studied in an older population.

Aims.—The objective of our study was to evaluate the association of CD with small bowel cancer in a population-based case–control study.

Methods.—All cases of small bowel cancer in persons 67 and older in the Surveillance, Epidemiology and End Results catchment area and in the Medicare claims data base were compared with cancer-free controls residing in the same geographic area. We used multivariable logistic regression models adjusted for demographic and other factors.

Results.—We identified 923 cases of small bowel cancer and 142,273 controls. Although we found a strong association between CD and small bowel cancer (OR = 12.07; 95% CI: 6.07–20.80; $P < 0.001$), the prevalence of CD in patients with small bowel cancer was low (1.6%).

Conclusions.—Although CD is a significant risk factor for small bowel cancers among individuals older than 67, the absolute risk is small.

Impact.—Older individuals with CD can be reassured that although there is an association between CD and small bowel cancer, the absolute risk remains small.

▶ Crohn disease (CD) is a well-established risk factor for small bowel adenocarcinoma. Although the odds of small bowel adenocarcinoma among patients with CD was increased 12-fold, this risk remains extremely small. The authors' conclusions are based on an analysis of Surveillance, Epidemiology and End Results (SEER)—Medicare. SEER is a program that captures cancer incidence and survival data from different regions in the United States. Linkage to Medicare claims data allows for analysis of patient characteristics that may affect cancer incidence and outcomes. The results, although interesting, were not surprising, and because of the small numbers of cases and the data sets used, further important details could not be determined. We are restricted to an elderly population. CD is a heterogeneous disease, and a breakdown of disease location would have been important. Most cases (41%) involved the duodenum compared with ileum (23%). Few patients with CD have duodenal involvement. It would also have been interesting to look at prescription data to determine whether previous use of immunomodulator or biologic agents affected risk in CD. If an increased risk was found, it may be associated with the drugs or possibly a worse disease course. Unfortunately, many questions remain, but we are reassured by the overall low risk. However, this article should serve as a reminder that, although rare, small bowel neoplasms should be considered among certain patients without a history of CD or with established disease refractory to medical therapy who present with small bowel pathology. Biopsy confirmation is essential in such patients.

M. F. Picco, MD

43 Nutrition and Celiac Disease

FERGIcor, a Randomized Controlled Trial on Ferric Carboxymaltose for Iron Deficiency Anemia in Inflammatory Bowel Disease
Evstatiev R, for the FERGI Study Group (Med Univ of Vienna, Austria; et al)
Gastroenterology 141:846-853, 2011

Background & Aims.—Iron deficiency anemia (IDA) is common in chronic diseases and intravenous iron is an effective and recommended treatment. However, dose calculations and inconvenient administration may affect compliance and efficacy. We compared the efficacy and safety of a novel fixed-dose ferric carboxymaltose regimen (FCM) with individually calculated iron sucrose (IS) doses in patients with inflammatory bowel disease (IBD) and IDA.

Methods.—This randomized, controlled, open-label, multicenter study included 485 patients with IDA (ferritin < 100 μg/L, hemoglobin [Hb] 7–12 g/dL [female] or 7–13 g/dL [male]) and mild-to-moderate or quiescent IBD at 88 hospitals and clinics in 14 countries. Patients received either FCM in a maximum of 3 infusions of 1000 or 500 mg iron, or Ganzoni-calculated IS dosages in up to 11 infusions of 200 mg iron. Primary end point was Hb response (Hb increase $\geq$ 2 g/dL); secondary end points included anemia resolution and iron status normalization by week 12.

Results.—The results of 240 FCM-treated and 235 IS-treated patients were analyzed. More patients with FCM than IS achieved Hb response (150 [65.8%] vs 118 [53.6%]; 12.2% difference, $P = .004$) or Hb normalization (166 [72.8%] vs 136 [61.8%]; 11.0% difference, $P = .015$). Both treatments improved quality of life scores by week 12. Study drugs were well tolerated and drug-related adverse events were in line with drug-specific clinical experience. Deviations from scheduled total iron dosages were more frequent in the IS group.

Conclusions.—The simpler FCM-based dosing regimen showed better efficacy and compliance, as well as a good safety profile, compared with the Ganzoni-calculated IS dose regimen (Fig 2 and Table 1).

▶ Anemia caused by iron deficiency is common in a number of chronic diseases. It is particularly common in inflammatory bowel disease and often affects as many as half of all patients. It has previously been recognized that correcting or improving the iron-deficiency anemia in these patients can result

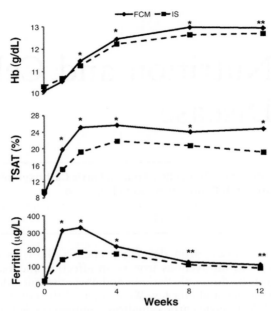

FIGURE 2.—Time courses of patients' Hb, TSAT, and ferritin levels show earlier and consistently better improvement of Hb and iron status with the FCM regimen compared with the IS regimen. *$P < .001$ and **$P \leq .015$ for changes vs baseline. (Reprinted from Gastroenterology, Evstatiev R, for the FERGI Study Group. FERGIcor, a randomized controlled trial on ferric carboxymaltose for iron deficiency anemia in inflammatory bowel disease. *Gastroenterology.* 2011;141:846-853. Copyright 2011, with permission from the AGA Institute.)

TABLE 1.—Total Iron Dose With the FCM Dose Regimen

Hb (g/dL)	Body Weight <70 kg	Body Weight ≥70 kg
≥10	1000 mg	1500 mg
7–10	1500 mg	2000 mg

NOTE. Total dosage was administered in single infusions of 500 mg or 1000 mg iron as FCM. For patients with a body weight <67 kg, single doses of 500 mg were given.

in significant improvement in quality of life. However, oral iron is often either ineffective or poorly tolerated in these patients. In addition, iron deficiency can be associated with thrombocytosis, and correcting this could theoretically reduce the risk of thrombosis in patients with inflammatory bowel disease. This study is a randomized, controlled, open-label trial of ferric carboxymaltose (FCM) in a total dose iron infusion determined by weight and hemoglobin (Table 1) compared with a calculated total iron need achieved with a series of iron sucrose (IS) injections utilizing an individually calculated dose—the Ganzoni formula[1]—total iron dose = (body weight × [target hemoglobin− actual hemoglobin]) × 2.4 + iron storage depot of 500 mg.

The primary endpoint was hemoglobin increase of ≥ 2 g/dL at 12 weeks compared with baseline as well as cost-effective analysis. A total of 485 subjects of 880 screened individuals were randomly assigned; most completed the study.

The subjects with ferric carboxymaltose achieved the primary endpoint 65% of the time, and those with iron sucrose 53.6% of the time, which was significantly different. In addition, normalization of hemoglobin was found more frequently in the FCM group than the IS group. Both treatment groups improved significantly with their Inflammatory Bowel Disease Questionnaire scores as well as Health Survey Short Form scores. Cost-effectiveness analysis also indicated earlier and consistently better improvement of hemoglobin and iron status with the FCM regimen compared with the IS regimen (Fig 2).

Iron-deficiency anemia is frequent in inflammatory bowel disease and can be corrected in the majority of patients with a total dose iron infusion using ferric carboxymaltose. It appears to be superior to the Ganzoni formula fractional administration with iron sucrose. The differences in efficacy may be because of the different total doses of iron given; the iron dose in the FCM protocol was 1377 ± 381 mg, whereas with IS it was 1160 ± 316 mg. This study demonstrates that it is practical to correct iron-deficiency anemia in patients with inflammatory bowel disease within a 12-week period utilizing total dose iron infusion. The standard formula for determining total dose iron infusion for iron sucrose is less effective. Both regimens appeared safe.

The availability of newer iron agents in the United States will require regulatory approval, but this approach is likely to generate more widespread treatment for iron-deficiency anemia in patients with inflammatory bowel disease. FCM is not currently available in the United States.

J. A. Murray, MD

Reference

1. Ganzoni AML. Intravenous iron-dextran: therapeutic and experimental possibilities. *Schweiz Med Wochenschr.* 1970;100:301-303.

Enteropathy-associated T-cell lymphoma: clinical and histological findings from the International Peripheral T-Cell Lymphoma Project
Delabie J, Holte H, Vose JM, et al (Univ Hosp of Oslo, Norway; Univ of Nebraska Med Ctr, Omaha; et al)
Blood 118:148-155, 2011

Few large, international series of enteropathy-associated T-cell lymphoma (EATL) have been reported. We studied a cohort of 62 patients with EATL among 1153 patients with peripheral T-cell or natural killer (NK)—cell lymphoma from 22 centers worldwide. The diagnosis was made by a consensus panel of 4 expert hematopathologists using World Health Organization (WHO) criteria. Clinical correlations and survival analyses were performed. EATL comprised 5.4% of all lymphomas in the study and was most common in Europe (9.1%), followed by North America (5.8%) and Asia (1.9%). EATL type 1 was more common (66%) than type 2 (34%), and was especially frequent in Europe (79%). A clinical diagnosis of celiac sprue was made in 32.2% of the patients and was associated with both EATL type 1 and type 2. The median overall survival was only 10 months, and the median failure-free survival was only 6 months. The International Prognostic Index (IPI) was not as good a predictor of survival as the Prognostic Index for Peripheral T-Cell Lymphoma (PIT). Clinical sprue predicted for adverse survival independently of the PIT. Neither EATL subtype nor other biologic parameters accurately predicted survival. Our study confirms the poor prognosis of patients with EATL and the need for improved treatment options.

▶ Celiac disease has classically been associated with enteropathy-associated T-cell lymphoma (EATL). Recently, celiac disease has been reported to be associated with both T-cell and B-cell lymphomas. This article documents an association between celiac disease and enteropathy-associated lymphoma in European and North American patients from this very large international Peripheral T-Cell Lymphoma Project, which incorporated 22 referral centers around the world. They found that celiac disease was associated with both EATL type 1 and type 2. There is a greater frequency of celiac disease in the European individuals with EATL than in North American, and both of these locations were much more frequently associated with celiac disease than Asia. In some of these subjects, the celiac disease diagnosis was available from clinical history. However, in others, the celiac disease was identified by examining the adjacent nonneoplastic intestinal epithelium (Fig 3 in original article).

This illustrates the importance of considering celiac disease in patients who present with proximal small intestinal tumors, a finding previously reported for adenocarcinoma of the small intestine.[1]

The clinical significance of this study is the high prevalence of celiac disease in patients with EATL, the fact that the celiac disease itself can be overlooked until EATL is diagnosed, and the relative rarity of this type of tumor among lymphomas in general.

Lastly, the survival of patients with EATL type 1 is substantially worse than in patients with celiac disease, and it appears to be related to failure of the EATL to respond to chemotherapy. The discovery of EATL in a patient with known celiac disease or celiac disease in a patient with newly diagnosed EATL should warrant prompt multidisciplinary and aggressive supportive management in order to effect improvement in outcome.

J. A. Murray, MD

Reference

1. Potter DD, Murray JA, Donohue JH, et al. The role of defective mismatch repair in small bowel adenocarcinoma in celiac disease. *Cancer Res.* 2004;64:7073-7077.

Duodenal Villous Atrophy: A Cause of Chronic Diarrhea After Solid-Organ Transplantation

Weclawiak H, Ould-Mohamed A, Bournet B, et al (CHU Rangueil, Toulouse, France; et al)

Am J Transplant 11:575-582, 2011

Persistent diarrhea is commonly observed after solid organ transplantation (SOT). A few cases of mycophenolate mofetil (MMF)-induced duodenal villous atrophy (DVA) have been previously reported in kidney-transplant patients with chronic diarrhea. Herein, we report on the incidence and characteristics of DVA in SOT patients with chronic diarrhea. One hundred thirty-two SOT patients with chronic diarrhea underwent an oesophago-gastroduodenoscopy (OGD) and a duodenal biopsy after classical causes of diarrhea have been ruled out. DVA was diagnosed in 21 patients (15.9%). It was attributed to mycophenolic acid (MPA) therapy in 18 patients (85.7%) (MMF [n = 14] and enteric-coated mycophenolate sodium [n = 4]). MPA withdrawal or dose reduction resulted in diarrhea cessation. The incidence of DVA was significantly higher in patients with chronic diarrhea receiving MPA compared to those who did not (24.6% vs. 5.1%, $p = 0.003$). DVA was attributed to a Giardia lamblia parasitic infection in two patients (9.5%) and the remaining case was attributed to azathioprine. In these three patients, diarrhea ceased after metronidazole therapy or azathioprine dose reduction. In conclusion, DVA is a frequent cause of chronic diarrhea in SOT recipients. MPA therapy is the most frequent cause of DVA. An OGD should be proposed to all transplant recipients who present with persistent diarrhea.

▶ It has long been known that a variety of medications can damage the intestine. These include drugs that are common causes of acute and chronic diarrhea, such as nonsteroidal anti-inflammatories and chemotherapeutic agents, among others. Solid organ transplantation is frequently complicated by gastrointestinal upset posttransplantation. Chronic diarrhea may affect as many as 20% of solid organ transplant recipients. This study examines and essentially establishes the role for mycophenolate mofetil as a cause of duodenal and villous atrophy in kidney transplant recipients. This was a systematic evaluation of consecutive patients seen with chronic diarrhea after kidney transplantation. The study identified 21 patients in whom duodenal villous was obtained. Other causes of villous atrophy, including celiac disease, were ruled out. Patients responded to withdrawal of the medication. The importance of this study is to bring to the attention the frequency with which this commonly used antirejection medication can cause severe injury to the intestine and chronic inflammation. Of course, other disorders, including infections of *Clostridium difficile*, *Campylobacter jejuni*, and *Giardia lambia*, are also important causes of diarrhea after transplantation.

J. A. Murray, MD

Collagenous Ileitis: A Study of 13 Cases

O'Brien BH, McClymont K, Brown I (Royal Brisbane and Women's Hosp, Queensland, Australia; Sullivan Nicolaides Pathology, Brisbane, Australia)
Am J Surg Pathol 35:1151-1157, 2011

Collagenous ileitis (CI), characterized by subepithelial collagen deposition in the terminal ileum, is an uncommon condition. The few cases reported to date have been associated with collagenous colitis (CC) or lymphocytic colitis. Thirteen cases of CI retrieved over a 9-year period were retrospectively studied. There were 7 female and 6 male patients, with an age range of 39 to 72 years (mean, 64 y). Two groups were identified: (1) CI associated with collagenous or lymphocytic disease elsewhere in the gastrointestinal tract and (2) CI as an isolated process. Diarrhea was the presenting symptom in 11 cases. Most patients had no regular medication use. Subepithelial collagen thickness ranged from 15 to 100 μm (mean, 32 μm) and involved 5% to 80% of the subepithelial region of the submitted biopsies. Six cases had > 25 intraepithelial lymphocytes (IELs)/100 epithelial cells, and villous blunting was observed in 11 cases. Chronic inflammation of the lamina propria was present in 9 cases, and focal neutrophil infiltration was identified in 3 cases. In biopsies taken from other sites, 7 of 13 colonic biopsies showed CC, 4 of 9 gastric biopsies showed collagenous gastritis, and 2 of 10 duodenal biopsies were abnormal with collagenous sprue (n = 1) and partial villous atrophy and increased IELs (n = 1) (both celiac disease related). Resolution of the subepithelial collagen deposition was found in the 1 case in which follow-up of terminal ileal biopsies were taken. There was partial or complete resolution of symptoms in 6 of 9 patients for whom follow-up information was available.

▶ Inflammatory conditions of the intestine associated with collagen deposition have long been recognized; however, they are rare, with the exception of collagenous colitis. Disorders, including collagenous gastritis[1] and collagenous sprue,[2,3] although rare, have been increasingly reported in adults. The etiology of these disorders is unclear, but associations with medications, autoimmune disorders, and celiac disease have been described. This study reviews findings in a series of patients with collagenous ileitis. Many of these patients had symptoms typical for inflammatory conditions, and a significant minority had inflammatory and often collagenous conditions elsewhere within the GI tract. The mechanism through which excess collagen is deposited in the intestinal tract is not well understood. A similar condition is that of chronic human immunodeficiency virus (HIV) enteropathy. In the context of patients who have chronic HIV infection managed by highly active antiretroviral therapy, chronic inflammation and collagen deposition in the intestinal lamina propria develop. This article by O'Brien et al brings together a series of patients with a relatively new entity of collagenous ileitis. The cause of collagenous ileitis is still an enigma in most of the patients presented. What is not known is the specific impact that collagenous ileitis has on patients, especially those who have other disorders. Also, treatment needs to be better defined. Anecdotal reports of benefits from steroids and immu-nosuppressives have been reported for collagenous sprue.[2]

J. A. Murray, MD

References

1. Leung ST, Chandan VS, Murray JA, Wu TT. Collagenous gastritis: histopathologic features and association with other gastrointestinal diseases. *Am J Surg Pathol.* 2009;33:788-798.
2. Rubio-Tapia A, Talley NJ, Gurudu SR, Wu TT, Murray JA. Gluten-free diet and steroid treatment are effective therapy for most patients with collagenous sprue. *Clin Gastroenterol Hepatol.* 2010;8:344-349.e3.
3. McCashland TM, Donovan JP, Strobach RS, Linder J, Quigley EM. Collagenous enterocolitis: a manifestation of gluten-sensitive enteropathy. *J Clin Gastroenterol.* 1992;15:45-51.

Natural History of Eosinophilic Gastroenteritis

de Chambrun GP, Gonzalez F, Canva J-Y, et al (Univ Lille Nord de France; UDSL, Lille, France)
Clin Gastroenterol Hepatol 9:950-956.e1, 2011

Background & Aims.—Eosinophilic gastroenteritis (EGE) is a rare gastrointestinal disorder; little is known about its natural history. We deter-mined the clinical features and long-term outcomes of patients with EGE.

Methods.—We reviewed files from 43 patients diagnosed with EGE who were followed from January 1988 to April 2009. The diagnosis was made according to standard criteria after other eosinophilic gastrointestinal disorders were excluded. We analyzed data on initial clinical presentation and long-term outcomes.

Results.—EGE was classified as mucosal, subserosal, or muscular in 44%, 39%, and 12% of cases, respectively. Disease location was mostly duodenal (62%), ileal (72%), or colonic (88%); it was less frequently esophageal (30%) or gastric (38%). Blood eosinophilia (numbers > 500/mm^3) was observed in 74% of cases. Spontaneous remission occurred in 40% of patients; the majority of treated patients (74%) received oral corti-costeroids, which were effective in most cases. After a median follow-up period of 13 years (0.8–29 years), we identified 3 different courses of disease progression: 18 patients (42%; 9 with subserosal disease) had an initial flare of the disease without relapse, 16 (37%) had multiple flares that were separated by periods of full remission (recurring disease), and 9 (21%) had chronic disease.

Conclusions.—The clinical presentation of EGE is heterogeneous and varies in histologic pattern; about 40% of patients resolve the disease spon-taneously, without relapse. Approximately 50% have a more complex dis-ease, which is characterized by unpredictable relapses and a chronic course.

▶ Eosinophilic gastroenteritis is a relatively rare disorder, and this group followed a consecutive series of 43 patients seen at a single center over

404 / The Digestive System

20 years. Slightly less than half of these had mucosal involvement, with subserosal or muscular involvement in 39% and 12% of patients, respectively. Most patients had colonic ileal or duodenal involvement, with upper gut involvement being less frequent, and a majority of patients had significant peripheral eosinophilia. Most patients responded to oral steroids, and a significant minority (40%) had spontaneous remission. In summary, eosinophilic gastroenteritis is a heterogeneous condition with a significant number of patients who will have a spontaneous remission, but in whom half will have unpredictable relapse or a chronic course of disease. In addition, peripheral eosinophilia seemed to predict the high likelihood of relapse.

J. A. Murray, MD

Repeat Stool Testing to Diagnose *Clostridium difficile* Infection Using Enzyme Immunoassay Does Not Increase Diagnostic Yield
Deshpande A, Pasupuleti V, Patel P, et al (Cleveland Clinic, OH; et al)
Clin Gastroenterol Hepatol 9:665-669.e1, 2011

Background & Aims.—*Clostridium difficile* infection (CDI) is a hospital-acquired infection with increasing incidence and severity. The most frequently used test to diagnose CDI is an enzyme immunoassay (EIA) for toxins A and B in stool samples. It is common to test 2 or more stool samples, based on the assumption that this detects CDI with greater sensitivity than analysis of 1 sample. We investigated whether repeat stool testing significantly improves the diagnostic yield for CDI.

Methods.—We performed a retrospective analysis of hospitalized patients who were tested for CDI using EIA. From year 2005 to 2008, 39,402 stool samples from 17,971 patients with 29,373 diarrhea episodes were tested. Transition probabilities were calculated based on results from repeated tests.

Results.—A total of 2692 diarrheal episodes (9.17%) were diagnosed with CDI. Based on results of 3 consecutive tests, 2675 (99.36%) were diagnosed with CDI. The first stool sample tested produced positive results for 90.7% of cases. When samples were tested consecutively, for the second and third time, an additional 6.6% and 2% patients had positive test results, respectively. If the first test result was negative, the probability of the second test result being positive was 2.7%. If the first 2 test results were negative, the probability of the third test result being positive was 2.3%.

Conclusions.—In patients who had multiple stool samples tested for CDI by EIA, almost 91% were accurately diagnosed based on the results of a single stool sample alone. Subsequent testing yielded a positive result in only 8.6% of patients. We therefore recommend that repeat testing not be done on a routine basis because it does not significantly improve diagnostic yield.

▶ *Clostridium difficile* has become an increasingly common hospital-acquired and community-acquired infection. In the hospital, it is associated with substantial morbidity and even mortality. The standard approach to evaluation has been the detection of toxins A and B using enzyme immunoassay. As a test, this is cost effective and technologically easy with a quick turnaround time. Sensitivities vary somewhat. A common practice is to test 3 consecutive stool samples; the variability of sensitivities reported for tests have largely driven this repeat test strategy. This large, retrospective study evaluates the experience of hospitalized patients who underwent successive testing. Over a 3-year period, almost 40 000 stool samples were tested for *C difficile*. Over 2600 episodes were characterized as *C difficile* infections. Most, over 90%, were positive on the first sample. In those negative on the first sample, the positive rate for subsequent samples was less than 3%, with a similarly low positive rate for patients with 2 successive negative samples. The sensitivity of 2 tests was over 97%, suggesting that persistent, repeat testing for *C difficile* may not provide any additional benefit. Although the strength of the study is largely the inclusion of all subjects, some lack of details on clinical correlation and correlation with Polymerase chain reaction (PCR) are also potentially important. Being able to refine these results for prediction of pretest prevalence by such factors as age, morbidities, immuno-compromise, and patients not on enteral feeding may be important. Also, whether patients had prior inflammatory bowel disease may also influence the pretest probability. However, this study shows that there seems to be little advantage to multiple repeat tests in patients who are initially negative, consistent with clinical practice guidelines published in 2010.[1] Exceptions may occur in patients with very high pretest prevalence, such as patients with toxic megacolon-type picture, and the use of additional novel testing methodologies such as PCR may be necessary.

J. A. Murray, MD

Reference

1. Cohen SH, Gerding DN, Johnson S, et al. Clinical practice guidelines for *Clostridium difficile* infection in adults: 2010 update by the Society for Healthcare Epidemiology of America (SHEA) and the Infectious Diseases Society of America (IDSA). *Infect Control Hosp Epidemiol.* 2010;31:431-455.

High Levels of Folate From Supplements and Fortification Are Not Associated With Increased Risk of Colorectal Cancer
Stevens VL, McCullough ML, Sun J, et al (American Cancer Society, Atlanta, GA)
Gastroenterology 141:98-105.e1, 2011

Background & Aims.—Folate intake has been inversely associated with colorectal cancer risk in several prospective epidemiologic studies. However, no study fully assessed the influence of the high levels of folate that are frequently consumed in the United States as a result of mandatory folate fortification, which was fully implemented in 1998, and the recent increase in use of folate-containing supplements. There is evidence that consumption of high levels of folic acid, the form of folate used for fortification and in supplements, has different effects on biochemical pathways than natural folates and might promote carcinogenesis.

Methods.—We investigated the association between folate intake and colorectal cancer among 43,512 men and 56,011 women in the Cancer Prevention Study II (CPS-II) Nutrition Cohort; 1023 were diagnosed with colorectal cancer between 1999 and 2007, a period entirely after folate fortification began. Cox proportional hazards regression was used to calculate multivariate hazards ratios (RR) and 95% confidence interval (CI).

Results.—Intake of high levels of natural folate ($RR_{Q5vsQ1} = 0.86$; 95% CI: 0.70−1.06; P trend = .12) or folic acid ($RR_{Q5vsQ1} = 0.84$; 95% CI: 0.68−1.03; P trend = .06) were not significantly associated with risk of colorectal cancer. Total folate intake was significantly associated with lower risk ($RR_{Q5vsQ1} = 0.81$; 95% CI: 0.66−0.99; P trend = .047).

Conclusions.—Intake of high levels of total folate reduces risk of colorectal cancer; there is no evidence that dietary fortification or supplementation with this vitamin increases colorectal cancer risk.

▶ Many epidemiologic studies have supported the conclusion that folate intake reduces the risk of colorectal cancer. However, the intake of folate, reflected by serum levels of folate in Americans, has more than doubled since mandatory folate supplementation was introduced in the late 1990s. This supplementation has led to a reduction in spina bifida and other neural tube defects. This high rate of folate consumption, mainly from artificial folic acid, has many potential effects on the pathways that could either retard or promote carcinogenesis. Concerns have been raised that such a high level of folate supplementation might actually increase carcinogenesis. This is based on observations in the Polyp Prevention Trial that individuals who received high levels of folate supplementation had a higher rate of development of advanced lesions in those with prior colorectal adenomas.[1] This very large prospective study followed almost 100 000 individuals for incidence cases of colorectal cancer following the introduction of mandatory folate supplementation. The estimated total folate ingestion combined natural folate as well as synthetic folic acid. Not only did these researchers confirm the beneficial effects of folic acid in reduction of colorectal carcinoma risk, but they also demonstrated that this benefit could be derived both from natural and synthetic folate. Most important, they showed no increase in the incidence of colorectal cancers. This study provides reassurance that folate supplementation of a level of 800 µg per day is quite safe and should not increase the risk of colorectal cancer while also having a substantial benefit in terms of reduced colorectal cancer occurrence over time. One caveat is the follow-up may not be of sufficient duration to fully understand all of the potential effects and likely benefits of a diet replete in folate.

J. A. Murray, MD

Reference

1. Cole BF, Baron JA, Sandler RS, et al; Polyp Prevention Study Group. Folic acid for the prevention of colorectal adenomas: a randomized clinical trial. *JAMA.* 2007; 297:2351-2359.

Diet and risk of diverticular disease in Oxford cohort of European Prospective Investigation into Cancer and Nutrition (EPIC): prospective study of British vegetarians and non-vegetarians

Crowe FL, Appleby PN, Allen NE, et al (Univ of Oxford, UK)
BMJ 343:d4131, 2011

Objective.—To examine the associations of a vegetarian diet and dietary fibre intake with risk of diverticular disease.

Design.—Prospective cohort study.

Setting.—The EPIC-Oxford study, a cohort of mainly health conscious participants recruited from around the United Kingdom.

Participants.—47 033 men and women living in England or Scotland of whom 15 459 (33%) reported consuming a vegetarian diet.

Main Outcome Measures.—Diet group was assessed at baseline; intake of dietary fibre was estimated from a 130 item validated food frequency questionnaire. Cases of diverticular disease were identified through linkage with hospital records and death certificates. Hazard ratios and 95% confidence intervals for the risk of diverticular disease by diet group and fifths of intake of dietary fibre were estimated with multivariate Cox proportional hazards regression models.

Results.—After a mean follow-up time of 11.6 years, there were 812 cases of diverticular disease (806 admissions to hospital and six deaths). After adjustment for confounding variables, vegetarians had a 31% lower risk (relative risk 0.69, 95% confidence interval 0.55 to 0.86) of diverticular disease compared with meat eaters. The cumulative probability of admission to hospital or death from diverticular disease between the ages of 50 and 70 for meat eaters was 4.4% compared with 3.0% for vegetarians. There was also an inverse association with dietary fibre intake; participants in the highest fifth (≥ 25.5 g/day for women and ≥ 26.1 g/day for men) had a 41% lower risk (0.59, 0.46 to 0.78; $P < 0.001$ trend) compared with those in the lowest fifth (< 14 g/day for both women and men). After mutual adjustment, both a vegetarian diet and a higher intake of fibre were significantly associated with a lower risk of diverticular disease.

Conclusions.—Consuming a vegetarian diet and a high intake of dietary fibre were both associated with a lower risk of admission to hospital or death from diverticular disease.

▶ Diverticulae of the colon are very common in the developed world, and complications are a relatively common cause of morbidity and occasionally mortality. It has been regarded as largely a disease of the developed world. Little is known about the dietary factors that predispose to the development or complications of colonic diverticulosis. This study of a large population of UK residents followed up for many years has shown a significant protective effect of high fiber or vegetarian diet, reducing the risk of complications of diverticular disease. We cannot tell, however, if it is a reduction in the development of diverticulosis or if it modifies the risk of complications occurring from such.

Nonetheless, it would support the broad adoption of a higher-fiber diet. What it does not tell us is if the intervention of increasing fiber in someone with already-established diverticular disease or even its complications will affect the risk of future complications.

J. A. Murray, MD

Enteral and Parenteral Nutrition in the Conservative Treatment of Pancreatic Fistula: A Randomized Clinical Trial
Klek S, Sierzega M, Turczynowski L, et al (Jagiellonian Univ Med College, Krakow, Poland)
Gastroenterology 141:157-163, 2011

Background & Aims.—Postoperative pancreatic fistula is the most common and potentially life-threatening complication after pancreatic surgery. Although nutritional support is a key component of conservative therapy in such cases, there have been no well-designed clinical trials substantiating the superiority of either total parenteral nutrition or enteral nutrition. This study was conducted to compare the efficacy and safety of both routes of nutritional intervention.

Methods.—A randomized clinical trial was conducted in a tertiary surgical center of pancreatic and gastrointestinal surgery. Seventy-eight patients with postoperative pancreatic fistula were treated conservatively and randomly assigned to groups receiving for 30 days either enteral nutrition or total parenteral nutrition. The primary end point was the 30-day fistula closure rate.

Results.—After 30 days, closure rates in patients receiving enteral and parenteral nutrition were 60% (24 of 40) and 37% (14 of 38), respectively ($P = .043$). The odds ratio for the probability that fistula closes on enteral nutrition compared to total parenteral nutrition was 2.571 (95% confidence interval [CI]: $1.031-6.411$). Median time to closure was 27 days (95% CI: $21-33$) for enteral nutrition, and no median time was reached in total parenteral nutrition ($P = .047$). A logistic regression analysis identified only 2 factors significantly associated with fistula closure, ie, enteral nutrition (odds ratio $= 6.136$; 95% CI: $1.204-41.623$; $P = .043$) and initial fistula output of ≤ 200 mL/day (odds ratio $= 12.701$; 95% CI: $9.102-47.241$; $P < .001$).

Conclusions.—Enteral nutrition is associated with significantly higher closure rates and shorter time to closure of postoperative pancreatic fistula.

▶ One of the most devastating complications of pancreatic surgery is the development of pancreatic fistula. Pancreatic fistula can result in substantial morbidity and indeed mortality, presenting challenges of fluid imbalance, electrolyte derangements, nutritional support, and septic complications, particularly in the abdominal wall. Management is difficult. Many attempts at treatment, including sealing fistulas with glues, endoscopic diversions, and inhibition of pancreatic secretions, have been attempted but without any confirmed efficacy. Nutritional support is a crucial part of the management. It has long been debated whether enteral feeding or parental feeding is more effective in this setting. With the recent acceptance of enteral feeding past the ligament of Treitz as being more effective in situations of the management of acute pancreatitis, this group undertook a randomized, controlled trial comparing enteral feeding with parenteral feeding in the management of postoperative pancreatic fistula. They clearly showed after 30 days a dominance of the enteral route. It is likely that parenteral nutrition is not as effective because, in the absence of luminal nutrition, there may be atrophy of the gut and other physiologic derangements that occur because of the lack of endoluminal nutrition. Not only was enteral feeding superior in speeding the probability of closure, but it also shortened the time of closure and was associated with significantly lower costs. Patients with the most severe fistulas as well as patients with very mild fistulas were excluded. This study establishes enteral feeding as the preferred method of nutritional support in the context of postoperative pancreatic fistula. It further expands the dominance of using the enteral route in many circumstances where parenteral nutrition had been preferred.

J. A. Murray, MD

A Team-Based Protocol and Electromagnetic Technology Eliminate Feeding Tube Placement Complications

Koopmann MC, Kudsk KA, Szotkowski MJ, et al (William S. Middleton Memorial Veterans Hosp, Madison, WI; et al)
Ann Surg 253:297-302, 2011

Objective.—To examine whether feeding tube placement into high-risk patients using a team-based protocol and electromagnetic tube tracking reduces complications associated with blind tube placement and to evaluate safety of blind tube placement in alert, low-risk patients.

Background.—Approximately $1 \cdot 2$ million feeding tubes with stylets are placed annually in the US. Serious complications during placement exceed the rates of retained sponges and wrong site surgery. Several suggested solutions to the problem have been proposed but none completely eliminate the serious complications and many are neither cost-effective nor practical.

Methods.—In a retrospective, single center study, we compared complications after bedside feeding tube placement using a blind technique in 2005 to a hospital protocol mandating tube placement in high-risk patients by a Tube Team in 2007 using electromagnetic tracking. Outcome variables included airway placement, pneumothorax, death, and radiology resource utilization.

Results.—The Tube Team protocol eliminated airway tube placement (0 of 1154 vs. 20 of 1822, $P < 0.001$), pneumothorax (0/715 vs. 11/1822, $P = 0.009$), and all mortality whereas improving placement (83.9% success vs. 60.5%, $P < 0.001$) in high-risk patients compared to the 2005 study. The number of X-rays obtained per tube (1.07 ± 0.01 vs. 1.49 ± 0.026,

$P < 0.001$) and need for fluoroscopy (2.1% vs. 10.9%, $P < 0.001$) significantly dropped with the Tube Team. A final comparison was made to low-risk patients considered acceptable for blind tube placement in 2007 due to their alertness and ability to cooperate and provide feedback during tube placement. Although no mortality occurred during blind placement in low risk, alert patients, blind placement resulted in significantly increased airway placement (3/143, $p = 0.001$) and pneumothorax (2 of 143, $P = 0.01$) compared to the Tube Team protocol. Most patients who would have required fluoroscopic placement of feeding tube due to failed blind technique had successful placement by the Team avoiding fluoroscopy.

Conclusion.—Feeding tube placement by a dedicated team using electromagnetic tracking eliminates the morbidity and mortality of this common hospital procedure. Blind placement is not acceptable in awake, alert patients.

▶ Feeding-tube placement is a common procedure in hospitals across the country. Although often considered a bedside procedure performed by a resident, physician's assistant, or nurse, morbidity can be significant. This study looks at outcomes in patients who underwent feeding-tube placement by a specially trained team compared with before such a team-based approach was used. The authors found a significant reduction in morbidity and mortality, improved success in placement, and decreased use of fluoroscopy when a dedicated team places these tubes. They also used an electromagnetic tracking system to facilitate the decreased reliance on fluoroscopy.

This is a single-center, retrospective cohort study analyzing the effect of a hospital-wide quality improvement protocol for small-bore feeding-tube placement into high-risk hospitalized patients on patient outcomes and resource utilization using electromagnetic tube placement technology and a dedicated Tube Team. They compared complications after bedside feeding tube placement using a blind technique in 2005 to a hospital protocol mandating tube placement in high-risk patients by the Tube Team in 2007. Outcome variables included airway placement, pneumothorax, death, and radiology resource utilization. The Tube Team protocol eliminated airway tube placement (0 of 1154 vs 20 of 1822, $P < .001$), pneumothorax (0/715 vs 11/1822, $P = .009$), and all mortality, while improving placement (83.9% success vs 60.5%, $P < .001$). Also, the number of x-rays obtained per tube (1.07-0.01 vs 1.49-0.026, $P < .001$) and need for fluoroscopy (2.1% vs 10.9%, $P < .001$). These same improvements were realized in low-risk patients.

I have selected this article for several reasons. First, feeding-tube placement is a common need in gastrointestinal (GI) practice. Although complications are infrequent, the sheer volume of these procedures taking place puts the overall consequence of misplacement or complications on par with other rare events such as retained foreign objects in surgery. Second, it highlights where we are going in medicine today—standardized, team-based care focusing on improving the value of health care (value = outcomes/cost). Although the authors did not perform a cost analysis, cost decrease by avoiding fluoroscopy and the improved outcomes should move the value equation positively. This appears to be something that could be easily adopted into GI practices where the management of the tube-fed patient often involves the GI service.

C. D. Smith, MD

A One-Year Randomized Trial of Lorcaserin for Weight Loss in Obese and Overweight Adults: The BLOSSOM Trial

Fidler MC, for the BLOSSOM Clinical Trial Group (Arena Pharmaceuticals, San Diego, CA; et al)
J Clin Endocrinol Metab 96:3067-3077, 2011

Context.—Lorcaserin is a novel selective agonist of the serotonin 2C receptor.

Objective.—Our objective was to evaluate the effects of lorcaserin on body weight, cardiovascular risk factors, and safety in obese and overweight patients.

Design and Setting.—This randomized, placebo-controlled, double-blind, parallel arm trial took place at 97 U.S. research centers.

Patients.—Patients included 4008 patients, aged 18–65 yr, with a body mass index between 30 and 45 kg/m^2 or between 27 and 29.9 kg/m^2 with an obesity-related comorbid condition.

Interventions.—Patients were randomly assigned in a 2:1:2 ratio to receive lorcaserin 10 mg twice daily (BID), lorcaserin 10 mg once daily (QD), or placebo. All patients received diet and exercise counseling.

Main Outcome Measures.—The ordered primary endpoints were proportion of patients achieving at least 5% reduction in body weight, mean change in body weight, and proportion of patients achieving at least 10% reduction in body weight at 1 yr. Serial echocardiograms monitored heart valve function.

Results.—Significantly more patients treated with lorcaserin 10 mg BID and QD lost at least 5% of baseline body weight (47.2 and 40.2%, respectively) as compared with placebo (25.0%, $P < 0.001$ vs. lorcaserin BID). Least squares mean (95% confidence interval) weight loss with lorcaserin BID and QD was 5.8% (5.5–6.2%) and 4.7% (4.3–5.2%), respectively, compared with 2.8% (2.5–3.2%) with placebo ($P < 0.001$ vs. lorcaserin BID; least squares mean difference, 3.0%). Weight loss of at least 10% was achieved by 22.6 and 17.4% of patients receiving lorcaserin 10 mg BID and QD, respectively, and 9.7% of patients in the placebo group ($P < 0.001$ vs. lorcaserin BID). Headache, nausea, and dizziness were the most common lorcaserin-related adverse events. U.S. Food and Drug Administration-defined echocardiographic valvulopathy occurred in 2.0% of patients on placebo and 2.0% on lorcaserin 10 mg BID.

Conclusions.—Lorcaserin administered in conjunction with a lifestyle modification program was associated with dose-dependent weight loss that was significantly greater than with placebo.

▶ Weight loss drugs have come and gone; however, few have as negative connotations as the serotonin 2C receptor agonists fenfluramine and dexfenfluramine. Although these agents, especially in combination, were effective at producing weight loss, they caused valvular heart disease. This trial studied a novel agent targeting the same receptor but in a selective fashion. It targets specifically the receptors in the hypothalamus that seem to regulate food intake. This trial studied 2 different doses of lorcaserin versus placebo, with all groups having the same dietary and behavioral interventions. They showed substantial benefit in terms of success of change in baseline weight that appear dose dependent (Fig 1 in the original article).

All patients underwent echocardiography and in all groups just 2% of patients and controls had valvulopathy that might meet Food and Drug Administration criteria.

This study is important in that it shows that an agent custom designed to reproduce the same benefit as prior drugs can apparently avoid the valvular heart disease complications. This drug, along with other novel approaches, is important in the war on obesity and appears to show benefit beyond weight change in terms of improvement in lean body mass, reduction of total body fat, and reduction in blood pressure.

J. A. Murray, MD

44 Liver Disease

A Randomized Trial Comparing Radiofrequency Ablation and Surgical Resection for HCC Conforming to the Milan Criteria

Huang J, Yan L, Cheng Z, et al (Sichuan Univ, Chengdu, China)
Ann Surg 252:903-912, 2010

Objective.—To compare the long-term outcomes of surgical resection and radiofrequency ablation for the treatment of small hepatocellular carcinoma (HCC).

Summary Background Data.—Radiofrequency ablation (RFA) is a promising, emerging therapy for small HCC. Whether it is as effective as surgical resection (RES) for long-term outcomes is still indefinite.

Methods.—Two hundred thirty HCC patients who met the Milan criteria and were suitable to be treated by either RES or RFA entered into a randomized controlled trial. The patients were regularly followed up after treatment for 5 years (except for those who died). The primary end point was overall survival; the secondary end points were recurrence-free survival, overall recurrence, and early-stage recurrence.

Results.—The 1-, 2-, 3-, 4- and 5-year overall survival rates for the RFA group and the RES group were 86.96%, 76.52%, 69.57%, 66.09%, 54.78% and 98.26%, 96.52%, 92.17%, 82.60%, 75.65%, respectively. The corresponding recurrence-free survival rates for the 2 groups were 81.74%, 59.13%, 46.08%, 33.91%, 28.69% and 85.22%, 73.92%, 60.87%, 54.78%, 51.30%, respectively. Overall survival and recurrence-free survival were significantly lower in the RFA group than in the RES group ($P = 0.001$ and $P = 0.017$). The 1-, 2-, 3-, 4-, and 5-year overall recurrence rates were 16.52%, 38.26%, 49.57%, 59.13%, and 63.48% for the RFA group and 12.17%, 22.60%, 33.91%, 39.13%, and 41.74% for the RES group. The overall recurrence was higher in the RFA group than in the RES group ($P = 0.024$).

Conclusions.—Surgical resection may provide better survival and lower recurrence rates than RFA for patients with HCC to the Milan criteria.

▶ This is a well-done and important study comparing radiofrequency ablation (RFA) with surgical resection for small hepatocellular carcinoma. It is a prospective, randomized, controlled trial, although not blinded. The authors present long-term data (5 years). The authors find that in terms of disease-free survival, overall survival, and recurrence, surgical resection is superior to RFA. On the other hand, surgical resection has greater morbidity, mortality, and overall length of hospital stay and cost. The authors conclude that RFA still plays an important role in HCC but should be limited to patients who are poor surgical candidates or decline surgery.

When assessing the impact of this article, it is important to acknowledge its limitations, and the authors have done a nice job of listing the major limitations, reproduced here:

1. A double-blind technique was not used. This directly resulted in 7 patients withdrawing their consent for RFA and choosing surgical resection (RES).

2. Histopathologic grading of HCC was not included in the analysis. The majority of patients in the RFA group (87/115) had no pathological diagnosis; moreover, there was significant difference in solitary tumor size between the 2 groups.

3. The rate of loss to follow-up was greater in the RES group than in the RFA group, being 15.6% (18/115) versus 6.1% (7/115; $P < .05$). Having that information would probably influence the comparison between 2 groups.

4. The authors accepted the suggestion from their ethics committee authorizing patients to choose second-time treatment when HCC recurred. This may influence overall survival of this study, but significant difference of recurrence-free survival between the 2 therapies was still robust.

Although these do call into question the strength of some of their conclusions, the analysis remains robust and relevant.

C. D. Smith, MD

45 Diabetes

Long-Term Effects of Intensive Glucose Lowering on Cardiovascular Outcomes
The Accord Study Group (McMaster Univ and Hamilton Health Sciences, Ontario, Canada; Wake Forest Univ School of Medicine, Winston-Salem, NC; Case Western Reserve Univ, Cleveland, OH)
N Engl J Med 364:818-828, 2011

Background.—Intensive glucose lowering has previously been shown to increase mortality among persons with advanced type 2 diabetes and a high risk of cardiovascular disease. This report describes the 5-year outcomes of a mean of 3.7 years of intensive glucose lowering on mortality and key cardiovascular events.

Methods.—We randomly assigned participants with type 2 diabetes and cardiovascular disease or additional cardiovascular risk factors to receive intensive therapy (targeting a glycated hemoglobin level below 6.0%) or standard therapy (targeting a level of 7 to 7.9%). After termination of the intensive therapy, due to higher mortality in the intensive-therapy group, the target glycated hemoglobin level was 7 to 7.9% for all participants, who were followed until the planned end of the trial.

Results.—Before the intensive therapy was terminated, the intensive-therapy group did not differ significantly from the standard-therapy group in the rate of the primary outcome (a composite of nonfatal myocardial infarction, nonfatal stroke, or death from cardiovascular causes) ($P = 0.13$) but had more deaths from any cause (primarily cardiovascular) (hazard ratio, 1.21; 95% confidence interval [CI], 1.02 to 1.44) and fewer nonfatal myocardial infarctions (hazard ratio, 0.79; 95% CI, 0.66 to 0.95). These trends persisted during the entire follow-up period (hazard ratio for death, 1.19; 95% CI, 1.03 to 1.38; and hazard ratio for nonfatal myocardial infarction, 0.82; 95% CI, 0.70 to 0.96). After the intensive intervention was terminated, the median glycated hemoglobin level in the intensive-therapy group rose from 6.4% to 7.2%, and the use of glucose-lowering medications and rates of severe hypoglycemia and other adverse events were similar in the two groups.

Conclusions.—As compared with standard therapy, the use of intensive therapy for 3.7 years to target a glycated hemoglobin level below 6% reduced 5-year nonfatal myocardial infarctions but increased 5-year mortality. Such a strategy cannot be recommended for high-risk patients with advanced type 2 diabetes. (Funded by the National Heart, Lung and Blood Institute; ClinicalTrials.gov number, NCT00000620.)

▶ Cardiovascular diseases are the main cause of death in people suffering from diabetes. It is, therefore, tempting to assume that an intensive glucose-lowering treatment might prevent cardiovascular events in diabetics. The aim of the Action to Control Cardiovascular Risk in Diabetes (ACCORD) trial was to investigate whether lowering glycated hemoglobin (HbA1c) level below 6.0% (corresponding to the normal range) would reduce cardiovascular events. Persons suffering from diabetes for a median of 10 years with HbA1c of 7.5% or higher and who had a high risk of cardiovascular diseases were enrolled. In this high-risk cohort, an intensive glucose-lowering treatment cannot be recommended because increased 5-year mortality was observed in the intensive-treatment group. The outcome of this trial suggests that starting an intensive glucose-lowering therapy after approximately 10 years of diabetes is too late. However, intensive therapy directly after diagnosing diabetes might still be beneficial.

E. Oetjen, MD

The duration of diabetes affects the response to intensive glucose control in type 2 subjects: the VA Diabetes Trial
Duckworth WC, for the Investigators of the VADT (Phoenix VA Health Care Ctr, AZ; et al)
J Diabetes Complications 25:355-361, 2011

Background.—The goal of the VA Diabetes Trial (VADT) was to determine the effect of intensive glucose control on macrovascular events in subjects with difficult-to-control diabetes. No significant benefit was found. This report examines predictors of the effect of intensive therapy on the primary outcome in this population.

Methods.—This trial included 1791 subjects. Baseline cardiovascular risk factors were collected by interview and the VA record. The analyses were done by intention to treat.

Findings.—Univariate analysis at baseline of predictors of a primary cardiovascular (CV) event included a prior CV event, age, insulin use at baseline, and duration of diagnosed diabetes (all $P < .0001$). Multivariable modeling revealed a U-shaped relationship between duration of diabetes and treatment. Modeled estimates for the hazard ratios (HRs) for treatment show that subjects with a short duration (3 years or less) of diagnosed diabetes have a nonsignificant increase in risk (HR > 1.0) after which the HR is below 1.0. From 7 to 15 years' duration at entry, subjects have HRs favoring intensive treatment. Thereafter the HR approaches 1.0 and over-21-years' duration approaches 2.0. Duration over 21 years resulted in a HR of 1.977 (CI 1.77–3.320, $P < .01$). Baseline c-peptide levels progressively declined up to 15 years and were stable subsequently.

Interpretation.—In difficult-to-control older subjects with type 2 DM, duration of diabetes altered the response to intensive glucose control.

Intensive therapy may reduce CV events in subjects with a duration of 15 years or less and may increase risks in those with longer duration.

▶ The findings of the Action to Control Cardiovascular Risk in Diabetes (ACCORD) Study Group were corroborated in the Veteran's Affairs Diabetes Trial (VADT), stating that an intensive glucose-lowering treatment failed to reduce major cardiovascular events significantly. In this post hoc analysis, the influence of the duration of diabetes on the response to intensive glucose-lowering treatment was analyzed in a difficult-to-control cohort. It should be noted that in this study, people were enrolled with mean glycated hemoglobin (HbA1c) levels of 9.4%. The mean HbA1c level in the standard treated group was 8.4%, that in the intensive treatment group was 6.9%. Both values are considerably higher than in the ACCORD study. However, the results of both studies are the same. Thus, an early intensive glucose-lowering therapy might be beneficial to prevent major cardiovascular events.

E. Oetjen, MD

Utility of Hemoglobin A_{1c} for Diagnosing Prediabetes and Diabetes in Obese Children and Adolescents
Nowicka P, Santoro N, Liu H, et al (Yale Univ School of Medicine, New Haven, CT; Yale Ctr for Clinical Investigation of Yale Univ School of Medicine, New Haven, CT)
Diabetes Care 34:1306-1311, 2011

Objective.—Hemoglobin A_{1c} (A1C) has emerged as a recommended diagnostic tool for identifying diabetes and subjects at risk for the disease. This recommendation is based on data in adults showing the relationship between A1C with future development of diabetes and microvascular complications. However, studies in the pediatric population are lacking.

Research Design and Methods.—We studied a multiethnic cohort of 1,156 obese children and adolescents without a diagnosis of diabetes (male, 40%/female, 60%). All subjects underwent an oral glucose tolerance test (OGTT) and A1C measurement. These tests were repeated after a follow-up time of ~2 years in 218 subjects.

Results.—At baseline, subjects were stratified according to A1C categories: 77% with normal glucose tolerance (A1C < 5.7%), 21% at risk for diabetes (A1C 5.7—6.4%), and 1% with diabetes (A1C > 6.5%). In the at risk for diabetes category, 47% were classified with prediabetes or diabetes, and in the diabetes category, 62% were classified with type 2 diabetes by the OGTT. The area under the curve receiver operating characteristic for A1C was 0.81 (95% CI 0.70—0.92). The threshold for identifying type 2 diabetes was 5.8%, with 78% specificity and 68% sensitivity. In the subgroup with repeated measures, a multivariate analysis showed that the strongest predictors of 2-h glucose at follow-up were baseline A1C and 2-h glucose, independently of age, ethnicity, sex, fasting glucose, and follow-up time.

Conclusions.—The American Diabetes Association suggested that an A1C of 6.5% underestimates the prevalence of prediabetes and diabetes in obese children and adolescents. Given the low sensitivity and specificity, the use of A1C by itself represents a poor diagnostic tool for prediabetes and type 2 diabetes in obese children and adolescents.

▶ Given that a prediabetic metabolic condition and diabetes do not hurt and that an early therapeutic intervention will retard the pathogenesis of diabetes-associated diseases, the identification of people suffering ignorantly from diabetes or being at risk for diabetes is important. This is especially true in obese children and adolescents. Because HbA1c usually reflects the glucose homeostasis of the previous 3 to 4 months, does not require fasting for accurate measurements, and has low intraindividual variability, its determination is considered a reliable marker and is recommended by the American Diabetes Association. However, this recommendation is based on studies in adults. In a multiethnic cohort of obese children and adolescents with a 2-year follow-up, the reliability of HbA1c to identify diabetics or persons at risk for diabetes was compared with that of an oral glucose tolerance test.

E. Oetjen, MD

Long-Term Persistence of Hormonal Adaptations to Weight Loss
Sumithran P, Prendergast LA, Delbridge E, et al (Univ of Melbourne, Victoria, Australia; La Trobe Univ, Melbourne, Victoria, Australia)
N Engl J Med 365:1597-1604, 2011

Background.—After weight loss, changes in the circulating levels of several peripheral hormones involved in the homeostatic regulation of body weight occur. Whether these changes are transient or persist over time may be important for an understanding of the reasons behind the high rate of weight regain after diet-induced weight loss.

Methods.—We enrolled 50 overweight or obese patients without diabetes in a 10-week weight-loss program for which a very-low-energy diet was prescribed. At baseline (before weight loss), at 10 weeks (after program completion), and at 62 weeks, we examined circulating levels of leptin, ghrelin, peptide YY, gastric inhibitory polypeptide, glucagon-like peptide 1, amylin, pancreatic polypeptide, cholecystokinin, and insulin and subjective ratings of appetite.

Results.—Weight loss (mean [± SE], 13.5 ± 0.5 kg) led to significant reductions in levels of leptin, peptide YY, cholecystokinin, insulin ($P < 0.001$ for all comparisons), and amylin ($P = 0.002$) and to increases in levels of ghrelin ($P < 0.001$), gastric inhibitory polypeptide ($P = 0.004$), and pancreatic polypeptide ($P = 0.008$). There was also a significant increase in subjective appetite ($P < 0.001$). One year after the initial weight loss, there were still significant differences from baseline in the mean levels of leptin ($P < 0.001$), peptide YY ($P < 0.001$), cholecystokinin ($P = 0.04$), insulin ($P = 0.01$), ghrelin ($P < 0.001$), gastric inhibitory polypeptide ($P < 0.001$), and pancreatic polypeptide ($P = 0.002$), as well as hunger ($P < 0.001$).

Conclusions.—One year after initial weight reduction, levels of the circulating mediators of appetite that encourage weight regain after diet-induced weight loss do not revert to the levels recorded before weight loss. Long-term strategies to counteract this change may be needed to prevent obesity relapse. (Funded by the National Health and Medical Research Council and others; ClinicalTrials.gov number, NCT00870259.)

▶ Nearly everyone has already experienced it: it is much easier to lose weight than keep the reduced weight. This is especially strenuous for obese people. The study by Sumithran et al conducted in 50 obese people sheds light on some of the underlying reasons—namely, that the circulating mediators of appetite are still increased 1 year after diet-induced weight reduction. Thus, inhibiting the effects of these mediators might help to prevent weight gain and relapse into obesity. It remains to be investigated whether mediators of appetite are also increased in people with a body mass index between 25 and 30 kg/m^2 and how long this increase persists. In addition, the duration of the obese state should be considered.

E. Oetjen, MD

Prospective Associations of Vitamin D With β-Cell Function and Glycemia: The PROspective Metabolism and ISlet cell Evaluation (PROMISE) Cohort Study

Kayaniyil S, Retnakaran R, Harris SB, et al (Univ of Toronto, Ontario, Canada; Univ of Western Ontario, London, Ontario, Canada; et al)
Diabetes 60:2947-2953, 2011

Objective.—To examine the prospective associations of baseline vitamin D [25-hydroxyvitamin D; 25(OH)D] with insulin resistance (IR), β-cell function, and glucose homeostasis in subjects at risk for type 2 diabetes.

Research Design and Methods.—We followed 489 subjects, aged 50 ± 10 years, for 3 years. At baseline and follow-up, 75-g oral glucose tolerance tests (OGTTs) were administered. IR was measured using the Matsuda index (IS$_{OGTT}$) and the homeostasis model assessment of IR (HOMA-IR), β-cell function was determined using both the insulinogenic index divided by HOMA-IR (IGI/IR) and the insulin secretion sensitivity index-2 (ISSI-2), and glycemia was assessed using the area under the glucose curve (AUC$_{glucose}$). Regression models were adjusted for age, sex, ethnicity, season, and baseline value of the outcome variable, as well as baseline and change in physical activity, vitamin D supplement use, and BMI.

Results.—Multivariate linear regression analyses indicated no significant association of baseline 25(OH)D with follow-up IS$_{OGTT}$ or HOMA-IR. There were, however, significant positive associations of baseline 25(OH) D with follow-up IGI/IR ($\beta = 0.005$, $P = 0.015$) and ISSI-2 ($\beta = 0.002$, $P = 0.023$) and a significant inverse association of baseline 25(OH)D with follow-up $AUC_{glucose}$ ($\beta = -0.001$, $P = 0.007$). Progression to dysglycemia (impaired fasting glucose, impaired glucose tolerance, or type 2 diabetes) occurred in 116 subjects. Logistic regression analyses indicated a significant reduced risk of progression with higher baseline 25(OH)D (adjusted odds ratio 0.69 [95% CI 0.53–0.89]), but this association was not significant after additional adjustment for baseline and change in BMI (0.78 [0.59–1.02]).

Conclusions.—Higher baseline 25(OH)D independently predicted better β-cell function and lower $AUC_{glucose}$ at follow-up, supporting a potential role for vitamin D in type 2 diabetes etiology.

▶ It is controversially discussed whether a vitamin D deficiency is associated with the development of the metabolic syndrome and diabetes. In the PROspective Metabolism and Islet cell Evaluation (PROMISE) Cohort Study it was found that a higher baseline vitamin D level predicted a better β-cell function at a 3-year follow-up. It should be noted, that vitamin D levels were measured only at baseline and not at the follow-up and that β-cell function and insulin resistance were determined by oral glucose tolerance tests. However, this cohort consisted of approximately 500 subjects with high risk for diabetes. Clearly, more prospective studies will be needed to evaluate whether vitamin D supplement might at least retard the development of diabetes type 2.

E. Oetjen, MD

Valsartan Improves β-Cell Function and Insulin Sensitivity in Subjects With Impaired Glucose Metabolism: A randomized controlled trial
van der Zijl NJ, Moors CCM, Goossens GH, et al (Vrije Univ Med Ctr, Amsterdam, The Netherlands; Maastricht Univ Med Ctr, The Netherlands)
Diabetes Care 34:845-851, 2011

Objective.—Recently, the Nateglinide and Valsartan in Impaired Glucose Tolerance Outcomes Research Trial demonstrated that treatment with the angiotensin receptor blocker (ARB) valsartan for 5 years resulted in a relative reduction of 14% in the incidence of type 2 diabetes in subjects with impaired glucose metabolism (IGM). We investigated whether improvements in β-cell function and/or insulin sensitivity underlie these preventive effects of the ARB valsartan in the onset of type 2 diabetes.

Research Design and Methods.—In this randomized controlled, double-blind, two-center study, the effects of 26 weeks of valsartan (320 mg daily; $n = 40$) or placebo ($n = 39$) on β-cell function and insulin sensitivity were assessed in subjects with impaired fasting glucose and/or impaired glucose tolerance, using a combined hyperinsulinemic-euglycemic and hyperglycemic clamp with subsequent arginine stimulation and a 2-h 75-g oral glucose tolerance test (OGTT). Treatment effects were analyzed using ANCOVA, adjusting for center, glucometabolic status, and sex.

Results.—Valsartan increased first-phase ($P = 0.028$) and second-phase ($P = 0.002$) glucose-stimulated insulin secretion compared with placebo, whereas the enhanced arginine-stimulated insulin secretion was comparable between groups ($P = 0.25$). In addition, valsartan increased the OGTT-derived insulinogenic index (representing first-phase insulin secretion after an oral glucose load; $P = 0.027$). Clamp-derived insulin sensitivity was significantly increased with valsartan compared with placebo ($P = 0.049$). Valsartan treatment significantly decreased systolic and diastolic blood pressure compared with placebo ($P < 0.001$). BMI remained unchanged in both treatment groups ($P = 0.89$).

Conclusions.—Twenty-six weeks of valsartan treatment increased glucose-stimulated insulin release and insulin sensitivity in normotensive subjects with IGM. These findings may partly explain the beneficial effects of valsartan in the reduced incidence of type 2 diabetes.

▶ Drugs interfering with the renin-angiotensin system, such as the inhibitors of the angiotensin-converting enzyme and the antagonists of the angiotensin 2 subtype 1 receptor (ARB), have been suggested to improve glucose homeostasis in patients with hypertensive diabetes. Furthermore, the Nateglinide and Valsartan in Impaired Glucose Tolerance Outcomes Research Trial demonstrated that treatment with the ARB valsartan for 5 years significantly reduced the incidence of diabetes type 2 in people with impaired glucose metabolism. The aim of the present study was to elucidate preventive effects of valsartan on glucose homeostasis. The study points to an improvement in insulin secretion and insulin sensitivity due to valsartan therapy. It remains to be investigated whether this is a compound or a class effect. Taken together, the present study strongly suggests that hypertensive patients with impaired glucose metabolism benefit from the treatment with ARB respective to their metabolic condition.

E. Oetjen, MD

46 Lipoproteins and Atherosclerosis

Coronary artery disease and cardiovascular outcomes in patients with non-alcoholic fatty liver disease
Wong VW-S, Wong GL-H, Yip GW-K, et al (The Chinese Univ of Hong Kong)
Gut 60:1721-1727, 2011

Objective.—Non-alcoholic fatty liver disease (NAFLD) is the hepatic manifestation of metabolic syndrome and is associated with cardiovascular risk. The aim of this study was to determine the role of fatty liver in predicting coronary artery disease and clinical outcomes in patients undergoing coronary angiogram.

Methods.—This was a prospective cohort study carried out in a University hospital. Consecutive patients who underwent coronary angiogram had ultrasound screening for fatty liver. Significant cardiovascular disease was defined as $\geq 50\%$ stenosis in at least one coronary artery. The primary outcome was a composite end point comprising cardiovascular deaths, non-fatal myocardial infarction and the need for further coronary intervention during prospective follow-up.

Results.—Among 612 recruited patients, 356 (58.2%) had fatty liver by ultrasonography, 318 (52.0%) had elevated serum alanine aminotransferase and 465 (76.0%) had significant coronary artery disease. Coronary artery disease occurred in 84.6% of patients with fatty liver and 64.1% of those without fatty liver ($p < 0.001$). After adjusting for demographic and metabolic factors, fatty liver (adjusted OR 2.31; 95% CI 1.46 to 3.64) and alanine aminotransferase level (adjusted OR 1.01; 95% CI 1.00 to 1.02) remained independently associated with coronary artery disease. At a mean follow-up of 87 ± 22 weeks, 30 (10.0%) patients with fatty liver and 18 (11.0%) patients without fatty liver reached the composite clinical end point ($p = 0.79$).

Conclusions.—In patients with clinical indications for coronary angiogram, fatty liver is associated with coronary artery disease independently of other metabolic factors. However, fatty liver cannot predict cardiovascular mortality and morbidity in patients with established coronary artery disease (Tables 1 and 2).

▶ The metabolic syndrome as defined by the National Cholesterol Education Program has been a useful clinical construct for helping to identify patients at

TABLE 1.—Baseline Characteristics of Patients with and Without Fatty Liver

Characteristics	All	Fatty liver	No fatty liver	p Value
n	612	356	256	
Age (years)	63±11	63±10	63±12	0.61
Male gender, n (%)	433 (70.8)	264 (74.2)	169 (66.0)	0.029
Smoking, n (%)				0.23
Current smoker	194 (31.7)	122 (34.3)	72 (28.1)	
Ex-smoker	115 (18.8)	67 (18.8)	48 (18.8)	
Non-smoker	303 (49.5)	167 (46.9)	136 (53.1)	
Alcohol, n (%)				0.84
Current drinker	93 (15.2)	54 (15.2)	39 (15.2)	
Ex-drinker	30 (4.9)	19 (5.3)	11 (4.3)	
Non-drinker	489 (79.9)	283 (79.5)	206 (80.5)	
Diabetes, n (%)	191 (31.2)	147 (41.3)	44 (17.2)	<0.001
Hypertension, n (%)	401 (65.5)	252 (70.8)	149 (58.2)	0.001
Systolic blood pressure (mm Hg)	137±22	140±22	132±21	<0.001
Diastolic blood pressure (mm Hg)	75±13	77±13	72±13	<0.001
Body mass index (kg/m^2)	24.7±3.9	25.7±4.0	23.2±3.1	<0.001
Male	24.3±3.3	25.2±3.4	23.0±2.8	<0.001
Female	25.5±4.9	27.2±5.2	23.6±3.7	<0.001
Waist circumference (cm)	90±9	93±8	87±9	<0.001
Male	91±8	93±8	88±8	<0.001
Female	89±11	93±9	84±10	<0.001
Fasting glucose (mmol/l)	6.2±2.1	6.4±2.2	6.0±2.0	0.021
Total cholesterol (mmol/l)	4.5±1.2	4.5±1.3	4.5±1.1	0.66
HDL-cholesterol (mmol/l)	1.2±0.3	1.1±0.3	1.2±0.4	<0.001
LDL-cholesterol (mmol/l)	2.6±0.9	2.6±0.9	2.6±0.9	0.50
Triglycerides (mmol/l)	1.4 (1.0, 1.9)	1.4 (1.0, 2.1)	1.2 (0.9, 1.8)	0.001
Creatinine (μmol/l)	89 (76, 105)	91 (78, 107)	87 (74, 104)	0.033
Alanine aminotransferase (IU/l)	26 (19, 40)	28 (19, 44)	24 (18, 38)	0.052
Drugs, n (%)				
Aspirin	523 (85.5)	323 (90.7)	200 (78.1)	<0.001
Clopidogrel	377 (61.6)	242 (68.0)	135 (52.7)	<0.001
β-Blockers	423 (69.1)	267 (75.0)	156 (60.9)	<0.001
Calcium channel blockers	133 (21.7)	87 (24.4)	46 (18.0)	0.056
ACE inhibitors	310 (50.7)	192 (53.9)	118 (46.1)	0.056
Angiotensin receptor antagonists	32 (5.2)	20 (5.6)	12 (4.7)	0.61
Statins	399 (65.2)	252 (70.8)	147 (57.4)	0.001
Metformin	77 (12.6)	62 (17.4)	15 (5.9)	<0.001
Thiazolidinedione	13 (2.1)	10 (2.8)	3 (1.2)	0.26
Sulfonylurea	111 (18.1)	83 (23.3)	28 (10.9)	<0.001
Insulin	25 (4.1)	19 (5.3)	6 (2.3)	0.065
Indication of coronary angiogram, n (%)				<0.001
Acute coronary syndrome or myocardial infarction	279 (45.6)	167 (46.9)	112 (43.8)	
Stable angina	273 (44.6)	173 (48.6)	100 (39.1)	
Valvular heart disease	46 (7.5)	10 (2.8)	36 (14.1)	
Others	14 (2.3)	6 (1.7)	8 (3.1)	
Follow-up duration (weeks)	87±22	89±19	85±25	0.055

Continuous variables were expressed as mean ± SD or median (IQR).
ACE, angiotensin-converting enzyme; HDL, high-density lipoprotein; LDL, low-density lipoprotein.

heightened risk for developing coronary artery disease (CAD) as well as diabetes mellitus.[1] Although not defined as a CAD risk equivalent, considerable evidence shows that the heightened risk for atherosclerotic disease is due to obesity, insulin resistance or hyperglycemia, dyslipidemia, hypertension, and heightened systemic inflammation. A frequent manifestation of insulin resistance is hepatic

TABLE 2.—Coronary Angiogram Findings of Patients with and Without Fatty Liver

Parameters	Fatty Liver	No Fatty Liver	p Value
Left main stem stenosis (%)	0 (0, 0)	0 (0, 0)	0.17
Left main stem steatosis ≥50%, n (%)	29 (8.1)	22 (8.6)	0.84
Left anterior descending artery stenosis (%)	80 (30, 90)	50 (0, 80)	<0.001
Left anterior descending artery stenosis ≥50%, n (%)	232 (65.2)	135 (52.7)	0.002
Left circumflex artery stenosis (%)	50 (0, 90)	0 (0, 70)	<0.001
Left circumflex artery stenosis ≥50%, n (%)	176 (49.4)	88 (34.4)	<0.001
Right coronary artery stenosis (%)	50 (0, 90)	20 (0, 80)	<0.001
Right coronary artery stenosis ≥50%, n (%)	188 (52.8)	95 (37.1)	<0.001
Stenosis ≥50% in any coronary artery, n (%)	301 (84.6)	164 (64.1)	<0.001
Triple vessel disease, n (%)	100 (28.1)	60 (23.4)	0.20

The percentage stenosis of each coronary artery with respect to its diameter was expressed as the median (IQR).

steatosis (ie, nonalcoholic fatty liver disease [NAFLD]). All forms of ectopic fat deposition are considered to be abnormal and pathogenic, including within the liver, pancreas, skeletal muscle, and pericardium or myocardium. NAFLD is associated with increased risk for both carotid atherosclerosis and CAD.[2-5] It has not been clear, however, whether NAFLD is an independent risk factor for CAD.

In this study, 612 patients, with and without NAFLD, who had clinical indications for coronary angiography were evaluated. NAFLD was documented by ultrasonography. Significant CAD was defined as a stenotic lesion that was at least 50% occlusive. Groups were not well matched by risk factor burden, metabolic features, and background pharmacologic therapies. A significant reason for this likely has to do with the fact that the 2 groups were mismatched for incidence of diabetes at 41% and 17% in the NAFLD and normal liver groups, respectively. Nevertheless, based on multivariate regression analysis, NAFLD was an independent predictor of significant CAD in all branches of the coronary tree, incurring an increased hazard for disease of 2.3-fold (95% confidence interval, 1.46—3.64; $P < .001$). NAFLD did not, however, predict risk for cardiovascular events (myocardial infarction, stroke, or death), possibly because of small sample size and relatively short duration of mean follow-up (87 weeks).

This study certainly introduces important implications and widens the toxicity associated with NAFLD. Larger studies will be needed to help confirm whether NAFLD should be considered a CAD risk factor and count in CAD risk scoring paradigms used around the world. At minimum, it can be stated that the finding that NAFLD increases risk for significant CAD makes sense and helps to identify patients with diabetes mellitus or metabolic syndrome who have higher CAD risk than their counterparts who do not have NAFLD. It will be important to determine if patients who successfully achieve resorption of intrahepatic fat through lifestyle modification and pharmacologic intervention also experience a reduction in risk for CAD or regression of coronary atherosclerotic plaques.

P. P. Toth, MD, PhD

References

1. Expert Panel on Detection, Evaluation, and Treatment of High Blood Cholesterol in Adults. Executive summary of the third report of the National Cholesterol

Education Program (ncep) expert panel on detection, evaluation, and treatment of high blood cholesterol in adults (adult treatment panel III). *JAMA.* 2001;285: 2486-2497.
2. Villanova N, Moscatiello S, Ramilli S, et al. Endothelial dysfunction and cardiovascular risk profile in nonalcoholic fatty liver disease. *Hepatology.* 2005;42: 473-480.
3. Mirbagheri SA, Rashidi A, Abdi S, Saedi D, Abouzari M. Liver: an alarm for the heart? *Liver Int.* 2007;27:891-894.
4. McKimmie RL, Daniel KR, Carr JJ, et al. Hepatic steatosis and subclinical cardiovascular disease in a cohort enriched for type 2 diabetes: the Diabetes Heart Study. *Am J Gastroenterol.* 2008;103:3029-3035.
5. Assy N, Djibre A, Farah R, Grosovski M, Marmor A. Presence of coronary plaques in patients with nonalcoholic fatty liver disease. *Radiology.* 2010;254:393-400.

Niacin in Patients with Low HDL Cholesterol Levels Receiving Intensive Statin Therapy

The AIM-HIGH Investigators (Univ at Buffalo, NY; Univ of Washington, Seattle; Univ of Calgary and Libin Cardiovascular Inst, Calgary, Alberta, Canada; et al)
N Engl J Med 365:2255-2267, 2011

Background.—In patients with established cardiovascular disease, residual cardiovascular risk persists despite the achievement of target low-density lipoprotein (LDL) cholesterol levels with statin therapy. It is unclear whether extended-release niacin added to simvastatin to raise low levels of high-density lipoprotein (HDL) cholesterol is superior to simvastatin alone in reducing such residual risk.

Methods.—We randomly assigned eligible patients to receive extended-release niacin, 1500 to 2000 mg per day, or matching placebo. All patients received simvastatin, 40 to 80 mg per day, plus ezetimibe, 10 mg per day, if needed, to maintain an LDL cholesterol level of 40 to 80 mg per deciliter (1.03 to 2.07 mmol per liter). The primary end point was the first event of the composite of death from coronary heart disease, nonfatal myocardial infarction, ischemic stroke, hospitalization for an acute coronary syndrome, or symptom-driven coronary or cerebral revascularization.

Results.—A total of 3414 patients were randomly assigned to receive niacin (1718) or placebo (1696). The trial was stopped after a mean follow-up period of 3 years owing to a lack of efficacy. At 2 years, niacin therapy had significantly increased the median HDL cholesterol level from 35 mg per deciliter (0.91 mmol per liter) to 42 mg per deciliter (1.08 mmol per liter), lowered the triglyceride level from 164 mg per deciliter (1.85 mmol per liter) to 122 mg per deciliter (1.38 mmol per liter), and lowered the LDL cholesterol level from 74 mg per deciliter (1.91 mmol per liter) to 62 mg per deciliter (1.60 mmol per liter). The primary end point occurred in 282 patients in the niacin group (16.4%) and in 274 patients in the placebo group (16.2%) (hazard ratio, 1.02; 95% confidence interval, 0.87 to 1.21; $P = 0.79$ by the log-rank test).

Conclusions.—Among patients with atherosclerotic cardiovascular disease and LDL cholesterol levels of less than 70 mg per deciliter (1.81 mmol per liter), there was no incremental clinical benefit from the addition of niacin to statin therapy during a 36-month follow-up period, despite significant improvements in HDL cholesterol and triglyceride levels. (Funded by the National Heart, Lung, and Blood Institute and Abbott Laboratories; AIM-HIGH ClinicalTrials.gov number, NCT00120289.) (Tables 1 and 4).

▶ Nicotinic acid (niacin) is a broad-spectrum lipid-modifying agent that reduces atherogenic lipoprotein burden (very low-density lipoprotein, low-density lipoprotein [LDL], Lp[a]) and is currently the best drug available for raising serum levels of high-density lipoprotein (HDL)-C. It has demonstrable efficacy for reducing risk of cardiovascular events in patients with established coronary artery disease (CAD) when used as monotherapy.[1] In a number of smaller trials, the addition of niacin to other lipid-lowering medications such as statins[2,3] and fibrates[4,5] yielded relatively large reductions in risk for acute cardiovascular events. The High-Density Lipoprotein Atherosclerosis Treatment Study 2 (HATS) was of particular interest because patients in this secondary prevention trial experienced an average 89% relative risk reduction in the primary composite endpoint of the study (myocardial infarction [MI], stroke, death, and need for revascularization). Unfortunately, each treatment arm of the study contained only approximately 40 patients. While the magnitude of risk reduction was certainly impressive, it was of interest to ascertain whether such a large risk reduction could be confirmed in a larger cohort of patients.

The Atherothrombosis Intervention in Metabolic Syndrome with Low HDL/High Triglycerides: Impact on Global Health Outcomes (AIM-HIGH) trial evaluated whether extended-release niacin added to intensive statin therapy compared with statin therapy alone would lower the risk of cardiovascular events in patients with CAD and atherogenic dyslipidemia and low levels of HDL-C and elevated triglyceride levels. The study randomly assigned 3414 patients. The primary composite endpoint included MI, stroke, coronary death, need for coronary or cerebral revascularization, and hospitalization for acute coronary syndromes. The average baseline HDL-C was 35 mg/dL, LDL-C was 71 mg/dL, triglyceride was 161 mg/dL, and non—HDL-C was 106 mg/dL. The target LDL-C in this study was 40 to 80 mg/dL. The groups were well matched by demographic criteria (Table 1). Baseline statin therapy was in excess of 90% in both groups, and background therapy with β-blockers, angiotensin-converting enzyme inhibitors, and aspirin was high (Table 1). Approximately 20% and 10% of the patients in the placebo and niacin groups, respectively, were also receiving adjuvant ezetimibe therapy to facilitate LDL-C goal attainment.

The addition of niacin to aggressive statin plus ezetimibe therapy did not beneficially impact any major cardiovascular outcome (Table 4). The Kaplan-Meier survival curves are essentially superimposable for the entire 3-year duration of the study. This is despite the fact that niacin increased HDL-C by 7 mg/dL (this was dampened by a 3-mg/dL increase in the placebo group relative to baseline), decreased triglycerides to 122 mg/dL, and decreased LDL-C to 65 mg/dL. The National Heart Lung and Blood Institute terminated the study due to futility as well as the possibility for harm because of a small, statistically nonsignificant trend for an increase in risk for ischemic stroke (29 vs 18 patients, $P = .11$). These

TABLE 1.—Baseline Demographic and Clinical Characteristics of the Study Patients*

Characteristic	Placebo Plus Statin (N = 1696)	Extended-Release Niacin Plus Statin (N = 1718)
Age		
Mean — yr	63.7 (8.7)	63.7 (8.8)
Distribution — no. (%)		
<65 yr	915 (54.0)	917 (53.4)
≥65 yr	781 (46.0)	801 (46.6)
Sex — no. (%)		
Female	251 (14.8)	253 (14.7)
Male	1445 (85.2)	1465 (85.3)
Race or ethnic group — no. (%)[†]		
White	1576 (92.9)	1572 (91.5)
Black	49 (2.9)	68 (4.0)
Asian	21 (1.2)	20 (1.2)
American Indian, Alaskan Native, or Aboriginal Canadian	11 (0.6)	11 (0.6)
Native Hawaiian or other Pacific Islander	5 (0.3)	7 (0.4)
Multiracial or other	33 (1.9)	40 (2.3)
Hispanic or non-Hispanic ethnic group — no. (%)[†]		
Non-Hispanic	1619 (95.5)	1654 (96.3)
Hispanic	77 (4.5)	63 (3.7)
Presenting history or diagnosis — no. (%)		
History of myocardial infarction	955 (56.3)	968 (56.3)
CABG	627 (37.0)	600 (34.9)
PCI	1044 (61.6)	1057 (61.5)
Stroke or cerebrovascular disease	362 (21.3)	358 (20.8)
Peripheral vascular disease	231 (13.6)	234 (13.6)
Metabolic syndrome	1353 (79.8)	1414 (82.3)
History of hypertension	1189 (70.1)	1250 (72.8)
History of diabetes	570 (33.6)	588 (34.2)
Laboratory values in patients with history of diabetes		
Glucose — mg/dl	126.4±27.1	126.9±26.9
Glycated hemoglobin — %	6.68±0.85	6.70±0.88
Insulin — μU/ml	25.63±31.09	25.32±29.23
Concomitant medications — no. (%)		
Statin		
Use at baseline	1601 (94.4)	1595 (92.8)
Duration of prior statin therapy[‡]		
<1 yr	190 (11.2)	202 (11.8)
1−5 yr	629 (37.1)	627 (36.5)
>5 yr	684 (40.3)	669 (38.9)
Previous use of niacin or Niaspan[§]	338 (19.9)	324 (18.9)
Beta-blocker	1342 (79.1)	1377 (80.2)
ACE inhibitor or ARB	1271 (74.9)	1258 (73.2)
Aspirin or other antiplatelet or anticoagulant agent	1654 (97.5)	1680 (97.8)

*Plus−minus values are means ± SD. There were no significant differences between the treatment groups at baseline in any of the baseline characteristics. To convert the values for glucose to millimoles per liter, multiply by 0.05551. ACE denotes angiotensin-converting enzyme, ARB angiotensin II−receptor blocker, CABG coronary-artery bypass grafting, and PCI percutaneous coronary intervention.

[†]Race or ethnic group was self-reported.

[‡]The duration of prior statin therapy was not ascertained in 204 patients (6.0%).

[§]Niacin and other lipid-modifying drugs except statins and ezetimibe were discontinued 30 days before enrollment.

findings most certainly did not reproduce the results of the HATS trial. However, in HATS, baseline LDL-C was 124 mg/dL, and combination statin/niacin therapy was compared with placebo. In AIM-HIGH, the baseline LDL-C was dramatically lower, and patients were aggressively treated with statin therapy or combination therapy (statin/ezetimibe). Apo B and non−HDL-C were also

TABLE 4.—Primary, Secondary, and Tertiary End Points

End Point	Placebo Plus Statin (N = 1696) Number of Patients (Percent)	Extended-Release Niacin Plus Statin (N = 1718) Number of Patients (Percent)	Hazard Ratio with Niacin (95% CI)	P Value*
Primary end point: death from coronary heart disease, nonfatal myocardial infarction, ischemic stroke, hospitalization for acute coronary syndrome, or symptom-driven coronary or cerebral revascularization	274 (16.2)	282 (16.4)	1.02 (0.87–1.21)	0.80
Individual primary-end-point events				
Death from coronary heart disease	26 (1.5)	20 (1.2)		
Nonfatal myocardial infarction	80 (4.7)	92 (5.4)		
Ischemic stroke	15 (0.9)	27 (1.6)		
Hospitalization for acute coronary syndrome	67 (4.0)	63 (3.7)		
Symptom-driven coronary or cerebral revascularization	86 (5.1)	80 (4.7)		
Secondary end points				
Death from coronary heart disease, nonfatal myocardial infarction, high-risk acute coronary syndrome, or ischemic stroke	158 (9.3)	171 (10.0)	1.08 (0.87–1.34)	0.49
Death from coronary heart disease, nonfatal myocardial infarction, or ischemic stroke	138 (8.1)	156 (9.1)	1.13 (0.90–1.42)	0.30
All deaths from cardiovascular causes†	38 (2.2)	45 (2.6)	1.17 (0.76–1.80)	0.47
Tertiary end points†				
Death from coronary heart disease	34 (2.0)	38 (2.2)	1.10 (0.69–1.75)	0.68
Death from any cause	82 (4.8)	96 (5.6)	1.16 (0.87–1.56)	0.32
Nonfatal myocardial infarction	93 (5.5)	104 (6.1)	1.11 (0.84–1.47)	0.46
Hospitalizations for acute coronary syndrome	82 (4.8)	72 (4.2)	0.87 (0.63–1.19)	0.38
Symptom-driven coronary or cerebral revascularizations	168 (9.9)	167 (9.7)	0.99 (0.80–1.22)	0.90
Ischemic stroke‡	18 (1.1)	29 (1.7)	1.61 (0.89–2.90)	0.11
Ischemic stroke or stroke of uncertain origin	18 (1.1)	30 (1.7)	1.67 (0.93–2.99)	0.09

*The P value is for the superiority of niacin therapy over placebo, adjusted for sex and history or no history of diabetes, with the use of a Cox proportional-hazards model to estimate the Wald statistic.
†The tertiary end point included all events, rather than just those that occurred as the first study event (which are listed in the category of individual primary-end-point events).
‡Three strokes in the niacin group were detected during a blinded re-review, after the database was locked, of cases of transient ischemic attack; these three events are not included in these analyses.

stringently controlled at 80 mg/dL and 106 mg/dL, respectively. The most likely explanation for these results is that: (1) niacin does not provide incremental risk reduction in patients with atherogenic dyslipidemia when the atherogenic lipoprotein burden of a patient with CAD is this stringently controlled and (2) increasing HDL-C with a net difference between groups of 4 mg/dL did not appear to impact risk for events when other lipids were already well controlled. Some caution is urged when applying these results to direct patient care, as the average AIM-HIGH patient likely represents less than 12% of patients with CAD. The lipids of the large majority of patients with CAD are not nearly this well controlled. The increased signal for ischemic stroke is somewhat puzzling, especially given the fact that stroke risk was reduced by niacin in the Coronary Drug Project.[1] Had the study been allowed to proceed longer, we could have perhaps gleaned a more precise quantitative assessment of stroke risk in response to niacin therapy.

The results of the Heart Protection Study-2: Treatment of HDL to Reduce the Incidence of Vascular Events (HPS2-THRIVE) are eagerly awaited to either affirm or nuance the findings of AIM-HIGH. HPS-2 THRIVE has enrolled more than 25 000 patients with a broad range of entry lipid parameters to help further define the role of niacin adjuvant therapy in patients with a variety of dyslipidemias, not just those with "atherogenic dyslipidemia." A large number of post-hoc analyses are expected from AIM-HIGH. One that will be of particular interest is to determine if niacin was beneficial in the patients in the lowest tertile for baseline HDL-C or the highest tertile for baseline triglycerides.

P. P. Toth, MD, PhD

References

1. Clofibrate and niacin in coronary heart disease. *JAMA.* 1975;231:360-381.
2. Brown BG, Zhao XQ, Chait A, et al. Simvastatin and niacin, antioxidant vitamins, or the combination for the prevention of coronary disease. *N Engl J Med.* 2001; 345:1583-1592.
3. Brown G, Albers JJ, Fisher LD, et al. Regression of coronary artery disease as a result of intensive lipid-lowering therapy in men with high levels of apolipoprotein B. *N Engl J Med.* 1990;323:1289-1298.
4. Whitney EJ, Krasuski RA, Personius BE, et al. A randomized trial of a strategy for increasing high-density lipoprotein cholesterol levels: effects on progression of coronary heart disease and clinical events. *Ann Intern Med.* 2005;142:95-104.
5. Carlson LA, Rosenhamer G. Reduction of mortality in the Stockholm Ischaemic Heart Disease Secondary Prevention Study by combined treatment with clofibrate and nicotinic acid. *Acta Med Scand.* 1988;223:405-418.

Risk of Incident Diabetes With Intensive-Dose Compared With Moderate-Dose Statin Therapy: A Meta-analysis
Preiss D, Seshasai SRK, Welsh P, et al (Univ of Glasgow, UK; Univ of Cambridge, UK; et al)
JAMA 305:2556-2564, 2011

Context.—A recent meta-analysis demonstrated that statin therapy is associated with excess risk of developing diabetes mellitus.

Objective.—To investigate whether intensive-dose statin therapy is associated with increased risk of new-onset diabetes compared with moderate-dose statin therapy.

Data Sources.—We identified relevant trials in a literature search of MEDLINE, EMBASE, and the Cochrane Central Register of Controlled Trials (January 1, 1996, through March 31, 2011). Unpublished data were obtained from investigators.

Study Selection.—We included randomized controlled end-point trials that compared intensive-dose statin therapy with moderate-dose statin therapy and included more than 1000 participants who were followed up for more than 1 year.

Data Extraction.—Tabular data provided for each trial described baseline characteristics and numbers of participants developing diabetes and experiencing major cardiovascular events (cardiovascular death, nonfatal myocardial infarction or stroke, coronary revascularization). We calculated trial-specific odds ratios (ORs) for new-onset diabetes and major cardiovascular events and combined these using random-effects model meta analysis. Between-study heterogeneity was assessed using the I^2 statistic.

Results.—In 5 statin trials with 32 752 participants without diabetes at baseline, 2749 developed diabetes (1449 assigned intensive-dose therapy, 1300 assigned moderate-dose therapy, representing 2.0 additional cases in the intensive-dose group per 1000 patient-years) and 6684 experienced cardiovascular events (3134 and 3550, respectively, representing 6.5 fewer cases in the intensive-dose group per 1000 patient-years) over a weighted mean (SD) follow-up of 4.9 (1.9) years. Odds ratios were 1.12 (95% confidence interval [CI], 1.04-1.22; $I^2 = 0\%$) for new-onset diabetes and 0.84 (95% CI, 0.75-0.94; $I^2 = 74\%$) for cardiovascular events for participants receiving intensive therapy compared with moderate-dose therapy. As compared with moderate-dose statin therapy, the number needed to harm per year for intensive-dose statin therapy was 498 for new-onset diabetes while the number needed to treat per year for intensive-dose statin therapy was 155 for cardiovascular events.

Conclusion.—In a pooled analysis of data from 5 statin trials, intensive-dose statin therapy was associated with an increased risk of new-onset diabetes compared with moderate-dose statin therapy.

▶ One new concern with stain therapy is an increased risk of new onset diabetes mellitus (DM), which was first identified in the Justification for the Use of Statins in Primary Prevention: An Intervention Trial Evaluating Rosuvastatin trial.[1] Two subsequent meta-analyses confirmed that statin therapy is associated with an increased risk for new onset type 2 DM, with no heterogeneity among the statins.[2,3] In the meta-analysis by Sattar et al, 255 patients would have to be treated for 4 years to observe 1 new case of DM (ie, 1 new case for every 1000 patient years of therapy). It is as yet unclear how statins may affect glucose homeostasis. Despite this risk, it is clear that statins reduce risk for cardiovascular events in both nondiabetic and diabetic patients to an approximately equal degree.[4,5] It is also clear that there is better risk reduction in patients treated with high-dose as opposed to low-dose or moderate-dose statins in the secondary prevention setting.[6] It is not clear, however, if there is a dose dependency to the capacity of statins to increase risk for DM.

This study examined this issue by performing an analysis of pooled data from 5 large statin trials, including the Treating to New Targets trial, the Incremental Decrease in End Points Through Aggressive Lipid Lowering trial, the Aggrastat to Zocor trial, the Pravastatin or Atorvastatin Evaluation and Infection Therapy—Thrombolysis in Myocardial Infarction trial, and the Study of the Effectiveness of Additional Reductions in Cholesterol and Homocysteine, which compared high doses and moderate doses of statins and their effects on cardiovascular outcomes. There were 18.9 cases per 1000 patient years of high-dose statin therapy and 16.9 cases per 1000 patient years, for an absolute difference of 2 cases per 1000 patient years of therapy and a number needed to harm of 498 per year (Fig 1 in the original article). No heterogeneity between study cohorts was detected. There was also no heterogeneity as a function of age, body mass index, high-density lipoprotein cholesterol, or fasting plasma glucose. Curiously, if triglycerides were below the median, this was an independent predictor of increased risk for statin-dependent DM. There is currently no explanation for this, although it may be attributed to play of chance (Fig 2 in the original article). In contrast, there were 6.5 fewer first cardiovascular events per 1000 patient years in patients who received high-dose as opposed to moderate-dose therapy, yielding a number needed to treat to prevent 1 cardiovascular event of 155 per year.

Despite the increased risk for DM, this analysis provides quantitative demonstration of net benefit with statin therapy when comparing moderate doses to high doses of statins. Much work remains to be done in this area. It will be important to elucidate the mechanism(s) by which statin therapy elevates the risk for DM. In the meantime, however, patients should not be discouraged from initiating statin therapy for dyslipidemia, as the benefits of their use still outweigh their risks.

P. P. Toth, MD, PhD

References

1. Ridker PM, Danielson E, Fonseca FA, et al. Rosuvastatin to prevent vascular events in men and women with elevated C-reactive protein. *N Engl J Med.* 2008;359:2195-2207.
2. Rajpathak SN, Kumbhani DJ, Crandall J, Barzilai N, Alderman M, Ridker PM. Statin therapy and risk of developing type 2 diabetes: a meta-analysis. *Diabetes Care.* 2009;32:1924-1929.
3. Sattar N, Preiss D, Murray HM, et al. Statins and risk of incident diabetes: a collaborative meta-analysis of randomised statin trials. *Lancet.* 2010;375:735-742.
4. Baigent C, Keech A, Kearney PM, et al. Efficacy and safety of cholesterol-lowering treatment: prospective meta-analysis of data from 90,056 participants in 14 randomised trials of statins. *Lancet.* 2005;366:1267-1278.
5. Kearney PM, Blackwell L, Collins R, et al. Efficacy of cholesterol-lowering therapy in 18,686 people with diabetes in 14 randomised trials of statins: a meta-analysis. *Lancet.* 2008;371:117-125.
6. Cannon CP, Steinberg BA, Murphy SA, Mega JL, Braunwald E. Meta-analysis of cardiovascular outcomes trials comparing intensive versus moderate statin therapy. *J Am Coll Cardiol.* 2006;48:438-445.

47 Obesity

Comparative Effectiveness of Weight-Loss Interventions in Clinical Practice
Appel LJ, Clark JM, Yeh H-C, et al (Johns Hopkins Univ, Baltimore, MD; et al)
N Engl J Med 365:1959-1968, 2011

Background.—Obesity and its cardiovascular complications are extremely common medical problems, but evidence on how to accomplish weight loss in clinical practice is sparse.

Methods.—We conducted a randomized, controlled trial to examine the effects of two behavioral weight-loss interventions in 415 obese patients with at least one cardiovascular risk factor. Participants were recruited from six primary care practices; 63.6% were women, 41.0% were black, and the mean age was 54.0 years. One intervention provided patients with weight-loss support remotely — through the telephone, a study-specific Web site, and e-mail. The other intervention provided in-person support during group and individual sessions, along with the three remote means of support. There was also a control group in which weight loss was self-directed. Outcomes were compared between each intervention group and the control group and between the two intervention groups. For both interventions, primary care providers reinforced participation at routinely scheduled visits. The trial duration was 24 months.

Results.—At baseline, the mean body-mass index (the weight in kilograms divided by the square of the height in meters) for all participants was 36.6, and the mean weight was 103.8 kg. At 24 months, the mean change in weight from baseline was −0.8 kg in the control group, −4.6 kg in the group receiving remote support only ($P < 0.001$ for the comparison with the control group), and −5.1 kg in the group receiving in-person support ($P < 0.001$ for the comparison with the control group). The percentage of participants who lost 5% or more of their initial weight was 18.8% in the control group, 38.2% in the group receiving remote support only, and 41.4% in the group receiving in-person support. The change in weight from baseline did not differ significantly between the two intervention groups.

Conclusions.—In two behavioral interventions, one delivered with in-person support and the other delivered remotely, without face-to-face contact between participants and weight-loss coaches, obese patients achieved and sustained clinically significant weight loss over a period of

24 months. (Funded by the National Heart, Lung, and Blood Institute and others; ClinicalTrials.gov number, NCT00783315.)

▶ Obesity is known to increase the risk for type 2 diabetes and cardiovascular disease, among many other comorbid conditions. The prevalence of obesity has risen sharply, mainly because of lifestyle changes. It is clear that to halt this epidemic, large-scale, population-based strategies should be implemented. It is also important that weight-loss counseling can be delivered in primary care centers, but there is a paucity of community-based weight-loss trials in which its effectiveness and reproducibility can be evaluated.

The purpose of the trial by Appel et al was to evaluate the long-term (24-month) effectiveness of 2 behavioral weight-loss interventions, differing in personal contact. A total of 415 obese patients were randomized to 3 groups. The control group had in-person individual sessions, the second group had in-person individual sessions plus group sessions, and the third group had in-person support delivered by electronic and telephone contact or a commercial call-center-directed group in which lifestyle interventions were delivered by telephone, Internet, or mail (remote support). The role of the primary care physicians (PCPs) was to support the patients with the weight-loss treatment. The weight loss was similar in the group that received in-person support and remote support, and both were superior to the control group (5.1 kg, 4.6 kg, and 0.8 kg, respectively; Fig 1 in the original article). Patients in both active groups lost more than 5% of initial weight compared with the control group (41% in the in-person group, 38% in the remote group, and 19% in the control group).

This study was one of the longest trials to evaluate remote (telephone, Web-based) interventions. Surprisingly, the effect of in-person and remote counseling yielded similar results. It is not clear if the in-person contact with the PCP influenced the clinical results. Previous studies have shown inferior weight loss in remote counseling compared with frequent in-person sessions.

Unfortunately, neither of the studies (by Wadden and the present study by Appel) were powered to evaluate change in cardiovascular risk factors, and there was no significant change in these parameters in both studies. Nevertheless, when dealing with an epidemic, the use of remote counseling enables providers to offer large-scale, more convenient counseling that can be easily implemented in clinical practice.

R. Ness-Abramof, MD

Hypertriglyceridemic waist: a simple clinical phenotype associated with coronary artery disease in women
Blackburn P, Lemieux I, Lamarche B, et al (Université du Québec à Chicoutimi, Saguenay, Canada; Centre de recherche de l'Institut universitaire de cardiologie et de pneumologie de Québec, Canada; Université Laval, Québec, Canada; et al)
Metabolism 61:56-64, 2012

The aim of the present study was to compare the ability of the hyper-triglyceridemic waist phenotype and the National Cholesterol Education

Program—Adult Treatment Panel III (NCEP-ATP III) clinical criteria to predict coronary artery disease (CAD) risk in a sample of women. We studied 254 women among whom the presence/absence of CAD was assessed by angiography. The *hypertriglyceridemic waist phenotype* was defined as having both a high waist circumference (≥ 85 cm) and increased fasting triglyceride levels (≥ 1.5 mmol/L), whereas the presence of at least 3 of the 5 NCEP-ATP III criteria was used as the "reference" screening approach to identify women with the features of the metabolic syndrome. Women with hypertriglyceridemic waist were characterized by higher adiposity indices as well as by a more disturbed fasting metabolic risk profile compared with women without this phenotype. Similar differences were observed when comparing the metabolic profile of women with vs without at least 3 of the NCEP-ATP III clinical criteria. Moreover, differences in the Framingham risk score were essentially similar when women were considered at low or high risk by either hypertriglyceridemic waist or by NCEP-ATP III clinical criteria ($P < .0001$). Finally, both clinical phenotypes were predictive of CAD (hypertriglyceridemic waist: relative odds ratio, 2.1; 95% confidence interval, 1.1-3.8; $P = .02$; NCEP-ATP III clinical criteria: relative odds ratio, 2.5; 95% confidence interval, 1.4-4.6; $P < .003$). These results suggest that hypertriglyceridemic waist is a simple screening tool to identify women with clustering metabolic abnormalities and at increased CAD risk.

▶ The metabolic syndrome comprises a cluster of risk factors that increase the risk for type 2 diabetes mellitus (type 2 DM) and cardiovascular disease. The risk factors include increased glucose levels, high blood pressure, elevated triglycerides, low high-density lipoprotein cholesterol, and a high waist circumference as a marker of obesity. Meeting 3 of 5 of the diagnostic criteria fulfills the diagnosis of the syndrome. The prevalence of the syndrome has been increasing worldwide due to the increasing prevalence of obesity.

The cutoff for waist circumference differs among ethnic groups and recommendations of different health organizations. The initial threshold for waist circumference by the American Heart Association/National Heart, Lung, and Blood Institute (AHA/NHLBI) was a waist circumference of 88 cm or more for women and 102 cm or more for men.[1] This cutoff was changed according to ethnic-specific cutoffs; for whites a cutoff of 80 cm or more for women and 94 cm or more for men has been recommended.[2] When using the AHA/NHLBI definition for the United States, the higher or lower waist circumference thresholds do not significantly change the diagnosis of the metabolic syndrome because of the high prevalence of the other components of the syndrome in the population and because of the high prevalence of obesity.

The metabolic syndrome criteria are not the only criteria proposed to identify high-risk patients. The hypertriglyceridemic waist, a combination of increased waist circumference and high fasting triglyceride level, has also been shown to identify high-risk patients for cardiovascular disease and type 2 DM and may be an easier way to screen in clinical practice.

This study compared the diagnostic ability of the hypertriglyceridemic waist phenotype and the National Cholesterol Education Program—Adult Treatment

Panel III (NCEP-ATP III) to predict coronary artery disease (CAD) risk in women referred for coronary angiography. The study enrolled 254 women, in which the diagnosis of the hypertriglyceridemic waist was a waist circumference of 85 cm or more and increased fasting triglyceride of 1.5 mmol/L or more (133 mg/dL). As expected, women with the hypertriglyceridemic waist had higher adiposity and increased metabolic abnormalities. There was no significant difference for the diagnosis of high-risk or low-risk women when comparing the hypertriglyceridemic waist and the NCEP-ATP III criteria, with both criteria encompassing a higher risk for CAD (hypertriglyceridemic waist: relative odds ratio, 2.1; 95% confidence interval, 1.1–3.8; $P = .02$; NCEP-ATP III clinical criteria: relative odds ratio, 2.5; 95% confidence interval, 1.4–4.6; $P < .003$). The hypertriglyceridemic waist and NCEP diagnosed different subgroups of high-risk patients, a result that is concordant with previous studies.

This study reinforces the hypertriglyceridemic waist as a way to identify high-risk patients using a relatively easy and accessible clinical tool.

R. Ness-Abramof, MD

References

1. Grundy SM, Brewer HB Jr, Cleeman JI, Smith SC Jr, Lenfant C, for the Conference Participants. NHLBI/AHA Conference Proceedings: definition of metabolic syndrome: report of the National Heart, Lung, and Blood Institute/American Heart Association conference on scientific issues related to definition. *Circulation.* 2004;109:433-438.
2. Alberti KG, Eckel RH, Grundy SM, et al. Harmonizing the metabolic syndrome: a joint interim statement of the International Diabetes Federation Task Force on Epidemiology and Prevention; National Heart, Lung, and Blood Institute; American Heart Association; World Heart Federation; International Atherosclerosis Society; and International Association for the Study of Obesity. *Circulation.* 2009;120: 1640-1645.

Two-year sustained weight loss and metabolic benefits with controlled-release Phentermine/Topiramate in obese and overweight adults (SEQUEL): a randomized, placebo-controlled, phase 3 extension study
Garvey WT, Ryan DH, Look M, et al (Univ of Alabama at Birmingham; Pennington Biomedical Res Ctr, Baton Rouge, LA; San Diego Sports Medicine, CA; et al)
Am J Clin Nutr 95:297-308, 2012

Background.—Obesity is a serious chronic disease. Controlled-release phentermine/topiramate (PHEN/TPM CR), as an adjunct to lifestyle modification, has previously shown significant weight loss compared with placebo in a 56-wk study in overweight and obese subjects with ≥ 2 weight-related comorbidities.

Objective.—This study evaluated the long-term efficacy and safety of PHEN/TPM CR in overweight and obese subjects with cardiometabolic disease.

Design.—This was a placebo-controlled, double-blind, 52-wk extension study; volunteers at selected sites continued with original randomly assigned treatment [placebo, 7.5 mg phentermine/46 mg controlled-release topiramate (7.5/46), or 15 mg phentermine/92 mg controlled-release topiramate (15/92)] to complete a total of 108 wk. All subjects participated in a lifestyle-modification program.

Results.—Of 866 eligible subjects, 676 (78%) elected to continue in the extension. Overall, 84.0% of subjects completed the study, with similar completion rates between treatment groups. At week 108, PHEN/TPM CR was associated with significant, sustained weight loss (intent-to-treat with last observation carried forward; $P < 0.0001$ compared with placebo); least-squares mean percentage changes from baseline in body weight were -1.8%, -9.3%, and -10.5% for placebo, 7.5/46, and 15/92, respectively. Significantly more PHEN/TPM CR—treated subjects at each dose achieved $\geq 5\%$, $\geq 10\%$, $\geq 15\%$, and $\geq 20\%$ weight loss compared with placebo ($P < 0.001$). PHEN/TPM CR improved cardiovascular and metabolic variables and decreased rates of incident diabetes in comparison with placebo. PHEN/TPM CR was well tolerated over 108 wk, with reduced rates of adverse events occurring between weeks 56 and 108 compared with rates between weeks 0 and 56.

Conclusion.—PHEN/TPM CR in conjunction with lifestyle modification may provide a well-tolerated and effective option for the sustained treatment of obesity complicated by cardiometabolic disease. This trial was registered at clinicaltrials.gov as NCT00796367.

▶ The prevalence of obesity in the United States has reached 35% and is associated with multiple adverse effects, including hypertension, hyperlipidemia, and diabetes.[1] A modest weight reduction of only 10% leads to improvement in obesity-related comorbidities; however, achieving and maintaining this degree of weight loss remains challenging. Currently, there are no definitive pharmacologic treatment options for obesity. Existing pharmacotherapy includes phentermine and orlistat. Phentermine, a sympathomimetic amine, achieves a weight loss of less than 10% and is only approved for short-term use. Orlistat, a gastric lipase inhibitor, shows a maximal weight loss of 7% and is often not tolerated because of its gastrointestinal side effects.[2] Thus, long-term, effective treatment options are needed to treat obesity.

The SEQUEL trial was a 2-year study that evaluated the efficacy and safety of a novel combination drug that combines phentermine plus topiramate for the treatment of obesity. Phentermine is a sympathomimetic amine that suppresses appetite and has been approved for short-term treatment of obesity (< 3 months). Topiramate was initially marketed as an anti-epileptic drug and was later approved for the prophylaxis of migraine headaches. In clinical trials, subjects using topiramate were noted to have dose-related weight loss. Subsequently, clinical trials evaluating topiramate for weight loss confirmed this effect. The rationale for combining topiramate with phentermine is 2-fold. First, the combination targets more than 1 pathway to satiety in the hopes of maximizing the weight loss effect. Second, lower doses of each drug are used to minimize the potential adverse effects.[3]

Initial data on the combination of phentermine plus topiramate were published in the CONQUER trial, which was a 52-week double-blind randomized controlled trial that assigned 2487 obese subjects with a body mass index of 27 to 45 kg/m^2 and 2 or more weight-related comorbidities to receive placebo, mid-dose (phentermine 7.5 mg plus topiramate 46 mg), or full-dose (phentermine 15 mg plus topiramate 92 mg) treatment for 52 weeks. Mean weight loss at 1 year was 7.8%, 9.8%, and 1.2% for mid-dose, full-dose, and placebo, respectively.[4] The SEQUEL trial was a 52-week extension of the CONQUER trial, with 78% of subjects electing to continue in the extension. Results from the SEQUEL show sustained weight loss at 2 years, with mean weight loss of 9.3%, 10.5%, and 1.8% for mid-dose, full-dose, and placebo, respectively. In addition to weight loss, treatment showed significant improvement in weight-related comorbidities, including lower fasting glucose and insulin values (compared with placebo) and improvement in both systolic and diastolic blood pressure as well as lipid parameters. Side effects of treatment include paresthesia, dry mouth, constipation, and headache. Serious adverse events were rare and occurred at similar rates for treatment versus placebo groups.

The SEQUEL trial demonstrates the effectiveness of long-term treatment with the novel combination of phentermine and topiramate. The magnitude of weight loss achieved may have a meaningful impact on treating or preventing obesity-related comorbidities. Although longer-term studies are needed to fully elucidate potential risks, this unique combination treatment may fill the current void in the pharmacologic treatment of obesity.

A. Powell, MD

References

1. Flegal KM, Carroll MD, Kit BK, Ogden CL. Prevalence of obesity and trends in the distribution of body mass index among US adults, 1999-2010. *JAMA.* 2012; 307:491-497.
2. Foxcroft DR, Milne R. Orlistat for the treatment of obesity: rapid review and cost-effectiveness model. *Obes Rev.* 2000;1:121-126.
3. Bray GA, Hollander P, Klein S, et al. A 6-month randomized, placebo-controlled, dose-ranging trial of topiramate for weight loss in obesity. *Obes Res.* 2003;11: 722-733.
4. Gadde KM, Allison DB, Ryan DH, et al. Effects of low-dose, controlled-release, phentermine plus topiramate combination on weight and associated comorbidities in overweight and obese adults (CONQUER): a randomized, placebo-controlled, phase 3 trial. *Lancet.* 2011;377:1341-1352.

Bariatric Surgery versus Intensive Medical Therapy in Obese Patients with Diabetes

Schauer PR, Kashyap SR, Wolski K, et al (Cleveland Clinic, OH; et al)
N Engl J Med 366:1567-1576, 2012

Background.—Observational studies have shown improvement in patients with type 2 diabetes mellitus after bariatric surgery.

Methods.—In this randomized, nonblinded, single-center trial, we evaluated the efficacy of intensive medical therapy alone versus medical therapy plus Roux-en-Y gastric bypass or sleeve gastrectomy in 150 obese patients with uncontrolled type 2 diabetes. The mean ($\pm$ SD) age of the patients was 49 ± 8 years, and 66% were women. The average glycated hemoglobin level was $9.2 \pm 1.5\%$. The primary end point was the proportion of patients with a glycated hemoglobin level of 6.0% or less 12 months after treatment.

Results.—Of the 150 patients, 93% completed 12 months of follow-up. The proportion of patients with the primary end point was 12% (5 of 41 patients) in the medical therapy group versus 42% (21 of 50 patients) in the gastric-bypass group ($P = 0.002$) and 37% (18 of 49 patients) in the sleeve-gastrectomy group ($P = 0.008$). Glycemic control improved in all three groups, with a mean glycated hemoglobin level of $7.5 \pm 1.8\%$ in the medical-therapy group, $6.4 \pm 0.9\%$ in the gastric-bypass group ($P < 0.001$), and $6.6 \pm 1.0\%$ in the sleeve-gastrectomy group ($P = 0.003$). Weight loss was greater in the gastric-bypass group and sleeve-gastrectomy group (-29.4 ± 9.0 kg and -25.1 ± 8.5 kg, respectively) than in the medical-therapy group (-5.4 ± 8.0 kg) ($P < 0.001$ for both comparisons). The use of drugs to lower glucose, lipid, and blood-pressure levels decreased significantly after both surgical procedures but increased in patients receiving medical therapy only. The index for homeostasis model assessment of insulin resistance (HOMA-IR) improved significantly after bariatric surgery. Four patients underwent reoperation. There were no deaths or life-threatening complications.

Conclusions.—In obese patients with uncontrolled type 2 diabetes, 12 months of medical therapy plus bariatric surgery achieved glycemic control in significantly more patients than medical therapy alone. Further study will be necessary to assess the durability of these results. (Funded by Ethicon Endo-Surgery and others; ClinicalTrials.gov number, NCT00432809.)

▶ The prevalence of type 2 diabetes mellitus (type 2 DM) has been increasing rapidly during the last 3 decades due to the increasing prevalence of obesity. More than 30% of the US population is obese with a body mass index (BMI) ≥ 30 kg/m^2. Currently, bariatric surgery is the most efficacious treatment yielding substantial and sustained weight loss. A recent meta-analysis by Buchwald et al, in which patients had a mean BMI of 47.9 kg/m^2, mean weight loss was 38.5 kg or 55.9% of excess body weight with 78% of the patients having complete resolution of diabetes and 86.6% having resolution or improvement in control of type 2 diabetes. Diabetes resolution and weight loss were greater for patients undergoing biliopancreatic diversion/duodenal switch, followed by gastric bypass and less in patients having banding procedures.[1]

There is an increasing interest in the effect of bariatric surgery in improving or even curing type 2 DM. Bariatric surgery is also referred to as *metabolic surgery*, with a trend in performing this surgery in diabetic patients with lower BMIs.

Recently, 2 prospective studies evaluating the effect of bariatric surgery versus intensive lifestyle changes in the control and resolution of type 2 diabetes were published.

The first study, by Schauer et al, included 150 patients with uncontrolled diabetes with a BMI range of 27 to 40 kg/m^2. The patients were randomly assigned to medical therapy, Roux-en-Y gastric bypass, or sleeve gastrectomy. The primary endpoint of the study was glycemic control at 1 year (proportion of patients achieving an A1c of 6% or less with or without diabetic medications); secondary endpoints included other parameters associated with cardiovascular risk factors, weight loss, and changes in medications. At the end of the first year, substantially more patients who had bariatric surgery had an A1c of 6% or less, had a greater decrease in A1c, and were taking fewer medications for glucose control (Fig 1 in the original article). Patients on the gastric bypass group who achieved an A1c of 6% or less did so without the need for medications, while 28% of the sleeve gastrectomy patients still required diabetic medications. There was no mortality during the study, with 4 patients requiring reoperation during this year.

It is known that longstanding diabetes and need for multiple glucose-lowering therapies, including insulin, will lower the rate of remission of type 2 diabetes after bariatric surgery. In this study, the mean duration of diabetes was 8 years, with an average use of 3 glucose-lowering medications and a high use of insulin therapy (44%). The strength of the study is the randomization of the patients with uncontrolled, longstanding diabetes to 3 treatment arms and the evaluation of 2 bariatric surgery techniques: gastric bypass and sleeve gastrectomy. The outcome between the 2 bariatric arms did not differ significantly concerning glucose control, although the study was not powered to compare between the 2 bariatric arms.

The improvement in glucose control was observed already 3 months after surgery, as has been reported in a previous study, probably due to changes in gut hormones in addition to weight loss.

As mentioned by the authors, the limitation of the study is that it was conducted in a bariatric surgery center in highly selected patients with a relatively low incidence of complications and, therefore, it is not clear if these results can be generalized. The long-term durability of the glycemic effect of surgery will be evaluated in a follow-up study. It is worth mentioning that aiming for normoglycemia (A1c < 6%) in high-risk patients with the use of hypoglycemic medications cannot be advocated after the results of the Action to Control Cardiovascular Risk in Diabetes study in which patients in the intensive therapy had a greater mortality risk, possibly due to hypoglycemia.[2]

We are just starting the era of metabolic surgery. Further studies should address the long-term effect of surgery in controlling or curing type 2 diabetes and specific patient characteristics for the choice of the right candidate for the appropriate surgical procedure.

R. N. Abramof, MD

References

1. Buchwald H, Estok R, Fahrbach K, et al. Weight and type 2 diabetes after bariatric surgery: systematic review and meta-analysis. *Am J Med.* 2009;122:248-256.e5.
2. Action to Control Cardiovascular Risk in Diabetes Study Group, Gerstein HC, Miller ME, Byington RP, et al. Effects of intensive glucose lowering in type 2 diabetes. *N Engl J Med.* 2008;358:2545-2559.

48 Thyroid

Outcome of Graves' Orbitopathy after Total Thyroid Ablation and Glucocorticoid Treatment: Follow-Up of a Randomized Clinical Trial
Leo M, Marcocci C, Pinchera A, et al (Univ of Pisa, Italy)
J Clin Endocrinol Metab 97:E44-E48, 2012

Context.—In a previous study, we found that total thyroid ablation (thyroidectomy plus ^{131}I) is associated with a better outcome of Graves' orbitopathy (GO) compared with thyroidectomy alone, as observed shortly (9 months) after glucocorticoid (GC) treatment.

Objective.—The objective of the study was to evaluate the outcome of GO in the same patients of the previous study over a longer period of time.

Design.—This was a follow-up of a randomized study.

Setting.—The study was conducted at a referral center.

Patients.—Fifty-two of 60 original patients with mild to moderate GO participated in the study.

Interventions.—Patients randomized into thyroidectomy (TX) or total thyroid ablation and treated with GC were reevaluated in 2010, namely 88.0 ± 17.7 months after GC, having undergone an ophthalmological follow-up in the intermediate period.

Main Outcome Measures.—The main outcome measures included the following: 1) GO outcome; 2) time to GO best possible outcome and to GO improvement; and 3) additional treatments.

Results.—GO outcome at the end of the follow-up was similar in the two groups. However, the time required for the best possible outcome to be achieved was longer in the TX group (24 *vs.* 3 months, $P = 0.0436$), as was the time required for GO to improve (60 *vs.* 3 months, $P = 0.0344$). Additional treatments were given to a similar proportion of patients in each group (TX, 28%, total thyroid ablation, 25.9%), but they affected GO beneficially more often in the TX group (28 *vs.* 3.7%, P: 0.0412).

Conclusions.—Compared with thyroidectomy alone, total thyroid ablation allows the achievement of the best possible outcome and an improvement of GO within a shorter period of time (Fig 1).

► Treatment of hyperthyroidism in patients with Graves' orbitopathy (GO) is controversial. A conservative strategy based on antithyroid drugs is favored by some, whereas others, based on a proposed pathogenetic link between thyroid and orbital tissues, advocate an ablative strategy because removal of thyroid antigens could be beneficial for GO. In this study, the authors investigated the same patients that have already been studied over a longer period

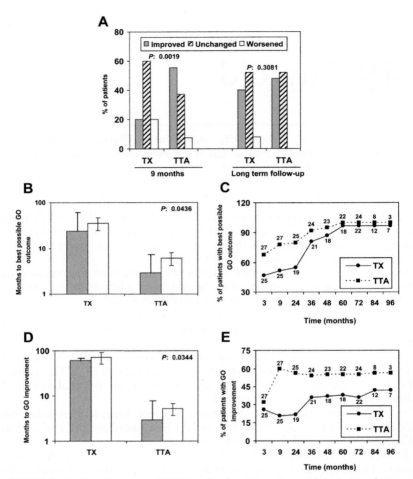

FIGURE 1.—A, Overall outcome of GO 9 months after the completion of glucocorticoid treatment and then in 2010 (long term follow-up), after a mean period of 88.0 ± 17.7 months (range 19–129). B, Median ± IQR (*gray columns*) and mean ± SD (*white columns*) time required to achieve the best possible outcome (the outcome observed at the end of the follow-up) of GO. C, Percent of patients reaching the best possible GO outcome over time. Number of patients available at each time point is indicated. D, Median ± IQR (*gray columns*) and mean ± SD (*white columns*) time required to reach an improvement of GO. E, Percent of patients with GO improvement over time. Number of patients available at each time point is indicated. (Reprinted from Leo M, Marcocci C, Pinchera A, et al. Outcome of Graves' orbitopathy after total thyroid ablation and glucocorticoid treatment: follow-up of a randomized clinical trial. *J Clin Endocrinol Metab*. 2012;97:E44-E48. Copyright 2012, The Endocrine Society.)

of time. Patients underwent a new evaluation on average approximately 7 years after glucocorticoid (GC) treatment, when GO outcome was similar, regardless of thyroid treatment. Nevertheless, this study shows that ablation may still have some advantages. Thus, the periods required to the best GO outcome and to GO improvement were shorter in total thyroid ablation (TTA). Whereas near-total thyroidectomy (TX) patients needed approximately 2 years to the best GO outcome and approximately 5 years to GO improvement, TTA patients needed only 3 months for both. The overlap concerning time to best outcome (Fig 1) should explain the relatively high, yet significant, *P* values. TSH receptor antibody (TRAb) reflect GO severity and activity. Thus, a shorter period would have been expected in TTA for TRAb to decrease or disappear. However, there was no difference with TX. In addition, approximately 25% of the patients still had detectable TRAb at the end of the follow-up, regardless of thyroid treatment, although the levels decreased over time. It may therefore be argued that the TTA advantages may not reflect a greater/faster attenuation of autoimmunity but rather other, unknown phenomena. Whatever the case, this study still shows some apparent advantages of ablation on the GO outcome, which may have clinical implications. To some extent, results in the long term reflected additional treatments, which were given to a similar proportion of patients in each group and affected GO favorably more often in TX. Nevertheless, additional treatments did not influence our conclusions, because GO outcome and time to improvement were not affected when the authors considered only patients who had not received these treatments.

Some issues and possible weaknesses of this study should be considered. First, the study cannot answer the question whether an ablative strategy is preferable to a conservative one. Second, patients were given GC, which certainly affected GO. Thus, it is not known whether ablation is beneficial in patients not given GC. Third, there was a 45-day difference between TX and TTA in terms of timing of GC administration. Whether this affected GO is unknown. Fourth, this evaluation was not part of the original protocol, and the frequency of visits might have been affected by GO severity.

M. Schott, MD, PhD
A. Thiel, MD

Simultaneous Occurrence of Subacute Thyroiditis and Graves' Disease
Hoang TD, Mai VQ, Clyde PW, et al (Natl Naval Med Ctr, Wisconsin, Bethesda, MD)
Thyroid 21:1397-1400, 2011

Background.—Rare cases of Graves' disease occurring years after subacute thyroiditis (SAT) have been reported. Here, we present the first known case of simultaneous occurrence of Graves' disease and SAT.

Patient Findings.—A 41-year-old woman presented with 10 days of neck pain, dysphagia, and hyperthyroid symptoms. Neck pain had initially started at the base of the right anterior neck and gradually spread to her upper chest, the left side of her neck, and bilateral ears. Physical examination revealed a heart rate of 110 beats/minute and a diffusely enlarged tender thyroid gland without evidence of orbitopathy. There was a resting tremor of the fingers and brisk deep tendon reflexes. Laboratory values: thyrotropin < 0.01 mcIU/mL (nL 0.39−5.33), free thyroxine 2.0 ng/dL (nL 0.59−1.60), free T3 6.6 pg/mL (nL 2.3−4.2), thyroglobulin 20.1 ng/mL (nL 2.0−35.0), thyroglobulin antibody 843 IU/mL (nL 0−80), thyroperoxidase antibody

130 IU/mL (nL 0–29), thyroid stimulating hormone receptor antibody 22.90 IU/L (nL < 1.22), thyroid stimulating immunoglobulins 299 units (nL < 140), erythrocyte sedimentation rate 120 mm/h (nL 0–20), and C-reactive protein 1.117 mg/dL (nL 0–0.5). Human leukocyte antigen (HLA) typing revealed DRB1, DR8, B35, B39, DQB1, DQ4, and DQ5. A thyroid ultrasound showed an enlarged heterogeneous gland with mild hypervascularity. Fine-needle aspiration (FNA) biopsies of both thyroid lobes revealed granulomatous thyroiditis. The thyroid scan showed a diffusely enlarged gland and heterogeneous trapping. There was a focal area of relatively increased radiotracer accumulation in the right upper pole. The 5-hour uptake (^{123}I) was 6.6% (nL 4–15). The patient was symptomatically treated. Over the next several weeks, she developed hypothyroidism requiring levothyroxine treatment.

Summary.—This case illustrates a rare simultaneous occurrence of Graves' disease and SAT. Previous case studies have shown that Graves' disease may develop months to years after an episode of SAT. A strong family history of autoimmune thyroid disorders was noted in this patient. Genetic predilection was also shown by HLA typing.

Conclusion.—Although the occurrence of SAT with Graves' disease may be coincidental, SAT-induced autoimmune alteration may promote the development of Graves' disease in susceptible patients. Genetically mediated mechanisms, as seen in this patient by HLA typing and a strong family history, may also be involved.

▶ Autoimmune alterations induced by subacute thyroiditis have been proposed to be causative in the development of Graves disease. The deferred occurrence of Graves disease in patients who suffered from subacute thyroiditis within an interval of 4 months to 8 years has been reported previously. In this case report, the authors introduce the simultaneous incidence of both diseases, thereby underlining the recently proposed pathophysiologic correlations.[1] The authors present a 41-year-old white woman with typical signs of hyperthyroidism combined with symptoms induced by subacute thyroiditis. Graves ophthalmopathy was clinically ruled out. Laboratory results, ultrasonography, and fine-needle aspiration confirmed the clinical diagnosis. During the course of disease, she eventually developed hypothyroidism, which was quite unusual, as only less than 1% of affected patients become hypothyroid subsequent to subacute thyroiditis. The incidence of Graves disease following subacute thyroiditis has been linked to stress on the immune system in predisposed patients, release or expression of autoantigens in susceptible patients, and, last but not least, to genetic susceptibility toward the disease. Risk factors leading to the induction of an acute thyroiditis were ruled out in this patient. However, interestingly, human leukocyte antigen typing revealed a genetic predilection for both Graves disease (HLADRB1, DQB1) and subacute thyroiditis (HLA-B35), supporting the theory of genetic susceptibility. Additionally, the authors propose autoimmunity induced by viral infection. Apart from the fact that the simultaneous appearance of both disorders might be coincidental, this case report reveals strong evidence for pathophysiologic interactions between subacute thyroiditis and Graves disease. Consequently, a regular monitoring for Graves disease seems reasonable in patients subsequent to recovery from subacute thyroiditis. Furthermore, the exact pathophysiologic process leading to these clinical findings is still nebulous and demands further clarification.

A. Thiel, MD

M. Schott, MD, PhD

Reference

1. Nakano Y, Kurihara H, Sasaki J. Graves' disease following subacute thyroiditis. *Tohoku J Exp Med.* 2011;225:301-309.

Serum TSH within the Reference Range as a Predictor of Future Hypothyroidism and Hyperthyroidism: 11-Year Follow-Up of the HUNT Study in Norway

Åsvold BO, Vatten LJ, Midthjell K, et al (Norwegian Univ of Science and Technology, Trondheim, Norway; Norwegian Univ of Science and Technology, Levanger, Norway; et al)
J Clin Endocrinol Metab 97:93-99, 2012

Context.—Serum TSH in the upper part of the reference range may sometimes be a response to autoimmune thyroiditis in early stage and may therefore predict future hypothyroidism. Conversely, relatively low serum TSH could predict future hyperthyroidism.

Objective.—The objective of the study was to assess TSH within the reference range and subsequent risk of hypothyroidism and hyperthyroidism.

Design and Setting.—This was a prospective population-based study with linkage to the Norwegian Prescription Database.

Subjects.—A total of 10,083 women and 5,023 men without previous thyroid disease who had a baseline TSH of 0.20—4.5 mU/liter and who participated at a follow-up examination 11 yr later.

Main Outcome Measures.—Predicted probabilities of developing hypothyroidism or hyperthyroidism during follow-up, by categories of baseline TSH, were estimated.

Results.—During 11 yr of follow-up, 3.5% of women and 1.3% of men developed hypothyroidism, and 1.1% of women and 0.6% of men developed hyperthyroidism. In both sexes, the baseline TSH was positively associated with the risk of subsequent hypothyroidism. The risk increased gradually from TSH of 0.50—1.4 mU/liter [women, 1.1%, 95% confidence interval (CI) 0.8—1.4; men, 0.3%, 95% CI 0.1—0.6] to a TSH of 4.0—4.5 mU/liter (women, 31.5%, 95% CI 24.6—39.3; men, 14.7%, 95% CI 7.7—26.2). The risk of hyperthyroidism was higher in women with a baseline TSH of 0.20—0.49 mU/liter (3.9%, 95% CI 1.8—8.4) than in women with a TSH of 0.50—0.99 mU/liter (1.4%, 95% CI 0.9—2.1) or higher (~1.0%).

Conclusion.—TSH within the reference range is positively and strongly associated with the risk of future hypothyroidism. TSH at the lower limit of the reference range may be associated with an increased risk of hyperthyroidism (Table 3).

▶ In this longitudinal population-based study, serum thyroid-stimulating hormone (TSH) within the reference range was positively and strongly associated with the risk of future hypothyroidism. The risk increased gradually from TSH of 0.50 to 1.4 mU/L to TSH of 4.0 to 4.5 mU/L (Fig 1 in the original article). The association of TSH with future hypothyroidism was essentially similar in women and men, but at any given TSH level, the absolute risk of hypothyroidism was higher in women than in men (Table 3). The risk of hyperthyroidism was higher in women with TSH of 0.20 to 0.49 mU/L than in women with higher TSH levels.

These results are of special importance. It has been suggested that the upper limit of the reference range for TSH should be lowered, in part based on the observation that people with TSH in the upper part of the reference range are at increased risk of hypothyroidism.[1] This study's results indicate, however, that

TABLE 3.—Age-Adjusted Predicted Probabilities (with 95% CI) of Hypothyroidism[a] at Follow-Up According to Categories of Baseline TSH in Women, by Age, Smoking, and BMI at Baseline[b]

TSH (mU/liter)	Hypothyroid, n/Total	Probability (%)	(95% CI)	Hypothyroid, n/Total	Probability (%)	(95% CI)
		20−49 yr of age			50−69 yr of age	
0.20−0.49	0/74	—		1/103	—	
0.50−1.4	28/2160	1.3	(0.9−1.9)	20/2371	0.8	(0.5−1.3)
1.5−1.9	25/1020	2.4	(1.7−3.6)	32/1398	2.3	(1.6−3.2)
2.0−2.4	23/575	4.0	(2.7−5.9)	26/821	3.2	(2.2−4.6)
2.5−2.9	24/305	7.8	(5.3−11.4)	38/454	8.3	(6.1−11.3)
3.0−3.4	23/164	13.9	(9.4−20.1)	26/231	11.2	(7.7−15.9)
3.5−3.9	13/83	15.7	(9.3−25.1)	28/171	16.4	(11.6−22.7)
4.0−4.5	21/56	37.3	(25.7−50.6)	27/97	27.8	(19.8−37.5)
		Nonsmokers			Smokers	
0.20−0.49	1/104	—		0/72	—	
0.50−1.4	31/2812	1.1	(0.8−1.6)	17/1704	1.0	(0.6−1.6)
1.5−1.9	32/1758	1.8	(1.3−2.6)	25/654	3.8	(2.5−5.5)
2.0−2.4	34/1113	3.0	(2.2−4.2)	15/279	5.3	(3.2−8.7)
2.5−2.9	41/609	6.7	(5.0−9.0)	21/146	14.5	(9.6−21.2)
3.0−3.4	33/322	10.2	(7.4−14.0)	16/73	21.8	(13.7−32.7)
3.5−3.9	34/222	15.4	(11.2−20.8)	7/32	21.7	(10.7−39.2)
4.0−4.5	35/121	28.9	(21.5−37.7)	13/31	40.5	(24.8−58.3)
		BMI <25.0 kg/m^2			BMI ≥25.0 kg/m^2	
0.20−0.49	0/77	—		1/100	—	
0.50−1.4	21/2067	1.0	(0.6−1.5)	27/2456	1.1	(0.7−1.6)
1.5−1.9	17/967	1.7	(1.1−2.7)	40/1446	2.7	(2.0−3.7)
2.0−2.4	22/546	3.9	(2.5−5.8)	27/849	3.2	(2.2−4.6)
2.5−2.9	24/263	8.7	(5.8−12.7)	38/495	7.7	(5.7−10.5)
3.0−3.4	19/148	12.3	(8.0−18.6)	30/247	12.3	(8.7−17.0)
3.5−3.9	15/82	18.2	(11.2−28.1)	26/172	15.3	(10.6−21.5)
4.0−4.5	19/52	35.4	(23.6−49.3)	29/101	29.2	(21.1−38.9)

Editor's Note: Please refer to original journal article for full references.
[a]Defined as prescription of levothyroxine, or TSH above 4.50 mU/liter combined with free T$_4$ below 9.0 pmol/liter, in people without a history of hyperthyroidism.
[b]Due to missing information on smoking or BMI, 31 and 15 women were excluded from the analyses by smoking and BMI, respectively.

most people with TSH between 2.5 and 4.5 mU/L did not develop hypothyroidism during 11 years of follow-up. Furthermore, the association of TSH with the risk of hypothyroidism appears to be gradual across the reference range, with no cutoff point that distinctly separates TSH levels that are associated with increased risk of hypothyroidism from TSH levels that are not. Nonetheless, a substantial proportion of people with TSH in the uppermost part of the reference range developed hypothyroidism, which gives support to the suggestion that follow-up of thyroid function in these individuals may be appropriate. In summary, this longitudinal population-based study shows that serum TSH concentrations within the reference range were positively and strongly associated with the risk of developing hypothyroidism during 11 years of follow-up in both women and men. Conversely, TSH at the lower limit of the reference range may be associated with an increased risk of hyperthyroidism.

A. Thiel, MD
M. Schott, MD, PhD

Reference

1. Wartofsky L, Dickey RA. The evidence for a narrower thyrotropin reference range is compelling. *J Clin Endocrinol Metab.* 2005;90:5483-5488.

Treatment of Amiodarone-Induced Thyrotoxicosis Type 2: A Randomized Clinical Trial
Eskes SA, Endert E, Fliers E, et al (Univ of Amsterdam, The Netherlands; et al)
J Clin Endocrinol Metab 97:499-506, 2012

Context.—Amiodarone-induced thyrotoxicosis (AIT) type 2 is self-limiting in nature, but most physicians are reluctant to continue amiodarone. When prednisone fails to restore euthyroidism, possibly due to mixed cases of AIT type 1 and 2, perchlorate (ClO_4) might be useful because ClO_4 reduces the cytotoxic effect of amiodarone on thyrocytes.

Objectives.—Our objectives were to demonstrate the feasibility of continuation of amiodarone in AIT type 2 and to evaluate the usefulness of ClO_4 (given alone or in combination with prednisone) in AIT type 2.

Design and Setting.—A randomized multicenter study was conducted in 10 Dutch hospitals.

Methods.—Patients with AIT type 2 were randomized to receive prednisone 30 mg/d (group A, n = 12), sodium perchlorate 500 mg twice daily (group B, n = 14), or prednisone plus perchlorate (group C, n = 10); all patients continued amiodarone and were also treated with methimazole 30 mg/d. Follow-up was 2 yr.

Main Outcome Measures.—Treatment efficacy (defined as TSH values ≥ 0.4 mU/liter under continuation of amiodarone) and recurrent thyrotoxicosis were evaluated.

Results.—Initial therapy was efficacious in 100, 71, and 100% of groups A, B, and C, respectively ($P = 0.03$). The 29% failures in group B became euthyroid after addition of prednisone. Neither the time to reach TSH of

0.4 mU/liter or higher [8 wk (4–20), 14 wk (4–32), and 12 wk (4–28) in groups A, B, and C respectively] nor the time to reach free T_4 of 25 pmol/liter or below [4 wk (4–20), 12 wk (4–20), and 8 wk (4–20) in groups A, B, and C)] were significantly different between groups (values as median with range). Recurrent thyrotoxicosis occurred in 8.3%.

Conclusion.—Euthyroidism was reached despite continuation of amiodarone in all patients. Prednisone remains the preferred treatment modality of AIT type 2, because perchlorate given alone or in combination with prednisone had no better outcomes (Table 2).

▶ Amiodarone-induced thyrotoxicosis (AIT) type 2 is caused by a destructive thyroiditis due to direct cytotoxic effects of the drug on thyrocytes. The nature of destructive thyroiditis is that of a self-limiting disease. The aim of this study was to demonstrate the feasibility of continuation of amiodarone in AIT type 2 and to evaluate the usefulness of perchlorate (given alone or in combination with prednisone) in AIT type 2. The authors could demonstrate that euthyroidism was reached despite continuation of amiodarone in all patients. Details are given in Table 2. The authors showed that prednisone remains the preferred treatment modality of AIT type 2, because perchlorate given alone or in combination with prednisone had no better outcomes.

This study is the first prospective, controlled trial indicating that discontinuation of amiodarone in AIT type 2 is not necessary for restoration of euthyroidism. One may argue that the time to normalize free thyroxine (T_4) and thyroid-stimulating hormone (TSH) is longer when amiodarone is continued. A recent

TABLE 2.—Treatment Outcomes in Patients with AIT Type 2

	Group A (n = 12) Prednisone + Methimazole	Group B (n = 14) Perchlorate + Methimazole	Group C (n = 10) Prednisone + Perchlorate + Methimazole
Efficacy of treatment[a]			
TSH ≥ 0.4 mU/liter on initial therapy	12 (100%)	10 (71%)	10 (100%)
TSH ≥ 0.4 mU/liter on additional therapy	NA	4 (29%)	NA
Time to FT₄ ≤ 25 pmol/liter (wk)[b]	4 (4–20)	12 (4 –20)	8 (4–20)
Time to TSH ≤ 0.4 mU/liter (wk)[b]	8 (4–20)	14 (4 –32)	12 (4 –28)
Amiodarone continued	12 (100%)	14 (100%)	10 (100%)
Recurrent thyrotoxicosis	1	0	2
Time of recurrence (wk)	24	NA	12 and 76
Time to TSH ≥ 0.4 mU/liter (wk)	8	NA	4
Follow-up			
Amiodarone continued until end of follow-up	12 (100%)	14 (100%)	10 (100%)
Follow-up < 2 yr	0	2[c]	1[d]
Follow-up 2 yr	12	12	9
TSH 0.4 –5.0 mU/liter at 2 yr	10	11	6
TSH > 5.0 mU/liter at 2 yr	2	1	3
On levothyroxine at 2 yr	3	1	1

NA, Not applicable.
[a]Defined as TSH of 0.4 mU/liter or higher while amiodarone is continued.
[b]Median (range).
[c]Sudden cardiac death and cardiac transplant.
[d]Agranulocytosis upon methimazole treatment of recurrent thyrotoxicosis.

retrospective study identified 8 patients with AIT type 2 assembled in the period 2003 through 2008 who were treated with prednisone under continuation of amiodarone. When compared with 32 matched controls with AIT type 2 treated with prednisone after discontinuation of amiodarone, median time to first normalization of thyroid hormone levels did not significantly differ between both groups (24 and 31 days, respectively).[1] Because of a higher rate of recurrences in patients continuing amiodarone, the median time for stably restoring euthyroidism was much longer in this group. To establish whether continuation of amiodarone in prednisone-treated AIT type 2 patients really affects cure time will require a randomized clinical trial comparing continuation of amiodarone with stopping amiodarone. Continuation of amiodarone carries a risk of recurrent thyrotoxicosis. The authors observed an incidence of 8.3% at 2-year follow-up. An open Japanese study reported 6% recurrences of AIT type 2 occurring 5 to 8 years after the first episode.[2] In agreement with that study, the recurrences in this study were also mild and responded quickly to therapy. In this study, there was a high incidence of hypothyroidism, which, although frequently transient in nature, persisted in many cases until the end of follow-up. One could argue that continuation of amiodarone would result in more cases of hypothyroidism. However, this appears unlikely because 17% of AIT type 2 patients in whom amiodarone was discontinued developed permanent hypothyroidism within 2 years after successful treatment with steroids.[3] This study had some limitations. As indicated, the authors did not apply color flow Doppler sonography to discriminate AIT types, because this method was not available in all centers. The number of patients in each treatment modality is rather small in the study. In view of this limited sample size, the results may not be generalized to all cases of AIT type 2, and, as indicated by the authors, they authors cannot exclude the possibility that in specific circumstances, discontinuation of amiodarone might be necessary.

A. Thiel, MD
M. Schott, MD, PhD

References

1. Bogazzi F, Bartalena L, Tomisti L, Rossi G, Brogioni S, Martino E. Continuation of amiodarone delays restoration of euthyroidism in patients with type 2 amiodarone-induced thyrotoxicosis treated with prednisone: a pilot study. *J Clin Endocrinol Metab*. 2011;96:3374-3380.
2. Sato K, Shiga T, Matsuda N, et al. Mild and short recurrence of type II amiodarone-induced thyrotoxicosis in three patients receiving amiodarone continuously for more than 10 years. *Endocr J*. 2006;53:531-538.
3. Bogazzi F, Dell'Unto E, Tanda ML, et al. Long-term outcome of thyroid function after amiodarone-induced thyrotoxicosis, as compared to subacute thyroiditis. *J Endocrinol Invest*. 2006;29:694-699.

PART EIGHT

ENDOCRINOLOGY, DIABETES, AND METABOLISM

DEREK LEROITH, MD, PHD

Introduction

The compilation of abstracts this year focuses primarily on diabetes, obesity, lipids, and to some degree, thyroid and bone disorders. These represent the majority of endocrine and metabolic disorders seen in academic or clinical practice. The outcome trials are of utmost importance for evidence-based medical practice. Numerous trials have been undertaken to assess the efficacy of drugs in diabetes, hyperlipidemia, osteoporosis, and other disorders. In the case of diabetes many have shown disappointing results, while bariatric surgery shows the most promise. Lipid-lowering drugs are very effective as are antiresorptives in the case of osteoporosis.

From the point of view of basic research, there are interesting studies on autoimmune thyroid disorders, providing a more in-depth understanding of the basic pathophysiology of diabetes, especially involving the beta cell dysfunction.

D. LeRoith, MD, PhD

49 Calcium and Bone Metabolism

Effect of Stopping Risedronate after Long-Term Treatment on Bone Turnover

Eastell R, Hannon RA, Wenderoth D, et al (Univ of Sheffield, UK; Warner Chilcott Deutschland GmbH, Weiterstadt, Germany; et al)
J Clin Endocrinol Metab 96:3367-3373, 2011

Context.—Determining how quickly bisphosphonate treatment effects begin to regress is crucial when considering termination of treatment.

Objective.—Our objective was to assess the effects of 1 yr discontinuation of risedronate use in postmenopausal women with osteoporosis who had previously received risedronate for 2 or 7 yr.

Design and Setting.—Before initiation of the current study, placebo/5-mg-risedronate patients had received placebo for 5 yr and risedronate for 2 yr, whereas 5-mg-risedronate patients had received risedronate for a total of 7 yr. Risedronate was then discontinued for 1 yr (yr 8).

Patients.—Postmenopausal women with osteoporosis who had previously completed the 3-yr Vertebral Efficacy with Risedronate Therapy Multi National (VERT-MN) pivotal trial, plus a 2-yr extension comparing risedronate or placebo for a total of 5 yr, followed by 2 yr of open-label risedronate treatment were enrolled in these trial extensions.

Main Outcome Measures.—Evaluations included changes in type I collagen cross-linked N-telopeptide (NTX)/creatinine (Cr) and bone mineral density (BMD) values, fracture incidence, and adverse events.

Results.—After 1 yr of risedronate discontinuation, NTX/Cr levels increased toward baseline in both patient groups vs. the values at the end of yr 7. In both treatment groups, off-treatment total hip and femoral trochanter BMD values decreased, whereas lumbar spine and femoral neck BMD were maintained or slightly increased. The adverse event profiles were similar between the two treatment groups during yr 8.

Conclusions.—One year of discontinuation of risedronate treatment in patients who had received 2 or 7 yr of risedronate therapy led to increases in NTX/Cr levels toward baseline and decreases in femoral trochanter and total hip BMD.

▶ Because of concerns regarding long-term safety and efficacy of bisphosphonate therapy, including risks related to jaw osteonecrosis and atypical subtrochanteric femoral fractures, the US Food and Drug Administration (FDA) has recommended that patients not be treated with continuous therapy with bisphosphonates for more than 5 years.[1] It has been assumed that all bisphosphonates share the same degree of long-term risk. Based on FLEX trial data with alendronate,[2,3] new HORIZON trial data with zoledronic acid,[4] and older data with risedronate,[5] it is assumed that most patients given a drug holiday after long-term treatment with bisphosphonate therapy should remain off treatment for at least 1, and perhaps as long as 5 years. No studies have addressed fracture risk after risedronate or ibandronate have been stopped.

This extension study gives insight into fracture risk in the first year after stopping risedronate after long-term therapy. Postmenopausal women with osteoporosis in the original VERT-MN pivotal fracture trial received treatment with risedronate for 3 years followed by a 2-year extension of risedronate treatment, and then 2 more years of open-label risedronate for a maximum cumulative exposure of 7 years, before they stopped treatment for 1 year.[6,7] The study showed that 24-hour urinary NTx-telopeptide recovered toward baseline over the year off treatment, suggesting wearing off of the antiresorptive effect of the previous long-term risedronate therapy. In addition, total hip and greater trochanteric bone mineral density (BMD) decreased, whereas lumbar spine and femoral neck BMD remained stable or slightly increased. Fractures did not increase during the year off treatment. The study concluded that stopping risedronate for 1 year after 2 to 7 years of continuous therapy led to urinary NTx-telopeptide increasing toward baseline after 1 year off therapy, with loss of total hip and greater trochanteric BMD, but without increased risk of fracture.

These findings suggest differences between the duration of antiresorptive effect of risedronate and longer-acting alendronate and zoledronic acid. The antiresorptive effect of longer-acting alendronate may take up to 5 years to wear off, whereas zoledronic acid takes at least 3 years to wear off. Why risedronate treatment effect appears to wear off so much more quickly is not clear, but it may have to do with avidity of binding of the drug to hydroxyapatite or other properties unique to risedronate. These findings reinforce the fact that not all bisphosphonates are the same, and that bone density protective effects of some bisphosphonates last longer than for other bisphosphonates.

B. L. Clarke, MD

References

1. Traynor K. FDA advisers uneasy about long-term bisphosphonate use. *Am J Health Syst Pharm.* 2011;68:2006-2008.
2. Black DM, Schwartz AV, Ensrud KE, et al; FLEX Research Group. Effects of continuing or stopping alendronate after 5 years of treatment: the Fracture Intervention Trial Long-term Extension (FLEX): a randomized trial. *JAMA.* 2006;296:2927-2938.
3. Schwartz AV, Bauer DC, Cummings SR, et al; FLEX Research Group. Efficacy of continued alendronate for fractures in women with and without prevalent vertebral fracture: the FLEX trial. *J Bone Miner Res.* 2010;25:976-982.
4. Black DM, Reid IR, Boonen S, et al. The effect of 3 versus 6 years of zoledronic acid treatment of osteoporosis: a randomized extension to the HORIZON-Pivotal Fracture Trial (PFT). *J Bone Miner Res.* 2012;27:243-254.
5. Watts NB, Chines A, Olszynski WP, et al. Fracture risk remains reduced one year after discontinuation of risedronate. *Osteoporos Int.* 2008;19:365-372.

6. Harris ST, Watts NB, Genant HK, et al. Effects of risedronate treatment on vertebral and nonvertebral fractures in women with postmenopausal osteoporosis: a randomized controlled trial. Vertebral Efficacy With Risedronate Therapy (VERT) Study Group. *JAMA*. 1999;282:1344-1352.
7. Reginster J, Minne HW, Sorensen OH, et al. Randomized trial of the effects of risedronate on vertebral fractures in women with established postmenopausal osteoporosis. Vertebral Efficacy with Risedronate Therapy (VERT) Study Group. *Osteoporos Int*. 2000;11:83-91.

Proton Pump Inhibitor Use and the Antifracture Efficacy of Alendronate

Abrahamsen B, Eiken P, Eastell R (Univ of Southern Denmark, Odense, Denmark; Hillerød Hosp, Denmark; Univ of Sheffield, England)
Arch Intern Med 171:998-1004, 2011

Background.—Proton pump inhibitors (PPIs) are widely used in elderly patients and are frequently coadministered in users of oral bisphosphonates. Biologically, PPIs could affect the absorption of calcium, vitamin B_{12}, and bisphosphonates and could affect the osteoclast proton pump, thus interacting with bisphosphonate antifracture efficacy. Moreover, PPIs themselves have been linked to osteoporotic fractures.

Methods.—Population-based, national register—based, open cohort study of 38 088 new alendronate sodium users with a mean duration of follow-up of 3.5 years. We related risk of hip fracture to recent pharmacy records of refill of prescriptions for alendronate.

Results.—For hip fractures, there was statistically significant interaction with alendronate for PPI use ($P<.05$). The treatment response associated with complete refill compliance to alendronate was a 39% risk reduction (hazard ratio [HR], 0.61; 95% confidence interval [CI], 0.52-0.71; $P<.001$) in patients who were not PPI users, while the risk reduction in concurrent PPI users was not significant (19%; HR, 0.81; 95% CI, 0.64-1.01; $P=.06$). The attenuation of the risk reduction was dose and age dependent. In contrast, there was no significant impact of concurrent use of histamine H_2 receptor blockers.

Conclusions.—Concurrent PPI use was associated with a dose-dependent loss of protection against hip fracture with alendronate in elderly patients. This is an observational study, so a formal proof of causality cannot be made, but the dose-response relationship and the lack of impact of prior PPI use provides reasonable grounds for discouraging the use of PPIs to control upper gastrointestinal tract complaints in patients treated with oral bisphosphonates.

▶ Previous studies have found increased hip fracture risk in patients taking proton pump inhibitors (PPIs).[1-5] Some of these studies have found dose-response relationships between PPI use and fracture risk. It has been presumed that PPIs decrease stomach acid secretion sufficiently to reduce intestinal absorption of calcium carbonate due to lack of solubilization of calcium carbonate tablets in reduced or minimal stomach acid.[1] PPIs may also possibly affect absorption of oral bisphosphonates by reducing conversion of bisphosphonate salts to bisphosphonate acids in stomach acid, as normally occurs. Finally, PPIs theoretically could have direct effects on osteoclast proton pumps, leading to decreased acidification of bone resorption lacunae.

This population-based national register open cohort study evaluated fracture risk in a large number of new alendronate sodium users over a mean follow-up of 3.5 years. National pharmacy records were used to verify alendronate prescription refills, and hip fractures were assessed based on national hospital discharge records. For subjects not taking PPIs who refilled all their alendronate prescriptions over the study interval, hip fracture risk was reduced by 39%, similar to previously published studies. For subjects who took PPIs concurrently and refilled all alendronate prescriptions, hip fracture risk reduction was only 19%, but this change was nonsignificant. The increase in hip fracture risk seen with PPI use was both dose dependent and age dependent, with elderly patients having the greatest loss of hip fracture protection from alendronate. This study also showed no effect on hip fracture reduction with histamine 2 receptor (H_2)-blockers. The study concluded that PPI use concurrent with oral bisphosphonate use may reduce hip fracture protection in the elderly.

These findings raise concern that hip fracture risk reduction associated with oral bisphosphonate therapy may be minimized by simultaneous PPI therapy. Because many patients taking oral bisphosphonates also take PPIs for gastro-esophageal reflux symptoms, it is possible that the bisphosphonate therapy is not benefiting these patients as much as previously thought. In some patients, PPI therapy has been prescribed to minimize gastroesophageal irritation resulting from bisphosphonate use. These findings suggest that patients requiring PPI therapy for treatment of gastroesophageal irritation may be better served by taking their bisphosphonate therapy by an intravenous route or by taking a nonbisphosphonate type of medication to treat their osteoporosis. Alternatively, H_2-blocker therapy might be considered in place of PPI therapy to reduce reflux symptoms in patients taking oral bisphosphonate therapy.

B. L. Clarke, MD

References

1. Yang YX, Lewis JD, Epstein S, Metz DC. Long-term proton pump inhibitor therapy and risk of hip fracture. *JAMA*. 2006;296:2947-2953.
2. Gray SL, LaCroix AZ, Larson J, et al. Proton pump inhibitor use, hip fracture, and change in bone mineral density in postmenopausal women: results from the Women's Health Initiative. *Arch Intern Med*. 2010;170:765-771.
3. Corley DA, Kubo A, Zhao W, Quesenberry C. Proton pump inhibitors and histamine-2 receptor antagonists are associated with hip fractures among at-risk patients. *Gastroenterology*. 2010;139:93-101.
4. Pouwels S, Lalmohamed A, Souverein P, et al. Use of proton pump inhibitors and risk of hip/femur fracture: a population-based case-control study. *Osteoporos Int*. 2011;22:903-910.
5. Ngamruengphong S, Leontiadis GI, Radhi S, Dentino A, Nugent K. Proton pump inhibitors and risk of fracture: a systematic review and meta-analysis of observational studies. *Am J Gastroenterol*. 2011;106:1209-1218.

Association of BMD and FRAX Score With Risk of Fracture in Older Adults With Type 2 Diabetes

Schwartz AV, for the Study of Osteoporotic Fractures (SOF), the Osteoporotic Fractures in Men (MrOS), and the Health, Aging, and Body Composition (Health ABC) Research Groups (Univ of California, San Francisco; et al)
JAMA 305:2184-2192, 2011

Context.—Type 2 diabetes mellitus (DM) is associated with higher bone mineral density (BMD) and paradoxically with increased fracture risk. It is not known if low BMD, central to fracture prediction in older adults, identifies fracture risk in patients with DM.

Objective.—To determine if femoral neck BMD T score and the World Health Organization Fracture Risk Algorithm (FRAX) score are associated with hip and nonspine fracture risk in older adults with type 2 DM.

Design, Setting, and Participants.—Data from 3 prospective observational studies with adjudicated fracture outcomes (Study of Osteoporotic Fractures [December 1998-July 2008]; Osteoporotic Fractures in Men Study [March 2000-March 2009]; and Health, Aging, and Body Composition study [April 1997-June 2007]) were analyzed in older community-dwelling adults (9449 women and 7436 men) in the United States.

Main Outcome Measure.—Self-reported incident fractures, which were verified by radiology reports.

Results.—Of 770 women with DM, 84 experienced a hip fracture and 262 a nonspine fracture during a mean (SD) follow-up of 12.6 (5.3) years. Of 1199 men with DM, 32 experienced a hip fracture and 133 a nonspine fracture during a mean (SD) follow-up of 7.5 (2.0) years. Age-adjusted hazard ratios (HRs) for 1-unit decrease in femoral neck BMD T score in women with DM were 1.88 (95% confidence interval [CI], 1.43-2.48) for hip fracture and 1.52 (95% CI, 1.31-1.75) for nonspine fracture, and in men with DM were 5.71 (95% CI, 3.42-9.53) for hip fracture and 2.17 (95% CI, 1.75-2.69) for nonspine fracture. The FRAX score was also associated with fracture risk in participants with DM (HRs for 1-unit increase in FRAX hip fracture score, 1.05; 95% CI, 1.03-1.07, for women with DM and 1.16; 95% CI, 1.07-1.27, for men with DM; HRs for 1-unit increase in FRAX osteoporotic fracture score, 1.04; 95% CI, 1.02-1.05, for women with DM and 1.09; 95% CI, 1.04-1.14, for men with DM). However, for a given T score and age or for a given FRAX score, participants with DM had a higher fracture risk than those without DM. For a similar fracture risk, participants with DM had a higher T score than participants without DM. For hip fracture, the estimated mean difference in T score for women was 0.59 (95% CI, 0.31-0.87) and for men was 0.38 (95% CI, 0.09-0.66).

Conclusions.—Among older adults with type 2 DM, femoral neck BMD T score and FRAX score were associated with hip and nonspine fracture risk; however, in these patients compared with participants without

DM, the fracture risk was higher for a given T score and age or for a given FRAX score.

▶ Previous studies have found increased fracture risk in adults with type 2 diabetes mellitus despite having higher bone mineral density (BMD) than age-matched controls.[1-3] These studies did not determine whether low BMD in adults with type 2 diabetes mellitus predicts fracture risk as it does in postmenopausal women or older men.[4-6]

This study evaluated whether femoral neck BMD T-score and the World Health Organization FRAX 10-year absolute fracture risk algorithm predict hip and nonvertebral fractures in older adults with type 2 diabetes mellitus. To do this, data from 3 prospective observational studies with adjudicated fracture outcomes were combined to obtain sufficient numbers of type 2 diabetic subjects. Data from the Study of Osteoporotic Fractures in postmenopausal women were obtained from December 1998 through July 2008; the Osteoporotic Fractures in Men Study from March 2000 through March 2009; and the Health, Aging, and Body Composition Study in women and men from April 1997 through June 2007. The analysis was done on 9449 community-dwelling women and 7436 community-dwelling men in the United States. Fractures identified by self-report were verified by radiology reports. In 770 women with type 2 diabetes mellitus, 84 hip fractures and 262 nonvertebral fractures were identified over 12.6 ± 5.6 years of follow-up. In 1199 men with type 2 diabetes mellitus, 32 hip fractures and 133 nonvertebral fractures were confirmed over 7.5 ± 2.0 years of follow-up. The age-adjusted hazard ratio for a 1.0-unit femoral neck BMD T-score decrease in women was 1.88 for hip fracture and 1.52 for nonvertebral fracture. Men had a similar hazard ratio of 5.71 for hip fracture, and 2.17 for nonvertebral fracture. The FRAX score correlated with fracture risk in the diabetic subjects. For a given T-score and age, or for a given FRAX score, subjects with type 2 diabetes mellitus had a higher fracture risk than those without type 2 diabetes. For similar fracture risk, diabetics had a higher T-score than subjects without diabetes. The study concluded that femoral neck BMD T-score and FRAX score were associated with hip and nonvertebral fracture risk in older adults with type 2 diabetes mellitus but that fracture risk was higher in diabetics than nondiabetics for a given T-score and age or for a given FRAX score.

These findings indicate that adults with type 2 diabetes mellitus, like those treated with glucocorticoid therapy, have increased fracture risk beyond that predicted by their femoral neck BMD T-score. In addition, adults with type 2 diabetes mellitus with the same fracture risk as nondiabetics have higher femoral neck BMD T-scores. These data imply that bone quality is decreased in adults with type 2 diabetes mellitus, perhaps because of accumulation of advanced glycation end products or other causes. Adult diabetics should be treated for osteoporosis more aggressively than adults without diabetes who have similar T-scores or FRAX scores.

B. L. Clarke, MD

References

1. Schwartz AV, Sellmeyer DE, Strotmeyer ES, et al; Health ABC Study. Diabetes and bone loss at the hip in older black and white adults. *J Bone Miner Res.* 2005;20: 596-603.
2. Strotmeyer ES, Cauley JA, Schwartz AV, et al. Nontraumatic fracture risk with diabetes mellitus and impaired fasting glucose in older white and black adults: the health, aging, and body composition study. *Arch Intern Med.* 2005;165:1612-1617.
3. de Liefde II, van der Klift M, de Laet CE, van Daele PL, Hofman A, Pols HA. Bone mineral density and fracture risk in type-2 diabetes mellitus: the Rotterdam Study. *Osteoporos Int.* 2005;16:1713-1720.
4. Johnell O, Kanis JA, Oden A, et al. Predictive value of BMD for hip and other fractures. *J Bone Miner Res.* 2005;20:1185-1194.
5. Hillier TA, Cauley JA, Rizzo JH, et al. WHO absolute fracture risk models (FRAX): do clinical risk factors improve fracture prediction in older women without osteoporosis? *J Bone Miner Res.* 2011;26:1774-1782.
6. Trémollieres FA, Pouillès JM, Drewniak N, Laparra J, Ribot CA, Dargent-Molina P. Fracture risk prediction using BMD and clinical risk factors in early postmenopausal women: sensitivity of the WHO FRAX tool. *J Bone Miner Res.* 2010;25: 1002-1009.

Effects of Antiresorptive Treatment on Nonvertebral Fracture Outcomes
Mackey DC, Black DM, Bauer DC, et al (California Pacific Med Ctr, San Francisco; Univ of California San Francisco; et al)
J Bone Miner Res 26:2411-2418, 2011

Various definitions of nonvertebral fracture have been used in osteoporosis trials, precluding comparisons of efficacy. Using only subgroups of nonvertebral fractures for trial outcomes may underestimate the benefits and cost-effectiveness of treatments. The objectives of this study were to determine (1) the effect of antiresorptive treatment on various nonvertebral fracture outcomes, (2) whether risk reduction from antiresorptive treatment is greater for nonvertebral fractures that have stronger associations with low BMD, and (3) sample size estimates for clinical trials of osteoporosis treatments. Study-level data were combined from five randomized fracture-prevention trials of antiresorptive agents that reduce the risk of nonvertebral fracture in postmenopausal women: alendronate, clodronate, denosumab, lasofoxifene, and zoledronic acid. Pooled effect estimates were calculated with random-effects models. The five trials included 30,118 women; 2997 women had at least one nonvertebral fracture. There was no significant heterogeneity between treatments for any outcome (all $p > 0.10$). Antiresorptive treatment had similar effects on all fractures (summary hazard ratio [HR] = 0.76, 95% CI 0.70−0.81), high-trauma fractures (HR = 0.74, 95% CI 0.57−0.96), low-trauma fractures (HR = 0.77, 95% CI 0.71−0.83), nonvertebral six (ie, hip, pelvis, leg, wrist, humerus, and clavicle) fractures (HR = 0.73, 95% CI 0.66−0.80), other than nonvertebral six fractures (HR = 0.78, 95% CI 0.70−0.87), and all fractures other than finger, face, and toe (HR = 0.75, 95% CI 0.70−0.81). Risk reduction was not greater for fractures with stronger associations with low BMD ($p = 0.77$). A trial of all nonvertebral fractures would require fewer participants ($n = 2641$ per arm) than one of a subgroup of six fractures ($n = 3289$), for example. In summary, antiresorptive treatments reduced all nonvertebral fractures regardless of degree of trauma or special groupings, supporting the use of all nonvertebral fractures as a standard endpoint of osteoporosis trials and the basis for estimating the benefits and cost-effectiveness of treatments.

▶ The large majority of low- to moderate-trauma osteoporotic fractures are nonvertebral fractures, yet clinical trials have focused on prevention of hip and vertebral fractures.[1-6] This has been necessary for a variety of reasons, including the fact that, in most cases, vertebral and hip fractures are easily verifiable clinically or by x-ray. Furthermore, different clinical trials have used different definitions for nonvertebral fractures, making direct comparisons of efficacy between the available therapeutic agents very difficult.

This study attempted to estimate the effect of antiresorptive treatment on nonvertebral fracture outcomes, determine whether fracture risk reduction is greater for nonvertebral fractures associated with low bone mineral density (BMD), and estimate sample sizes required to show treatment efficacy for nonvertebral fractures in osteoporosis clinical trials. Data from 5 randomized fracture prevention trials with alendronate, clodronate, zoledronic acid, denosumab, and lasofoxifene that showed efficacy for nonvertebral fractures were pooled to derive efficacy estimates using random effects models. These 5 trials included 30 118 postmenopausal women, of whom 2997 had at least 2 nonvertebral fractures. The analysis showed that each agent reduced all nonvertebral fractures by 24% on average, and reduced high- or low-trauma fractures, 6 common types of nonvertebral fractures (hip, pelvis, leg, wrist, humerus, and clavicle), nonvertebral fractures other than the 6 most common types, and all fractures other than finger, toe, or face fractures. These agents did not cause greater risk reduction of nonvertebral fractures associated with lower BMD. Clinical trials of drug efficacy for all nonvertebral fractures would require 2641 subjects per arm, whereas proving efficacy in a subgroup of nonvertebral fractures would require more subjects. The study concluded that these 5 antiresorptive agents reduced all nonvertebral fractures regardless of severity of trauma or subcategorization of fractures.

These important findings show that several currently available antiresorptive agents effectively reduce nonvertebral fractures of all types, albeit with reduced efficacy compared with vertebral or hip fractures. In addition, future clinical trials should assess efficacy of new agents for reduction of all nonvertebral fractures rather than subsets of nonvertebral fractures unique to each clinical trial to allow direct comparison of efficacy between agents.

B. L. Clarke, MD

References

1. Watts NB, Geusens P, Barton IP, Felsenberg D. Relationship between changes in BMD and nonvertebral fracture incidence associated with risedronate: reduction in risk of nonvertebral fracture is not related to change in BMD. *J Bone Miner Res.* 2005;20:2097-2104.

2. Hochberg MC, Greenspan S, Wasnich RD, Miller P, Thompson DE, Ross PD. Changes in bone density and turnover explain the reductions in incidence of non-vertebral fractures that occur during treatment with antiresorptive agents. *J Clin Endocrinol Metab.* 2002;87:1586-1592.
3. Siris ES, Harris ST, Eastell R, et al; Continuing Outcomes Relevant to Evista (CORE) Investigators. Skeletal effects of raloxifene after 8 years: results from the continuing outcomes relevant to Evista (CORE) study. *J Bone Miner Res.* 2005; 20:1514-1524.
4. Langsetmo LA, Morin S, Richards JB, et al; CaMos Research Group. Effectiveness of antiresorptives for the prevention of nonvertebral low-trauma fractures in a population-based cohort of women. *Osteoporos Int.* 2009;20:283-290.
5. Cadarette SM, Katz JN, Brookhart MA, Stürmer T, Stedman MR, Solomon DH. Relative effectiveness of osteoporosis drugs for preventing nonvertebral fracture. *Ann Intern Med.* 2008;148:637-646.
6. McCloskey EV, Beneton M, Charlesworth D, et al. Clodronate reduces the incidence of fractures in community-dwelling elderly women unselected for osteoporosis: results of a double-blind, placebo-controlled randomized study. *J Bone Miner Res.* 2007;22:135-141.

Diets Higher in Dairy Foods and Dietary Protein Support Bone Health During Diet- and Exercise-Induced Weight Loss in Overweight and Obese Premenopausal Women

Josse AR, Atkinson SA, Tarnopolsky MA, et al (McMaster Univ, Hamilton, Ontario, Canada)

J Clin Endocrinol Metab 97:251-260, 2012

Context.—Consolidation and maintenance of peak bone mass in young adulthood may be compromised by inactivity, low dietary calcium, and diet-induced weight loss.

Objective.—We aimed to determine whether higher intakes of dairy foods, dietary calcium, and protein during diet- and exercise-induced weight loss affected markers of bone health.

Participants.—Participants included premenopausal overweight and obese women.

Design/Intervention.—Ninety participants were randomized into three groups (n = 30 per group): high protein and high dairy (HPHD), adequate protein and medium dairy (APMD), and adequate protein and low dairy (APLD), differing in dietary protein (30, 15, or 15% of energy, respectively), dairy foods (15, 7.5, or < 2% of energy from protein, respectively), and dietary calcium (~ 1600, ~ 1000, or < 500 mg/d, respectively).

Outcome Measures.—Serum and urine bone turnover biomarkers, serum osteoprotegerin (OPG), receptor activator of nuclear factor-κB ligand (RANKL), PTH, 25-hydroxyvitamin D, leptin, and adiponectin measured at 0 and 16 wk.

Results.—All groups lost equivalent body weight ($P < 0.05$). N-telopeptide, C-telopeptide (CTX), urinary deoxypyridinoline, and osteocalcin increased in APLD ($P < 0.01$), whereas in HPHD, osteocalcin and procollagen 1 amino-terminal propeptide (P1NP) increased ($P < 0.05$), and all resorption markers remained unchanged. P1NP to CTX and OPG to RANKL ratios increased in HPHD ($P < 0.005$), and P1NP to CTX ratio decreased in APLD ($P < 0.05$). PTH decreased in HPHD and APMD *vs.* APLD ($P < 0.005$), and 25-hydroxyvitamin D increased in HPHD ($P < 0.05$), remained unchanged in APMD, and decreased in APLD ($P < 0.05$). Leptin decreased and adiponectin increased in APMD and HPHD only ($P < 0.001$).

Conclusions.—Hypoenergetic diets higher in dairy foods, dietary calcium, and protein with daily exercise, favorably affected important bone health biomarkers *vs.* diets with less of these bone-supporting nutrients.

▶ Adult bone mass is accrued in the teenage years and between the second and third decade of life. Establishing peak bone mass and maintaining it throughout life is important to prevent osteoporosis. Greater bone mass is achieved with higher body weight persons. However, weight loss after restriction of calories can adversely affect bone health. Remedies to restrict or improve bone loss during weight loss programs would be a great benefit. Diet, supplements, calcium, and vitamin D are some factors that have been recommended to achieve the goal of minimizing bone loss.[1-5] Josse and associates investigated a diet high in dairy foods and protein in supporting bone health in premenopausal women during diet- and exercise-induced weight loss. While weight loss was comparable between the groups, bone health was superior in the high dairy group based on assessment with bone formation and desorption markers. Long-term studies are needed to confirm that bone mineral density would corroborate the apparent benefits based on bone markers.

A. W. Meikle, MD

References

1. Josse AR, Atkinson SA, Tarnopolsky MA, Phillips SM. Diets higher in dairy foods and dietary protein support bone health during diet- and exercise-induced weight loss in overweight and obese premenopausal women. *J Clin Endocrinol Metab.* 2012;97:251-260.
2. Hirota T, Hirota K. Diet for lifestyle-related diseases to maintain bone health. *Clin Calcium.* 2011;21:730-736.
3. Thorpe MP, Jacobson EH, Layman DK, He X, Kris-Etherton PM, Evans EM. A diet high in protein, dairy, and calcium attenuates bone loss over twelve months of weight loss and maintenance relative to a conventional high-carbohydrate diet in adults. *J Nutr.* 2008;138:1096-1100.
4. Huth PJ, DiRienzo DB, Miller GD. Major scientific advances with dairy foods in nutrition and health. *J Dairy Sci.* 2006;89:1207-1221.
5. Bowen J, Noakes M, Clifton P. High dairy-protein versus high mixed-protein energy restricted diets - the effect on bone turnover and calcium excretion in overweight adults. *Asia Pac J Clin Nutr.* 2003;12:S52.

Is Vitamin D a Determinant of Muscle Mass and Strength?

Marantes I, Achenbach SJ, Atkinson EJ, et al (Mayo Clinic, Rochester, MN)
J Bone Miner Res 26:2860-2871, 2011

There remains little consensus on the link between vitamin D levels and muscle mass or strength. We therefore investigated the association of serum 25-hydroxyvitamin D (25(OH)D), 1,25-dihydroxyvitamin D

(1,25(OH)$_2$D), and parathyroid hormone (PTH) levels with skeletal muscle mass and strength. We studied 311 men (mean age, 56 years; range, 23–91 years) and 356 women (mean age, 57 years; range, 21–97 years) representing an age-stratified, random sample of community adults. Multivariate linear regression models were used to examine the association of skeletal muscle mass (by total body dual-energy X-ray absorptiometry) and strength (handgrip force and isometric knee extension moment) with each of 25(OH)D, 1,25(OH)$_2$D, and PTH quartiles, adjusted for age, physical activity, fat mass, and season. We found no consistent association between 25(OH)D or PTH and any of our measurements of muscle mass or strength, in either men or women. However, in subjects younger than 65 years, there was a statistically significant association between low 1,25(OH)$_2$D levels and low skeletal mass in both men and women and low isometric knee extension moment in women, after adjustment for potential confounders. Modestly low 25(OH)D or high PTH levels may not contribute significantly to sarcopenia or muscle weakness in community adults. The link between low 25(OH)D and increased fall risk reported by others may be due to factors that affect neuromuscular function rather than muscle strength. The association between low 1,25(OH)$_2$D and low skeletal mass and low knee extension moment, particularly in younger people, needs further exploration.

▶ Vitamin D deficiency has been associated with osteoporosis and fall risk. Studies have shown a moderate correlation between low vitamin D levels and decreased postural stability and poor functional performance that could lead to falls.[1,2] It is not yet clear how vitamin D levels might affect fall risk directly. The vitamin D receptor was previously reported to be found in human skeletal muscle,[3] but a more recent study has disputed this finding.[4] Genotypic variations in the vitamin D receptor have been associated with differences in muscle strength.[5,6] One potential mechanism by which vitamin D might prevent falls is by improving muscle mass and strength.

This study correlated skeletal muscle mass and strength with serum 25-hydroxyvitamin D, 1,25-dihydroxyvitamin D, and parathyroid hormone (PTH) levels in an age-stratified population-based sample of 311 men age 23–91 years and 356 women age 21–97 years living in the community. Skeletal muscle mass was assessed by total body dual-energy X-ray absorptiometry and muscle strength by handgrip force and isometric knee extension moment. Vitamin D deficiency was present in 42% of study subjects. The overall results showed no consistent association between muscle mass or strength and quartiles of either form of vitamin D or PTH after adjustment for age, physical activity, fat mass, and season. However, subjects younger than 65 years showed a significant correlation between low serum 1,25-dihydroxyvitamin D level and low skeletal muscle mass in men and women, and low isometric knee extension moment in women, after adjustment for potential confounders. The study showed no association between mildly decreased serum 25-hydrxoyvitamin D and increased PTH levels and muscle weakness. The study concluded that the previously reported association between low serum 25-hydroxyvitamin D and fall risk may be due to factors other than muscle strength, and that the association between low serum 1,25-dihydroxyvitamin D and low skeletal muscle mass and decreased knee extension requires further investigation.

These findings failed to confirm an association between serum 25-hydroxyvitamin D and muscle mass or strength in an adult community—dwelling, population-based sample of men and women. However, an association was found between low serum 1,25-dihydroxyvitamin D and decreased skeletal muscle mass in men and women and decreased knee strength in women, although a clear threshold below which muscle mass or strength was lower was not identified. One other study has reported a modest association between low serum 1,25-dihydroxyvitamin D levels and low muscle strength,[7] but others have not.[8,9] Further investigation will be necessary to clarify the relative contributions of 25-hydroxyvitamin D and 1,25-dihydroxyvitmain D levels to muscle mass, muscle strength, and fall risk.

B. L. Clarke, MD

References

1. Bischoff-Ferrari HA, Dawson-Hughes B, Staehelin HB, et al. Fall prevention with supplemental and active forms of vitamin D: a meta-analysis of randomised controlled trials. *BMJ.* 2009;330:b3692.
2. Bischoff-Ferrari HA, Dietrich T, Orav EJ, et al. Higher 25-hydroxyvitamin D concentrations are associated with better lower-extremity function in both active and inactive persons aged ≥60 y. *Am J Clin Nutr.* 2004;80:752-758.
3. Bischoff HA, Borchers M, Gudat F, et al. In situ detection of 1,25-dihydroxyvitamin D3 receptor in human skeletal muscle tissue. *Histochem J.* 2001;33:19-24.
4. Wang Y, DeLuca HF. Is the vitamin D receptor found in muscle? *Endocrinology.* 2011;152:354-363.
5. Windelinckx A, De Mars G, Beunen G, et al. Polymorphisms in the vitamin D receptor gene are associated with muscle strength in men and women. *Osteoporos Int.* 2007;18:1235-1242.
6. Grundberg E, Brändstrom H, Ribom EL, Ljunggren O, Mallmin H, Kindmark A. Genetic variation in the human vitamin D receptor is associated with muscle strength, fat mass and body weight in Swedish women. *Eur J Endocrinol.* 2004; 150:323-328.
7. Houston DK, Cesari M, Ferrucci L, et al. Association between vitamin D status and physical performance: the InCHIANTI study. *J Gerontol A Biol Sci Med Sci.* 2007;62:440-446.
8. Boonen S, Lysens R, Verbecke G, et al. Relationship between age-associated endocrine deficiencies and muscle function in elderly women: a cross-sectional study. *Age Ageing.* 1998;27:449-454.
9. Mowé M, Haug E, Bøhmer T. Low serum calcidiol concentration in older adults with reduced muscular function. *J Am Geriatr Soc.* 1999;47:220-226.

50 Adrenal Cortex

Bone Mineral Density Is Not Significantly Reduced in Adult Patients on Low-Dose Glucocorticoid Replacement Therapy

Koetz KR, Ventz M, Diederich S, et al (Charité Univ Medicine Berlin, Germany; Endokrinologikum, Berlin, Germany)
J Clin Endocrinol Metab 97:85-92, 2012

Context.—Patients with primary adrenal insufficiency (PAI) and patients with congenital adrenal hyperplasia (CAH) receive glucocorticoid replacement therapy, which might cause osteoporosis.

Objectives.—Questions addressed by this study were: 1) Is bone mineral density (BMD) reduced in PAI and CAH on lower glucocorticoid doses than previously reported? 2) Is BMD in PAI influenced by the type of glucocorticoid used? and 3) Does DHEA treatment affect BMD in PAI women?

Design and Patients.—We conducted a prospective, cross-sectional study including 81 PAI patients and 41 CAH patients.

Main Outcome Measures.—BMD was measured by dual-energy x-ray absorptiometry. Serum levels of bone turnover markers, minerals, vitamins, hormones, and urinary crosslinks were measured.

Results.—PAI and CAH patients received average daily hydrocortisone doses of 12.0 ± 2.7 mg/m^2 (range, 4.9–19.1) and 15.5 ± 7.8 mg/m^2 (range, 5.7–33.7), respectively. BMD varied within the normal reference range (-2 to $+2$) in both cohorts. However, lower Z-scores for femoral neck and Ward's region were found in CAH compared to PAI women, but not in men. Prednisolone treatment showed significant lower osteocalcin levels and lower Z-scores for lumbar spine and femoral neck compared to PAI patients on hydrocortisone. PAI women treated with DHEA had significantly lower urinary collagen crosslinks and bone alkaline phosphatase, and significantly higher Z-scores in lumbar spine and femoral Ward's region compared to non-DHEA-treated women.

Conclusions.—Adult PAI and CAH patients on low glucocorticoid doses showed normal BMD within the normal reference range. The use of longer acting prednisolone resulted in significantly lower BMD in PAI. In addition, DHEA treatment may have a beneficial effect on bone in Addison's women.

▶ Osteopenia or osteoporosis is a frequent complication of long-term corticosteroid therapy or severe Cushing syndrome. The mechanism for the decrease in bone mass is complex and involves the loss of bone matrix because of the protein catabolic effect of glucocorticoids (GC), interference with intestinal calcium absorption because of the inhibitory effect of GC on vitamin D intestinal action, and direct effects of GC on osteoblasts and osteocytes, possibly inducing apoptosis.[1] These effects are clearly encountered in patients on chronic pharmacological doses of corticosteroids but are not definitive in patients on replacement doses. Patients with primary adrenal insufficiency (PAI) are usually replaced with physiological doses of hydrocortisone or prednisone, and patients with congenital adrenal hyperplasia (CAH) are replaced with doses of prednisone sufficient to suppress excessive androgen production and compensate for limited cortisol secretion. There have been reports that many of these patients develop osteoporosis after several years of corticosteroid treatment, but it is likely that this depends on the dose of steroid received. The authors conducted a prospective cross-sectional study of 81 patients with PAI and 41 patients with CAH. They measured bone mineral density (BMD) by dual-energy x-ray densitometry (DEXA) and biomarkers of bone turnover, including osteocalcin, β-crosslaps, and bone resorption marker collagen cross-link N-telopeptide. Their results were interesting and important. Patients treated with low glucocorticoid doses showed normal BMD compared with patients who received higher doses, even within the "physiological" replacement range. The message is that we use too generous a dose of GC replacement in PAI, and that patients probably need no more than 12 to 20 mg of hydrocortisone for adequate replacement. Normal cortisol production rates by isotopic dilution are 12 to 22 mg per day. Patients with CAH, who frequently receive borderline high doses of GC for suppression of adrenal androgens, are more likely to develop lower osteocalcin levels and Z scores for lumbar spine and femoral neck than those with PAI on hydrocortisone. Replacement with prednisolone, a GC with more prolonged half-life than hydrocortisone, is also associated with higher risk of decreased BMD. Men with PAI and CAH on corticosteroid replacement appear to be more protected than women with these conditions because of their androgen production. Similarly, the administration of dehydroepiandrosterone, an adrenal androgen, seems to have a bone protective effect in women with PAI on GC replacement therapy.

D. E. Schteingart, MD

Reference

1. Xia X, Kar R, Gluhak-Heinrich J, et al. Glucocorticoid-induced autophagy in osteocytes. *J Bone Miner Res.* 2010;25:2479-2488.

51 Reproductive Endocrinology

Cardiovascular Disease and Risk Factors in PCOS Women of Postmenopausal Age: A 21-Year Controlled Follow-Up Study
Schmidt J, Landin-Wilhelmsen K, Brännström M, et al (Univ of Gothenburg, Göteborg, Sweden)
J Clin Endocrinol Metab 96:3794-3803, 2011

Context.—Polycystic ovary syndrome (PCOS) is associated with the metabolic syndrome and, consequently, with a potentially increased risk of cardiovascular disease (CVD) and related mortality later in life. Studies regarding CVD and mortality in PCOS women well into the postmenopausal age are lacking.

Objective.—Our objective was to examine whether postmenopausal PCOS women differ from controls regarding cardiovascular risk factors, myocardial infarction (MI), stroke and mortality.

Design and Setting.—We conducted, at a university hospital, a prospective study of 35 PCOS women (61–79 yr) and 120 age-matched controls. The study was performed 21 yr after the initial study.

Participants.—Twenty-five PCOS women (Rotterdam criteria) and 68 controls participated in all examinations. Data on morbidity were based on 32 of 34 PCOS women and on 95 of 119 controls.

Interventions.—Interventions included reexamination, interviews, and data from the National Board of Health and Welfare and from the Hospital Discharge Registry.

Main Outcome Measures.—Blood pressure, glucose, insulin, triglycerides, total cholesterol, high- and low-density lipoprotein, apolipoprotein A1 and B, fibrinogen, and plasminogen activator inhibitor antigen were studied. Incidences of MI, stroke, hypertension, diabetes, cancer, cause of death, and age at death were recorded.

Results.—PCOS women had a higher prevalence of hypertension ($P = 0.008$) and higher triglyceride levels ($P = 0.012$) than controls. MI, stroke, diabetes, cancer, and mortality prevalence was similar in the two cohorts with similar body mass index.

Conclusions.—The well-described cardiovascular/metabolic risk profile in pre- and perimenopausal PCOS women does not entail an evident increase in cardiovascular events during the postmenopausal period.

▶ Polycystic ovary syndrome (PCOS) is the most common endocrine disorder in women and is characterized by oligomenorrhea, hyperandrogenism, infertility, and polycystic ovaries. The metabolic syndrome is commonly observed in them as is insulin resistance, hyperglycemia, waist/hip ratio, and elevated triglycerides.[1-5] Schmidt et al followed up with women with PCOS for 21 years to assess their risk of cardiovascular disease (CVD) and metabolic risk factors. Despite having risk factors more commonly for CVD than controls, they were not at increased risk for myocardial infarction, stroke, or dying from CVD. The explanation for the failure to observe expected increased risk of CVD was that the PCOS women had higher concentrations of high-density lipoprotein than in later life. Serum testosterone concentrations are lower in men at risk for CVD, and the authors speculate that hyperandrogenism might be protective for CVD in women with PCOS. A limitation of the study was the small sample size, which might preclude detection of more subtle difference between controls and PCOS women.

A. W. Meikle, MD

References

1. Bentley-Lewis R, Seely E, Dunaif A. Ovarian hypertension: polycystic ovary syndrome. *Endocrinol Metab Clin North Am.* 2011;40:433-449. ix-x.
2. de Groot PC, Dekkers OM, Romijn JA, Dieben SW, Helmerhorst FM. PCOS, coronary heart disease, stroke and the influence of obesity: a systematic review and meta-analysis. *Hum Reprod Update.* 2011;17:495-500.
3. Sasaki A, Emi Y, Matsuda M, et al. Increased arterial stiffness in mildly-hypertensive women with polycystic ovary syndrome. *J Obstet Gynaecol Res.* 2011;37:402-411.
4. Lambrinoudaki I. Cardiovascular risk in postmenopausal women with the polycystic ovary syndrome. *Maturitas.* 2011;68:13-16.
5. Tomlinson J, Millward A, Stenhouse E, Pinkney J. Type 2 diabetes and cardiovascular disease in polycystic ovary syndrome: what are the risks and can they be reduced? *Diabet Med.* 2010;27:498-515.

High Serum Testosterone Is Associated With Reduced Risk of Cardiovascular Events in Elderly Men: The MrOS (Osteoporotic Fractures in Men) Study in Sweden

Ohlsson C, Barrett-Connor E, Bhasin S, et al (Univ of Gothenburg, Sweden; Univ of California San Diego, La Jolla; Boston School of Medicine and Boston Med Ctr, MA; et al)
J Am Coll Cardiol 58:1674-1681, 2011

Objectives.—We tested the hypothesis that serum total testosterone and sex hormone—binding globulin (SHBG) levels predict cardiovascular (CV) events in community-dwelling elderly men.

Background.—Low serum testosterone is associated with increased adiposity, an adverse metabolic risk profile, and atherosclerosis. However, few prospective studies have demonstrated a protective link between endogenous testosterone and CV events. Polymorphisms in the SHBG gene are associated with risk of type 2 diabetes, but few studies have addressed SHBG as a predictor of CV events.

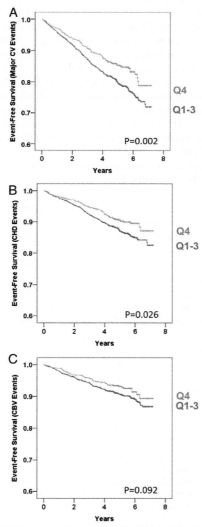

FIGURE 2.—Kaplan-Meier Plots by Testosterone Levels. Kaplan-Meier curves of event-free survival by serum testosterone for major CV events (**A**) CHD events (**B**), and CBV events (**C**). In quartile 4 of serum testosterone (**green lines**) or quartiles 1 to 3 (**blue lines**). p value assessed by logrank test. Abbreviations as in Figure 1 in the original article. For interpretation of the references to color in this figure legend, the reader is referred to web version of this article. (Reprinted from the [initial] Journal of the American College of Cardiology, Ohlsson C, Barrett-Connor E, Bhasin S, et al. High serum testosterone is associated with reduced risk of cardiovascular events in elderly men: the MrOS (osteoporotic fractures in men) study in Sweden. *J Am Coll Cardiol*. 2011;58:1674-1681. Copyright 2011, with permission from the American College of Cardiology.)

Methods.—We used gas chromatography/mass spectrometry to analyze baseline levels of testosterone in the prospective population-based MrOS (Osteoporotic Fractures in Men) Sweden study (2,416 men, age 69 to 81 years). SHBG was measured by immunoradiometric assay. CV clinical outcomes were obtained from central Swedish registers.

Results.—During a median 5-year follow-up, 485 CV events occurred. Both total testosterone and SHBG levels were inversely associated with the risk of CV events (trend over quartiles: $p = 0.009$ and $p = 0.012$, respectively). Men in the highest quartile of testosterone (≥ 550 ng/dl) had a lower risk of CV events compared with men in the 3 lower quartiles (hazard ratio: 0.70, 95% confidence interval: 0.56 to 0.88). This association remained after adjustment for traditional CV risk factors and was not materially changed in analyses excluding men with known CV disease at baseline (hazard ratio: 0.71, 95% confidence interval: 0.53 to 0.95). In models that included both testosterone and SHBG, testosterone but not SHBG predicted CV risk.

Conclusions.—High serum testosterone predicted a reduced 5-year risk of CV events in elderly men (Fig 2).

▶ Low testosterone has recently been associated with increased risk of death and higher risk of type 2 diabetes, but high-dose testosterone produced adverse cardiovascular (CV) events in aging men.[1,2] Thus, conflicting reports on the effects of testosterone on CV risk have been reported.[2-5] Testosterone has metabolic actions in men, such as favorable body composition, improved insulin sensitivity, and improved lipid metabolism. These actions might be expected to reduce CV mortality. Insulin resistance and obesity are associated with low sex hormone binding globulin. Ohlsson et al observed that high serum testosterone was associated with reduced risk of CV events in elderly men during a 5-year follow-up. While total testosterone was associated with CV risk benefit, free testosterone was weakly and not significantly associated with CV risk. There are limitations in the study, such as single measurement of sex steroids and sex hormone—binding globulin and it was not an interventional study. Large interventional trials are needed to confirm their observations.

A. W. Meikle, MD

References

1. Corona G, Rastrelli G, Forti G, Maggi M. Update in testosterone therapy for men. *J Sex Med.* 2011;8:639-654.
2. Lin JW, Lee JK, Wu CK, et al. Metabolic syndrome, testosterone, and cardiovascular mortality in men. *J Sex Med.* 2011;8:2350-2360.
3. Jones TH. Cardiovascular risk during androgen deprivation therapy for prostate cancer. *BMJ.* 2011;342:d3105.
4. Jones TH, Arver S, Behre HM, et al. Testosterone replacement in hypogonadal men with type 2 diabetes and/or metabolic syndrome (the TIMES2 study). *Diabetes Care.* 2011;34:828-837.
5. Basaria S, Coviello AD, Travison TG, et al. Adverse events associated with testosterone administration. *N Engl J Med.* 2010;363:109-122.

Effects of Simvastatin and Metformin on Polycystic Ovary Syndrome after Six Months of Treatment

Banaszewska B, Pawelczyk L, Spaczynski RZ, et al (Poznan Univ of Med Sciences, Poland; et al)
J Clin Endocrinol Metab 96:3493-3501, 2011

Context.—A randomized trial on women with polycystic ovary syndrome (PCOS) compared simvastatin, metformin, and a combination of these drugs.

Objective.—The aim of the study was to evaluate long-term effects of simvastatin and metformin on PCOS.

Design.—Women with PCOS (n = 139) were randomized to simvastatin (S), metformin (M), or simvastatin plus metformin (SM) groups. Evaluations were performed at baseline and at 3 and 6 months.

Setting.—The study was conducted at a university medical center.

Primary Outcome.—We measured the change of serum total testosterone.

Results.—Ninety-seven subjects completed the study. Total testosterone decreased significantly and comparably in all groups: by 25.6, 25.6, and 20.1% in the S, M, and SM groups, respectively. Both simvastatin and metformin improved menstrual cyclicity and decreased hirsutism, acne, ovarian volume, body mass index, C-reactive protein, and soluble vascular cell adhesion molecule-1. Dehydroepiandrosterone sulfate declined significantly only in the S group. Total cholesterol and low-density lipoprotein cholesterol significantly declined only in the S and SM groups. Ongoing reduction of ovarian volume, decreased hirsutism, acne and testosterone were observed between 0 and 3 months as well as between 3 and 6 months. Improvement of lipid profile, C-reactive protein, and soluble vascular cell adhesion molecule-1 occurred only during the first 3 months of treatment, with little change thereafter. Treatments were well tolerated, and no significant adverse effects were encountered.

Conclusions.—Long-term treatment with simvastatin was superior to metformin. Improvement of ovarian hyperandrogenism continued throughout the duration of the study.

► Polycystic ovary syndrome (PCOS) affects about 10% of women of the reproductive age and is characterized by hyperandrogenism, oligomenorrhea, insulin resistance, the metabolic syndrome, obesity, infertility, and polycystic ovaries. It is associated with a familial risk, but a genetic cause has been elusive. Treatment has been directed at correcting the clinical and laboratory abnormalities, which included agents to improve insulin responsiveness, with agents such as metformin, and suppression of hyperandrogenism, with androgen blockers such as spironolactone.[1-5] Banaszewska et al compared the effectiveness of simvastatin, metformin, and the combination of simvastatin and metformin on various biochemical and clinical aspects of PCOS.[6,7] Hyperandrogenism improved in all treatment groups, but no placebo group was included in the study. Simvastatin improved free and total testosterone.

A. W. Meikle, MD

References

1. Raval AD, Hunter T, Stuckey B, Hart RJ. Statins for women with polycystic ovary syndrome not actively trying to conceive. *Cochrane Database Syst Rev.* 2011;(10): CD008565.
2. Ortega I, Cress AB, Wong DH, et al. Simvastatin reduces steroidogenesis by inhibiting Cyp17a1 gene expression in rat ovarian theca-interstitial cells. *Biol Reprod.* 2012;86:1-9.
3. Economou F, Xyrafis X, Christakou C, Diamanti-Kandarakis E. The pluripotential effects of hypolipidemic treatment for polycystic ovary syndrome (PCOS): dyslipidemia, cardiovascular risk factors and beyond. *Curr Pharm Des.* 2011;17:908-921.
4. Kaya C, Pabuccu R, Cengiz SD, Dünder I. Comparison of the effects of atorvastatin and simvastatin in women with polycystic ovary syndrome: a prospective, randomized study. *Exp Clin Endocrinol Diabetes.* 2010;118:161-166.
5. Kazerooni T, Shojaei-Baghini A, Dehbashi S, Asadi N, Ghaffarpasand F, Kazerooni Y. Effects of metformin plus simvastatin on polycystic ovary syndrome: a prospective, randomized, double-blind, placebo-controlled study. *Fertil Steril.* 2010;94:2208-2213.
6. Banaszewska B, Pawelczyk L, Spaczynski RZ, Duleba AJ. Comparison of simvastatin and metformin in treatment of polycystic ovary syndrome: prospective randomized trial. *J Clin Endocrinol Metab.* 2009;94:4938-4945.
7. Banaszewska B, Spaczynski RZ, Ozegowska K, Pawelczyk L. The influence of lowdose oral contraceptive pill on clinical and metabolic parameters in young women with polycystic ovary syndrome. *Ginekol Pol.* 2011;82:430-435.

52 Pediatric Endocrinology

Effect of oxandrolone and timing of pubertal induction on final height in Turner's syndrome: randomised, double blind, placebo controlled trial
Gault EJ, on behalf of the British Society for Paediatric Endocrinology and Diabetes (Royal Hosp for Sick Children, Glasgow, UK; et al)
BMJ 342:d1980, 2011

Objective.—To examine the effect of oxandrolone and the timing of pubertal induction on final height in girls with Turner's syndrome receiving a standard dose of growth hormone.

Design.—Randomised, double blind, placebo controlled trial.

Setting.—36 paediatric endocrinology departments in UK hospitals.

Participants.—Girls with Turner's syndrome aged 7-13 years at recruitment, receiving recombinant growth hormone therapy (10 mg/m^2/week).

Interventions.—Participants were randomised to oxandrolone (0.05 mg/kg/day, maximum 2.5 mg/day) or placebo from 9 years of age. Those with evidence of ovarian failure at 12 years were further randomised to oral ethinylestradiol (year 1, 2 µg daily; year 2, 4 µg daily; year 3, 4 months each of 6, 8, and 10 µg daily) or placebo; participants who received placebo and those recruited after the age of 12.25 years started ethinylestradiol at age 14.

Main Outcome Measure.—Final height.

Results.—106 participants were recruited, of whom 14 withdrew and 82/92 reached final height. Both oxandrolone and late pubertal induction increased final height: by 4.6 (95% confidence interval 1.9 to 7.2) cm ($P = 0.001$, n = 82) for oxandrolone and 3.8 (0.0 to 7.5) cm ($P = 0.05$, n = 48) for late pubertal induction with ethinylestradiol. In the 48 children who were randomised twice, the effects on final height (compared with placebo and early induction of puberty) of oxandrolone alone, late induction alone, and oxandrolone plus late induction were similar, averaging 7.1 (3.4 to 10.8) cm ($P < 0.001$). No cases of virilisation were reported.

Conclusion.—Oxandrolone had a positive effect on final height in girls with Turner's syndrome treated with growth hormone, as did late pubertal induction with ethinylestradiol at age 14 years. However, these effects were not additive, so using both had no advantage. Oxandrolone could, therefore, be offered as an alternative to late pubertal induction for increasing final height in Turner's syndrome.

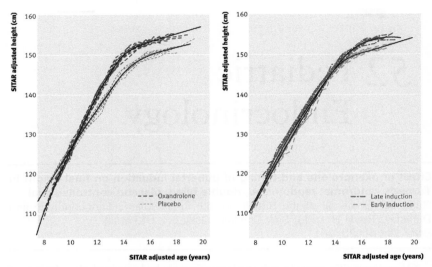

FIGURE 3.—SITAR fitted summary height curves by trial arm for randomisation 1 (left) and randomisation 2 (right). (Reproduced from Gault EJ, on behalf of the British Society for Paediatric Endocrinology and Diabetes. Effect of oxandrolone and timing of pubertal induction on final height in Turner's syndrome: randomised, double blind, placebo controlled trial. *BMJ.* 2011;342:d1980, with permission from BMJ Publishing Group Ltd.)

Trial Registration.—Current Controlled Trials ISRCTN50343149 (Fig 3).

▶ Although randomized placebo-controlled trials are relatively rare in pediatrics, no fewer than 3 rigorously designed prospective studies involving long-term outcomes in girls with Turner syndrome (TS) have been published this year alone. In this particular case, comparisons of the 2 separate randomizations (oxandrolone vs placebo; early vs late pubertal induction) as well as a combinatorial effect yield useful information that can readily be applied to the clinical setting. As seen in Fig 3, both oxandrolone and late pubertal induction were associated with greater gains in height. However, no additional benefit was observed from pursuing both. Several other aspects of the study are worth noting. One is the use of a low and slow protocol for estrogen replacement, which is supported by several other studies demonstrating better height outcomes in girls with TS when this approach is followed. Another point is that even the "early pubertal induction" group in whom E2 was initiated at age 12 was in fact "late" compared with the average age of pubertal onset in the general population. Because later pubertal induction has been associated with lower quality of life in young adults with TS, consideration should be given to starting estrogen therapy at an even younger age. Lastly, many clinicians who prescribe oxandrolone to girls with TS typically discontinue it once sex steroid replacement is underway. This study suggests that continuing oxandrolone throughout pubertal induction may in fact optimize height without undo side effects. On balance, this elegantly conducted multicenter study represents a significant contribution to the care of girls with TS.

E. Eugster, MD

Thyroid function in the nutritionally obese child and adolescent
Reinehr T (Univ of Witten/Herdecke, Datteln, Germany)
Curr Opin Pediatr 23:415-420, 2011

Purpose of Review.—In recent years, there has been an increasing focus on thyroid function in obese children. There is controversy concerning whether the changes in the levels of thyroid hormones and thyroid-stimulating hormone (thyrotropin − TSH) in obesity are causes or consequences of weight status and whether these subtle differences merit treatment with thyroxine. This review aimed to study the prevalence of disturbed thyroid hormone and TSH values in childhood obesity and the underlying pathophysiologic mechanisms linking obesity to thyroid function.

Recent Findings.—In the past 18 months, four studies demonstrated moderate elevation of TSH concentrations in 10−23% of obese children, which was associated with normal or slightly elevated thyroxine and triiodothyronine values. Two studies reported ultrasonographic hypoechogenicity of the thyroid in obese children with hyperthyrotropinemia, which was not caused by autoimmune thyroiditis; therefore, the authors hypothesized a link to chronic inflammation in obesity. Weight loss led to a normalization of elevated TSH levels in two studies. The adipokine leptin is the most promising link between obesity and hyperthyrotropinemia since leptin stimulates the hypothalamic−pituitary−thyroid.

Summary.—The elevated TSH levels in obesity seem a consequence rather than a cause of obesity. Therefore, treatment of hyperthyrotropinemia with thyroxine seems unnecessary in obese children (Fig 1).

▶ Pediatric endocrine clinics are inundated with referrals for abnormal thyroid function tests in obese children. These typically consist of a minimally elevated thyrotropin (TSH) with a normal total or free thyroxine. More often than not, the family has been given the message that this biochemical abnormality is the cause of the child's difficulty with weight control and that consequently the endocrinologist holds the key to fixing it. Sadly, much of our time is spent in correcting this misconception and in educating parents about the interplay between energy intake and energy utilization. Despite long-standing recognition of the childhood obesity epidemic, the increased incidence of an elevated TSH in this setting has only recently been established. This article is a concise and informative review of recent literature in this area that addresses prevalence, radiographic and laboratory features, pathophysiology, and clinical implications. As shown in Fig 1, the putative mechanism for an elevated TSH in obesity involves leptin, which is known to stimulate the hypothalamic-pituitary-thyroid axis, and the postulated etiology is an adaptive increase in energy expenditure to avoid additional weight gain. In fact, as the author points out, the decrease in TSH that

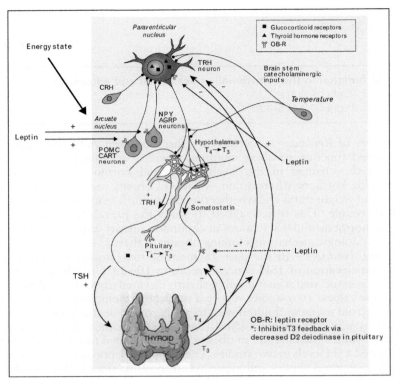

FIGURE 1.—Relationship between leptin and thyroid hormone synthesis. AGRP, agouti-related peptide; CART, cocaine and amphetamine-regulated transcript; CRH, corticotropin-releasing hormone; NPY, neuropeptide γ; TRH, thyrotropin-releasing hormone; TSH, thyroid-stimulating hormone. Adapted from [27]. *Editor's Note*: Please refer to original journal article for full references. (Reprinted from Reinehr T. Thyroid function in the nutritionally obese child and adolescent. *Curr Opin Pediatr.* 2011;23:415-420, with permission from Lippincott Williams & Wilkins.)

accompanies initial weight loss may in part explain the notorious difficulty in maintaining weight control and progressively shedding pounds that is encountered by many individuals. Regardless, ample evidence now exists to support a policy of lifestyle counseling rather than levothyroxine therapy in obese children with a mildly elevated TSH and no evidence of thyroid autoimmunity.

E. Eugster, MD

Article Index

Chapter 1: Rheumatoid Arthritis

Chapter 2: Systemic Lupus Erythematosus

Chapter 3: Vasculitis

Chapter 9: Bacterial Infections

Chapter 10: Fungal Infections

Chapter 11: Miscellaneous

Chapter 15: Cancer Prevention

Chapter 16: Chemotherapy: Mechanisms and Side Effects

Chapter 17: Gastrointestinal

Chapter 18: Genitourinary

Chapter 19: Gynecology

Chapter 20: Supportive Care

Chapter 21: Thoracic Cancer

Chapter 22: Chronic Kidney Disease and Clinical Nephrology

Chapter 23: Mediators and Modifiers of Renal Injury

Chapter 24: Diabetes

Chapter 25: Selected Issues in Acute Kidney Injury

Chapter 31: Pleural, Interstitial Lung, and Pulmonary Vascular Disease

Chapter 32: Sleep Disorders

Chapter 33: Critical Care Medicine

Chapter 34: Cardiac Arrhythmias, Conduction Disturbances, and Electrophysiology

Chapter 35: Cardiac Surgery

Chapter 36: Coronary Heart Disease

Chapter 37: Hypertension

Chapter 38: Non-Coronary Heart Disease in Adults

Chapter 39: Pediatric Cardiovascular Disease

Chapter 40: Esophagus

Chapter 44: Liver Disease

Chapter 45: Diabetes

Chapter 46: Lipoproteins and Atherosclerosis

Chapter 47: Obesity

Chapter 48: Thyroid

Chapter 49: Calcium and Bone Metabolism

Chapter 50: Adrenal Cortex

Chapter 51: Reproductive Endocrinology

Chapter 52: Pediatric Endocrinology

Author Index

Printed and bound by CPI Group (UK) Ltd, Croydon, CR0 4YY

08/05/2025

01864678-0016